ADAPTOGENETIC
Medicine

THE NEW
PARADIGM FOR
SYNERGISTIC HEALING

Justin D. Adair, Integrative Specialist
Jessica Bacon, D.O.

Adaptogenetic Medicine
The New Paradigm for Synergistic Healing

ISBN: 978-1-7956-7506-2
(also available for Kindle)

Book design and layout: Lighthouse24
Cover art: Kim Anton

CONTENTS

To the reader:

We hope you benefit from, and tremendously enjoy this book! If you or your loved ones are sick of the "one size fits all" model of western medicine and would like to know more about some of the therapies described in these chapters, as well as how they could possibly help you, feel free to check out our website and/or contact us at:

OrthoAdaptiveWellness.com

CHAPTER 1
INTRODUCTION –
BELIEVING IN WHAT WORKS

I believe in what works. My philosophy is simple. If it works, if it heals, if it brings my patients positive results, I'll learn about it and find a way to integrate it into my practice. This means that I'm always open to new ideas. It allows for 'good/better/best' scenarios to unfold... i.e. 'ok this modality worked adequately for the patient for a while but now we can supplant it with something far superior and more effective.' This also means that I'm open to saying "I was wrong" when better information than I initially had becomes available. The human body is a highly individualized, highly adaptive organism, why isn't our philosophy of medicine? Why are we so averse to the concept of dynamic, continually evolving treatments?

It is not the intent of this book to try to introduce a new type of medicine (although new discoveries are always a welcome side effect). It is not the intent of this book to try to persuade the reader that one form of medicine is superior to another. The most optimal treatment for any given patient doesn't necessarily have to exclusively fall under what we know to be either 'traditional' or 'alternative.' And it is most certainly not the intent of this book to demonize allopathic medicine (although some of its more deleterious shortcomings will be addressed). The intent of this book is point out the single biggest obstacle we as a society, as a culture, and as homo sapiens face with regard to the advancement of medicine and medical care as a whole. That obstacle isn't science; the science is there (and is continuing to advance daily). The obstacle isn't money, the funding is there, as is the technology. The obstacle isn't even information; we have an aggregate of information that encompasses at least 6,000 years of human history, most of it readily available to those who seek it. No, the greatest hindrances we have are obstructionist philosophy and willful ignorance. It is the ego, plain and simple. It is imperative that we have the collective realization that as human beings we possess a predilection towards extremism, polarization and bias. If ever we were able to zero out our need to have such rigidly inflexible and dogmatic *opinions*, perhaps we could begin to see (and leverage) the merit and power and synergy of using *all* forms of healing...together. That is the singular pursuit of this book...to create an entirely new thought form...to create a new paradigm where we can incept and grow an emerging community of practitioners who begin to diagnose and heal from the space of neutrality and totality (i.e. mind, body, and spirit), without the innate conflicts of interest that currently plague and permeate the entire system. We are going to foster a more dynamic mindset where the focus from peer review is to be able to rapidly **adapt**, instead of trying to double down on defending firmly entrenched 50 year-old draconian or obsolete protocols. We are going to enter into a new realm where holistic/integrative medicine and allopathic medicine don't necessarily hold such an utterly antagonistic superposition to each other.

This sort of predisposition is philosophically foreign to a lot of physicians and most institutions of medical training. It isn't safe. It isn't static. It isn't comfortable. It wasn't what they teach in med school and it isn't firmly established data with decades of PubMed studies behind it. This mindset is an outright threat to the crusty old construct and paradigm of how things are 'supposed' to work and how patients are 'supposed' to be treated. The old institution and its constituency are not interested in being wrong or out of their depth or moving past the one-size-fits-all mindset, or the comfortable profit margins. They aren't interested in *adaptive* medicine. They don't have time for a moving target. No, the very concept of continuous individualization, integration, and adaption makes the hardline allopathic institution and its disciples shudder in discomfort.

But that's where the growth is. That's where the event horizon of advancement is. Being uncomfortable is what both facilitates and acts as a catalyst for new understanding of how to treat patients, and more importantly, how to heal the human body. It allows for ancient knowledge to be relearned, it allows for brand new knowledge and new insight to be discovered, and for the new frontier of medicine to be explored. That *doesn't* mean being careless or haphazard or using snake oil or playing God with needlessly dangerous experiments. What that means is using wisdom, experience, intelligence and a sense of pragmatic discernment to ascertain the viability of emerging medicine(s) and technology and thus holding the space for new breakthroughs to occur. It means potentiating an unbiased scientific process (a surprisingly huge barrier). It means upholding the Hippocratic Oath without standing in the way of or impeding progress. It means taking the very best ancient knowledge and wisdom of the ages and augmenting it with the bleeding-edge state of the art technological, genetic, biochemical, and spiritual break-throughs that we are witnessing happen every day. It means leveraging the synergistic effect and benefits of different, sometimes completely unrelated modalities and not 'hanging our hat' on a singular protocol. But most importantly, it means advancing medicine as a whole *without conflicts of interest.*

To give example, there was a time in ancestral China when everyone in an entire village would pay the local doctor a monthly stipend as a de facto insurance policy. The only time an individual would *stop* paying the doctor was *if the individual got sick.* Let that sink in for a moment. In that model of medicine, the practitioner held a *vested interest in actually healing the patient.* Why isn't that sort of thinking our primary directive now? It would be a win-win scenario for everyone. Physicians everywhere would ostensibly retain more consistent streams of income, patients would actually have their health issues addressed on an individual basis instead of being herded through the system like cattle, and patient compliance would likely drastically improve, ensuring optimal outcomes. This very old way of thinking may very well be, and should be our only answer for the future of medicine. It should be, and most likely will be what replaces the current, broken system once it inevitably collapses. It is what will allow us as a human race to usher in the 22nd century of medicine, now.

CHAPTER 2

THE STATE AND FUTURE OF DIAGNOSTIC MEDICINE

Specialists and specialization of medicine are important. I wouldn't want a podiatrist to suddenly get thrown into the realm of having to make decisions about my heart (nor would I want a cardiologist attempting to do a procedure on my feet!). But we as a community of health care practitioners have got to stop biasing idiopathic disease, and the diagnosis/treatment thereof. It is a well-worn joke in the medical field that if you are experiencing symptoms of an unknown cause and you go to a psychiatrist first, your condition will be psychosomatic, if you go to a chiropractor, your condition will be related to subluxations of the spine, and if you go to a gastro-enterologist, it's going to be because you're full of shit! The funny thing is that they could all three be correct in their assessment!

We need to be a little less isolated and a little more cooperative, coordinated, and communicative with each other as practitioners in our efforts to accurately assess and properly treat patients, and greatly reduce errors and oversights.

We also need to better share the scope of knowledge and wisdom that can be garnered from learning different diagnostic methods. Blood serum assay reference intervals need to stop being based on a sick population and need to start being more comprehensive and updated to reflect what the optimal values would be in a healthy person. Saliva and Urine labs need to be better understood and more commonly utilized. The science and wealth of information provided by 'alternative' diagnostic measures like Applied Kinesiology (which functions by measuring muscle response to the same bio-electric pathways we discuss in the acupuncture chapter), live/dry blood cell analysis, and dark-field microscopy needs to be validated and integrated into primary care. And more importantly, we need to be forward-thinking enough to be ready to give up things like blood serum draws altogether as they become obsolete and give way to newer emerging 'instant read' technologies. Even now, at the time of this writing in 2017, scientists are developing the equivalent of a Star Trek style medical 'tri-corder,' and I imagine it will come to the forefront with undeniable viability after a few more years of evolution and refinement. Let's welcome that with open arms when it finally gets here instead of going kicking and screaming. (It would make Dr. McCoy and Dr. Crusher proud!)

It is the intent of the author in the following chapters to present the reader with information that will lead to a greater understanding of true healing modalities, as well as to provide access to a wealth of previously scattered but now unified data regarding complimentary and synergistic therapies, both allopathic and alternative. It is meant to start intelligent dialogues and augment our relationships with our health care practitioners—not replace them. It is intended to encourage the reader to take charge of their own health (and by proxy, their own healthcare) while still integrating the watchful guidance of informed healthcare practitioners.

From here on, the is continuity is only in theme, not necessarily in chapter order, and the reader is invited to jump around to different sections of the book if he or she so chooses. This work is meant to act as a helpful resource with some of the best current meta-data on the planet, not as a manifesto or a cure-all. It's best read with an *open mind*, and it is written with the intent that you, the reader, are encouraged to take what you want and leave the rest. It is my greatest hope that within the next 25 years this book will be rendered nearly, or perhaps even completely obsolete with regard to the treatments mentioned herein, because the *mindset* set forth in this writing was able to take hold in the collective human consciousness and usher in a new era of healing beyond our wildest dreams....

(and a big nod and thank you once again to Gene Roddenberry for showing us what those dreams may very well one day look like...)

CHAPTER 3

ALLOPATHIC MEDICINE

I'll reiterate my earlier sentiment with respect to my hardline allopathic friends; the purpose of this book is not to bash western medicine. Mainstream medical care has its shortcomings and failings, as does our healthcare system in its entirety. I don't really think there are too many people out there who would argue against that. But western medicine does have a place. It saves lives. If I (God forbid) find myself mangled and bleeding after a bad car accident, I don't want someone rushing over to render first aid with an herbal tincture or enchanted crystals. I want to be taken to the E.R., to have my vitals stabilized, to have any broken bones set, to be given any necessary blood transfusions, anti-biotics, intubation, and any other life-saving measures (and please throw some morphine/dilaudid in there while you're at it so that I'm not suffering in agony from my injuries). What I *don't* want to do is go to my primary care physician and be put on a statin drug for the rest of my life or be given a flu shot.

That's the dichotomy, and that's the problem. Most people either drink the kool-aid or they don't. I'm arguing that we take a more pragmatic approach. Let's un-deify the implied infallibility of what they teach at Harvard Medical. PubMed studies aren't sacrosanct. There are conflicts of interest when board members of the FDA also have either a history, a future job opportunity, or currently sit on the board of a member of big Pharma like Merck or Pfizer. (In a governing medical entity, a vested interest is *always* a conflict of interest.) It's a known fact pharmaceutical drugs kill people every day, and that's just counting the ones that are *correctly* prescribed and *correctly* taken.

Let's keep flip flopping though (because it's fun and I can do that if I want because it's my book!) ...If I have an allergic reaction, I'm going to reach for the Benedryl, or if it's a severe anaphylactic reaction, I really hope there's an Epi-pen close by. I'm not going to pretend like I don't use Aleve *every now and then* when I can't get acute inflammation under control from a sports injury as quickly as I would like from R.I.C.E. (rest, ice, compression, elevation), arnica gel, and turmeric/curcumin. But therein lies the appropriate (and in my mind, only) time and place for this modality: in an acute setting.

People don't get headaches because they have a Tylenol deficiency. The optimal number of drugs to be on is *zero*. But if that was the aim, if that was the goal, what would our doctors have left to do? Nutrition is an *optional elective* one semester class in med school, as opposed to the foundation and bedrock of becoming a physician as it should be. They aren't trained in the art and science of *healing*, they are instead very well educated and thoroughly trained in the game of *treatments* and *symptom management through the prescription of drugs*. Get enough doctors and specialists in the mix and before long you have patients that are literally prescribed 25 to 30 medications to take daily. That's not an exaggeration, I've seen it, and everything about it is wrong. There is no way in hell that the human liver and kidneys are designed to process all that, nor can they be expected to come out unscathed or even maintain homeostasis in the long run. It's nothing more than a slow kill, it's a death sentence.

Worse than that (and without trying to get overly technical), most maintenance medications create a condition called a "negative feedback loop mechanism." That's another way of saying, "When you stop taking this drug, the symptoms you're currently experiencing from the original problem are going to get worse."

Let's give a very common example: heartburn/acid reflux medication. The class of medication used to treat this condition is known as 'Proton Pump Inhibitors' or PPI's for short, and it includes well-known names like Nexium, Protonix, Prilosec, Omeprazole, Aciphex, etc. PPI's work by shutting down proton pumps (i.e. acid producers) in the gastrointestinal tract. This does work quite effectively at arresting the very unpleasant feeling of having a brick in your chest and/or having acid burn your esophagus...but it's also the equivalent of shoving a potato in the exhaust pipe of your car or putting a piece of black tape over the 'check engine' light and acting like the problem is fixed. The problem is *not* fixed; it's creating a recipe for disaster. Most physicians don't realize that the symptoms of having 'too much acid' can be *identical* to when the body doesn't have enough acid. Throw a PPI in the mix and now the body goes into a silent panic mode—it already didn't have enough acid to begin with, and now it has to spool up even more acid production to compensate for the drug that's actively trying to thwart its normal process of being able to digest heavy foods and keep the pH low enough in the stomach to keep out opportunistic infections like H.pylori, which is what can take hold when the gut gets too alkaline. PPI's have also been associated with an increased risk of vitamin and mineral deficiencies, most notably magnesium, B12, vitamin C, calcium, and iron. (*See PubMed study here: https://www.ncbi.nlm.nih.gov/pmc/articles/PMC4110863/)

A truly versed healer would be able to provide a better answer. Instead of using anti-secretory therapy to block the acid/proton pumps, why not *add* a little acid? This seems counterintuitive at first pass, but not when you understand how the human body actually works. The homo sapien is an absolute marvel of engineering, and the ultimate testament to Intelligent Design. Give the body what it needs, and it can and will *heal itself*. In the case of heartburn, swallow a big mouthful of Bragg's Apple Cider Vinegar, and watch how quickly the symptoms disappear. Take it every day (in addition to positive dietary changes) and watch how the symptoms never or almost never come back. But what did we do there? We gave the body what it needed. We gave it a little *more* acid and in real time, it begins to relax the proton response. The body goes 'oh, hey, I've got plenty of acid now, maybe I can chill out and shut down the pumps.' It's an intelligent, highly sentient biological response that immediately springs into action to restore a homeostatic equilibrium once it's simply given the right tools/substances/resources with which to work. This is the way it's *supposed* to work.

This isn't just my opinion; it actually happens this way. It's easily duplicable and provable a thousand times over. And yet there may never be a peer reviewed double-blind study of any notoriety proving this remedy as a scientific fact, or as being anything more than 'anecdotal.' (Who the hell would fund it anyways?) But you know what? I don't care. This is the real world, not the soulless confines of Academia, where everything happens in a vacuum or on a piece of paper with formulas. It works, it always has worked, and it always will work. ACV has no harmful side effects. It's been used for millennia.

> Let they food be thy medicine and medicine be thy food.
> –Hippocrates, 431 B.C.

The Hippocratic Oath to 'first do no harm' is sworn by every doctor graduating from medical school, perhaps it's time we start actually heeding the rest of his teachings and wisdom. Maybe we could learn a thing or two.

This is a fervent call to all our allopathic friends who know only western medicine. The totality of true healing and all those of us who practice 'alternative' modalities are not your enemy, nor are we enemies of science. We need you. You represent the very best and the very brightest and most capable members of the human race. Your intellect is often unsurpassed. Your intention to become a physician and help fellow human beings is the highest of callings and you should be commended for that. But it is imperative for you to raise your consciousness and *spiritual* awareness and realize that the conflicts of interest are real. There are clear and present dangers with blindly accepting the *religion* of Big Pharma and its funding of Harvard Medical. There is evil in our midst. There is a blatant and malevolent agenda to profit from the illness of human beings. Cancer is a billion-dollar (with a 'B') *industry*. If there was a cancer cure (and there are several) that was announced from the front lawn of the White House tomorrow, most oncologists would happily hang up their white lab coats and go into a different area of medicine...but not the companies who produce the chemo drugs, they would *violently* suppress it. This isn't a conspiracy theory, and doctors aren't the enemy. The problem isn't science. The problem is once again philosophy. Follow me down the rabbit hole here for a moment. Most doctors have about them an altruistic nature--that's what makes them want to do what they do. They've allowed the *good* within themselves to shine through in an effort to carry out *service to others*, which is what the true meaning of life is all about and the real reason we've been put here on this planet. An altruistic natured person wants to see good done in the world, and they want to find the good in everyone. An altruistic natured person however, usually can't fathom...or at the very least doesn't want to acknowledge the concept of living in a world where the very institutions who are designed to look out for our best interests, i.e. the government, the medical research institutions, the pharmaceutical companies, the vaccine manufacturers etc.., have a clear and malevolent underlying mandate to do us harm. If that was the case, then nearly everything they've ever learned becomes invalidated, and they have to face the real possibility that they themselves have violated their Hippocratic oath and caused patients harm. That's a tough pill to swallow (pun intended). That is a startling, unnerving, disconcerting, blisteringly painful realization. That's the very definition of raw emotion.......to come to that actualization and stare at yourself as a practitioner in the mirror and say, 'I've caused harm.' Even the best, brightest, and most capable doctors I've known would have an impossibly hard time having that conversation with themselves. And yet, it's a necessary one to have. Intellect and having a high I.Q. do not equate to having *raised consciousness* and *awareness*. Realize the capacity you possess to harm (even by following your training) and you begin to develop the ability to truly heal. Raise your consciousness and realize that there is true evil in the world, and use the collective power of your true abilities as a healer to combat that evil. If people perish due to lack of knowledge, then even more perish due to misinformation. This is a call to know, a call to act, a call to no longer blindly accept incorrect information at the expense of the human race. We as wearers of the white coat owe ourselves and our patients better. In fact, we owe them the very best, which is the synthesis and synergy of all of our modalities and knowledge and wisdom, both eastern and western, ancient and modern, combined.

Though we have certain commonalities as humans, one size does not fit all, and every single patient is unique. Every patient has a unique mind, a unique soul, a unique spirt, a unique body, a unique biochemistry, and a unique DNA. If our DNA is adaptive and unique, why isn't our medicine? Friends let us cast off the blinders of sterile absolutism and join hands together to begin a new chapter in true, profound healing.

CHAPTER 4

ADRENALS/STRESS/ADAPTOGENS/ AYURVEDA and CAFFEINE TOXICITY

We begin this chapter with a modern take on one of the key principles of Ayurvedic Medicine, which originated from India more than 3,000 years ago. The word Ayurveda comes from the combination of the Sanskrit words *ayur* (life) and *veda* (knowledge/science), hence "the science of life," This concept of medicine is based on interconnectedness and the philosophy of individualized treatments for patients which address mind, body, and spirit as an integrated unit. It also very specifically observes the notion that different types of people thrive and flourish in different conditions...and that realizing one's unique proclivities, traits, tendencies, predispositions, and constitution can make it easier to compensate for our inherent strengths and weaknesses in health and allow us to lead the best life possible.

The key principle which we borrow and integrate into modern holistic/integrative practice is Adaptogenic therapy, which utilizes the group of herbs known as Adaptogens. Adaptogenic herbs come from a group of plants that have the ability to increase the body's resilience and resistance to the negative side effects of physical, mental, and emotional stress. They can increase energy production, stamina, endurance, and mental clarity, but their main use in holistic medicine is to support adrenal function—this function being the primary mechanism the body uses to modulate stress. (The adrenal glands sit directly on top of the kidneys and signal the secretion of stress hormones like adrenaline and cortisol when we need it.) Unfortunately, our modern lifestyles have a tendency to drastically over-tax that system on a regular basis and we often need help to undo the damage caused by this perpetual death spiral of *chronic* stress. The human body was *not* designed to handle chronic stress. It was designed to handle *acute* stress quickly and efficiently, and then return to a state of rest.

The really cool thing about Adaptogens though is how they work. They have the versatility to be 'multi-directional,' based upon what you need as an individual. Think of them like the thermostat in your house which can down-regulate the temperature if it's too hot or up-regulate the temperature if it's too cold. Stress affects different people differently, it crashes some people to a point where they can't get out of bed in the morning and it winds other people up so much that they become insomniacs and can't fall asleep. This is why the multi-directional nature of adaptogenic herbs is so key. They have unique properties like the ability to give you an energy boost and a measure of calm simultaneously. They help the body eliminate cellular waste. They balance the entire axis. They provide the raw materials to play into and amplify the intelligent homeostatic and self-regulatory cogs/gears of the human body. The mechanism(s) of action of Adaptogens do something that pharmaceutical drugs cannot do, which is increase the *balance* quotients and gradients of multiple bodily functions by normalizing them—most notably energy levels, blood glucose metabolism, inflammation response, immune response, neurotransmitter production, stress hormone production, nervous system response, and several others. These types of adaptogenic benefits—and the availability of these benefits—is relatively unknown and completely outside the realm of consciousness of the majority of the western workforce and its corporate structures. Everyone gets locked into a vicious cycle of getting this huge initial spike from slamming coffee/caffeine and pastries/sugar in the morning, only to suffer an epic crash a few hours later. It then becomes a habitual game of 'chasing the dragon.' One must consume even more caffeine and sugary junk at lunch time to once again get that temporary surge of 'dirty' energy in order to maintain productivity. People become drug addicts. It's just that caffeine happens to not carry the social stigma associated with other psychoactive drugs because, well...*everyone's* on it). Notice I mentioned that caffeine is a psychoactive drug. Caffeine itself is a methylxanthine alkaloid produced by multiple plants as a *pesticide used to paralyze and kill certain insects that feed on them.*

In this uncredited but widely circulated (circa 2017) article, "The Coffee Deception: 13 Little Known Facts About Coffee", there are some eye opening statements made that should give us pause before firing up that Keurig in the morning:

> 1. Caffeine is an alkaloid that the coffee plant uses to kill bugs, which eat its seeds.
>
> The coffee plant also uses caffeine in the coffee pods to kill surrounding plants, so the coffee plant can attain more sunlight and grow larger. Caffeine is a pesticide, which causes genetic termination in [certain] living cells that come into contact with it.
>
> 2. MRI images taken before and after 1 cup of coffee showed a decrease in blood flow to the brain by 45%. When the blood flow reduction was measured exactly, it was actually 52% less blood flow to the brain, after just one small cup of coffee.
>
> 3. Brain imaging studies of chronic coffee drinkers showed they presented the same degradation of their brains as chronic alcoholics, cigarette smokers, Parkinson's patients and marijuana users.
>
> 4. Coffee can cause an urge to move ones' bowels because this is one way the body tries to eliminate poison from the

system. The sudden urge to "poo" after drinking coffee is one of the body's defense mechanisms to poison.

5. Coffee increases energy via the human fight or flight metabolic response, because the body is afraid of the caffeine-based poison. Coffee doesn't give energy, it removes it from the body.

The energy a person feels when they drink coffee is the body going into overdrive because caffeine is a poison and all poisons activate an energy release in the body. (fight or flight)

Coffee removes energy from the system, leaving the person progressively more and more exhausted each day that passes, therefore setting up the world's most dangerous energy stimulation addiction... coffee dependence for energy.

6. When the fight or flight response is triggered in the body, the lower IQ centers of the brain are activated as well as hormonal systems in control of aggression, violence, irrational and illogical decision making, jealousy, rage, anger, fear and paranoia.

Coffee generates lower end mental functioning with a side of every negative emotional response the body can generate.

7. When measured, 1 coffee activated the fight and flight response for 3 consecutive weeks, even though no other caffeine was consumed after that 1 cup of coffee. One cup of coffee poisons the body for 3 consecutive weeks, on a decreasing scale.

8. When coffee (caffeine) is consumed, the limbic part of the brain is hyper activated and the higher learning centers of the mind inhibited. The limbic part of the brain is only concerned with sex, reproduction, protection of territory, food acquisition and personal safety.

The limbic portion of the brain is the most primitive and least developed portion of the mind complex. When you want to out-smart or dominate another person, it's best that their limbic system is activated, because it brings them to a mental state equal to that of a child.

9. The birth control pill inhibits clearing of ingested caffeine. This effect is increased dramatically by alcohol or pain killer use, therefore causing many cases of caffeine poisoning, which get treated as other things once the person reaches the hospital.

10. Coffee is proven to cause an enlarged prostate, high anxiety, insomnia, depression, birth defects, pain syndromes, unnatural breathing patterns, brain damage, hyperactivity, learning disorders (from the brain damage) behavior disorders, fatigue, certain types of cancer, Crohns, IBS, colitis, carpel tunnel, ulcers, low iron, heart disease, headaches, PMS, increased incidence of muscle and tendon injury, joint pain, heart attack, stroke, TIA's (mini strokes)... and that's a short list.

11. Coffee causes fat gain and cellulite because by triggering the body's flight or fight system (which any poison or threat does). This eventually changes the body's primary fuel source requirement to one of fat.

When the body is threatened, it prefers fat as its primary fuel source, over sugar or protein.

Constant activation of the body's fight or flight system (via the daily ingestion of caffeine poison) aids in a metabolic shift to fat storage and fat conservation, because again the body prefers fat as a fuel source when fighting any toxic intruder... because fat contains 9 calories per gram for the fight, as opposed to 4 calories per gram housed by sugar and protein.

Welcome to the land of coffee (caffeine) induced fat gain, weight gain and cellulite. Coffee also destroys muscle, as the body purposely flushes muscle, when it's poisoned, to facilitate additional fat storage.

12. Coffee (caffeine) blocks iron absorption and is a significant factor in the vast majority of anemia today.

The entire threat of caffeine in general includes caffeine teas, chocolates, caffeine based energy drinks, caffeine based pre-workout drinks and over 2000 over-the-counter and prescription medications that PURPOSELY include caffeine.

13. An investigation conducted by the author of the most extensive book on coffee ever written (*Caffeine Blues: Wake Up to the Hidden Dangers of America's #1 Drug* by Stephen Cherniske, M.S.), reviewed almost every scientific research piece regarding coffee and his conclusion was that there's absolutely no scientific evidence whatsoever that coffee provides any health benefits to the human body, on any level, in anyway.

He openly declares that any positive promotion of coffee consumption is a blatant lie, doing grave harm to our entire society. The publication of any positive effects of coffee are false and all can be traced back to a very powerful, covert and secret "coffee lobby," which has both commercial and ruling family origins.

The human body is not designed for this type of abuse. These relentlessly violent peaks and troughs of the insulin/glucose see-saw are one of the major reasons we have such an overwhelming epidemic of diabetes and obesity, and it must stop if we are ever going to improve the health of our society. Furthermore, when you compound poor dietary fuel with the external stresses, the resulting biochemical responses, and the drugs we then take to medicate and mask those negative responses, we end up with what you would expect...cancer, coronary events, strokes, chronic illness and inflammation. We end up with cascade failure in one form or another, and most victims don't even fully realize it's by their own hand. If people perish due to lack of knowledge, we as a culture have somehow managed to compound that by being willfully ignorant, even in the face of overwhelming scientific data. As a collective we embody the proverbial 'train wreck in slow motion.' Stress itself, whether internal or external, poisons every square inch of the human body. It cripples the immune system, disturbs fragile hormonal balances, impedes digestion, and creates a massive amount of systemic inflammation. The non-stop adrenaline we run on is *corrosive* to our arteries.

This is where adaptogenic herbs can come to the rescue! The body has a type of master on/off sentinel response mechanism that reacts in a defensive nature when introduced to external dangers like radiation, stress, environmental toxins, etc. This single mechanism controls over 500 genes that, when expressed, trigger inflammation. Adaptogenic herbs like ginseng help turn off this mechanism and make sure it stays off, thereby greatly reducing the overall inflammatory response.

In the 1960's and 1970's, Soviet Union scientists conducted over a thousand published studies on Adaptogenic herbs, and while doing so established the three criteria an herb must adhere to be admitted to the category:

1) It must be non-toxic.
2) Its benefits are nonspecific, it has to improve the entire body's resistance to stress, not just one particular organ or system.
3) It balances bodily functions, regardless of where the disruption may originate.

To take an article quote from science writer Catherine Guthrie:

What sets Adaptogens apart from other medicinal plants is their ability to nudge our bodies toward optimal health, or homeostasis. The best way to appreciate this nuance is to compare adaptogens with pharmaceuticals. Drugs are typically designed to block or replace something. For instance, Celebrex lessens arthritis pain by inhibiting COX-2, an enzyme that causes inflammation. But COX-2 also shields the body from heart disease and stroke. Obstructing it brings on a two- to three-fold increase in heart attacks and strokes, according to an FDA alert. Many conventional drugs are anti-this and anti-that. In contrast, adaptogens enhance the body's overall ability to adapt in ways that maintain optimal functionality.

Are we not doing ourselves a huge disservice by missing the boat on these amazing herbs?

So what are the most well-known and widely used adaptogens?

- Ginseng (American, Asian, and Siberian/Eleuthero strains)
- Maca
- Ashwaganda
- Rhodiola
- Holy Basil
- Astragalus
- Milk Thistle
- Aloe Vera
- Water Hyssop
- Omija (Schisandra berry)
- Rosemary
- Gotu Kola
- Moringa
- Bacopa
- Licorice Root
- Kratom

- Cordyceps
- Sarsparilla
- Tribulus (Puncturevine)
- Jiaogulan (Gynostemma)
- Reishi Mushrooms
- Rhaponticum
- Sea Buckthorn (which contains rare Omega 7 fatty acid)

There are many more herbs as well which could qualify under the Adaptogenic criteria, but these are the most commonly used worldwide and have the most known benefits. At our clinic we carry a few different adaptogenic formulas as well as some of them individually, but for general stress/fatigue/adrenal support, our favorite formula so far has been "**Adaptocrine**" by Apex Energetics. To balance the other side of the equation, we can also introduce a form of *glandular* support in order to replenish a true insufficiency. Our favorite formula for that is **Thyro Complex** by Professional Formulas, which contains lyophilized thyroid, adrenal, pituitary, spleen, thymus, and hypothalamus tissue(s). (There are a few other excellent formulas available on the market for adaptogenic and glandular support, these just happen to be the ones we are well-acquainted with and have confidence in.)

It is the intent of this chapter to let the reader know that there are many superior forms of stress management out there than the normalized self-destruction we've integrated into our lifestyles via poor diet and substance abuse (whether it's prescribed or not) ...and it's the hope of the writer of this chapter that the reader will do some of his or her own personal research into those better forms, whether or not adaptogenic herbs come into play. They are certainly a good starting point though. You deserve better and your body deserves better.

For an extremely comprehensive guide on the full spectrum of Adaptogenic herbs and essential oils—the real, therapeutically effective oils that actually work (not the crap your Aunt Brenda peddles from her MLM pyramid scheme), the reader is invited to read the book: *Adaptogens in Medical Herbalism: Elite Herbs and Natural Compounds for Mastering Stress, Aging, and Chronic Disease* by Donald R. Yance, CN, MH, RH(AHG).

CHAPTER 5

ALLERGIES

We have all been there. Your eyes are red and itchy, your nose is either stuffed up or it's running like a water faucet, you can't stop sneezing your head off, you have "cotton mouth," and at night when you're trying to get some rest, the post nasal drip is running down the back of your throat causing a nagging, hacking cough. You don't really feel sick, and you still have a reasonable amount of energy, you just feel really *irritated* and stuffy. This is your body's histamine response trying to protect you from what it perceives as foreign invaders. Typically, the more taxed/over-worked the immune system is, the more likely it is to mount this response on a continual basis, even against the most innocuous seeming items on a potential allergen list. But what if we could cool off that response and address the underlying root cause without drugging ourselves into oblivion with anti-histamines like Benedryl), corticosteroids (like Prednisone), and leukotriene receptor antagonists (like Singulair) all the time? That would be an improvement would it not?

So let's do just that—let's address it in short order. This chapter is going to be short and sweet.

- Step 1) The body that is overloaded with toxins is going to be more prone to inflammation, cytokine/immune response, mucous production, and histamine/leukotriene response. I highly suggest investing $6 and purchasing a copy of *The Master Cleanser* (by Stanley Burroughs). You can find a copy on Amazon.com. Getting through this cleanse (preferably under the supervision of a physician) will eliminate an overwhelming majority of the immediate toxins in your body. Lowering the toxin levels = lowering the strain on the immune system = lowering mucous/histamine production = drastically reduced allergy symptoms.

- Step 2) After completing the cleanse, adapt a healthier eating routine and eliminate the primary *distractors* from your diet, at least temporarily. Primary distractors include four major items which are known to cause mucous production, inflammation, and histamine response. Those four are **Sugar, Dairy, Gluten,** and **Alcohol**. Yes, yes, I know, those are all the things we love. When you (at least temporarily) cut them out and switch to a primarily plant-based diet, you may feel like you're dying of unhappiness, but you're really not, and you'll feel better in roughly 3 days. (Also, see the Dental clean-up chapter of this book, this an essential part of calming the overall immune response.)

- Step 3) It can be quite helpful to do *food-intolerance testing* in order to ascertain and eliminate any additional foods (if any) that you might have a severe intolerance to in addition to the 'major four." At our clinic we have enjoyed good success using the **ALCAT** 100 Food Panel Assay. The ALCAT (by Cell Science Systems) is also helpful in that we can scale it up or down based on the patient needs, but the 100 Food Panel is usually sufficient.

- Step 4) Remove pet dander as a distractor. We all love our pets as members of the family, but sometimes our immune systems don't love the dander/allergenic component that routinely sheds from their skin/glands/fur/hair. One of the single unhealthiest things you can do allergy-wise is to let a cat or a dog sleep in the bed with you. To the people that do this, you'll get no judgment from me, I grew up with a miniature dachshund named Precious who slept in the bed every night (and acted as an excellent foot warmer during the winter months), but I do want to point this out as something to consider removing from the equation, especially if you suffer severe allergies. You can't reasonably expect to not have some sort of immune response if you're sleeping in bed linens every night that are soiled by pet hair, dander, and whatever bugs/dirt/feces/urine/grass/pollen that your kitty Mr. Jingles tracked in from outside. If you do have inside pets, I also highly recommend purchasing a couple of Ionic Comfort Quadra air purifiers (from SharperImage.com). They make a significant difference when it comes to reducing airborne allergens, regardless if those allergens are pet-sourced or not.

- Step 5) If you have tried these methods, have found some moderate success, yet still have a significant or severe seasonal allergy attack on a regular basis, or if you accidentally petted your neighbor's cat and you find yourself a snotty, sneezy mess, even after taking a shower, it's time to bring in a little conventional help.

I personally have to deal with this on occasion, but only when I visit family in New Mexico during a very specific time-frame. Apparently I have a severe reaction to some vengeful and spiteful plant that blooms in that specific region from approximately February 1st through about the middle of April. It's like clockwork, even when I'm healthy and cleansed, my histamine response goes into overdrive and has a fit from whatever god-awful, anthrax-like pollen/toxin that this angry little shrub/tree/plant releases into the air around that time. And it only seems to affect me. So here are the counter measures I deploy:

For 3 days, I alternate the anti-histamines Allegra and Zyrtec every 12 hours to aggressively get the histamine response under control. (I'll also sparingly use Afrin nasal spray if I need it for sinus congestion, as well as either Visine-A or Zaditor anti-histamine eye drops.) I eliminate the 'big 4' (sugar/dairy/gluten/alcohol). I use my Nettie pot for saline sinus rinsing religiously. I also begin to simultaneously consume a daily helping of local honey. Consuming local honey seems to have an adaptogenic effect and helps provide your immune system with the resources, raw materials, and *information* it needs to acclimate to the local flora. This concept has been known to folk medicine for centuries, although I will admit that it's purely anecdotal. I don't have any studies to back it up, maybe I'll do one myself in the future, but for now it just seems to make sense from a biochemical perspective, and it seems to have significantly helped me and a lot of friends/family over the years who are seasonal allergy sufferers. (Being consistent with this book's theme, use your critical thinking skills, see if it resonates and works for you, it's damn sure not going to hurt anything.) Lastly, and most importantly, I add in a *natural* anti-histamine formula from day 1 (the same day as I begin the anti-histamines.) My favorite one that I've found so far is **AllerDHQ** from Xymogen. It's practitioner-grade and has a powerful herbal support formula which includes Quercetin, Stinging Nettle, Bromelain, Rutin, Dihydroquercetin, and more.

Most importantly, what I've found is that if I aggressively treat the seasonal allergies for 2 or 3 days with the Allegra/Zyrtec combo, and simultaneously begin the local honey and AllerDHQ, I can get the initial histamine/symptom surge under control pretty easily. About the Day 3 point, the honey and natural ingredients from AllerDHQ have built up enough in my system to where I can *completely discontinue* the Allegra/Zyrtec combo, and yet still be asymptomatic.

To me this is an effective, proper solution with each form of medicine playing its role. Allopathic (Allegra/Zyrtec) are used in a very short term (2 to 3 day) setting for acute/emergency-basis symptom management, meanwhile we remove any distractors to the best of our ability and let the natural remedies slowly build up enough in our system to take over so that we can discontinue any pharmaceutical drugs. This is a vastly superior and healthier option than living on a combination of Kenalog/Cortisone injections to reduce inflammation, Advair/ProAir to breathe, Afrin/Sudafed to decongest, Benedryl to dry up mucous/snot, Singulair to chronically manage leukotrienes, NyQuil to stop coughing and to sleep, etc. Some people live in a drug induced fog this way on and off for the whole year, and that's a very poor solution.

Let's give our body the support it needs to cleanse, detox, and manage whatever minor allergy symptoms head our way as opposed to drugging it to death indefinitely and just hoping for the best. The Cox-II/cytokine/histamine/etc response is, in truth, an absolute marvel of engineering. It's designed to keep us alive and protect us from injury and pathogenic invasion. It's not a bad thing, nor should it be classified as such. But an overactive immune system is indicative of a more serious underlying issue, and calls for us to address that issue by cleansing, removing any distractors, and helping the body itself lower the immune response, *naturally*.

CHAPTER 6

ARTERIAL HEALTH

Blood flow is the key to life. Without it we would die in minutes. Without blood flow, the oxygen, nutrients, and bioelectric currents cannot reach our tissues and organs to keep them alive. Our blood vessels consist of arteries, which carry freshly oxygenated blood away from the heart to where it's needed, and of veins, which return oxygen- depleted blood back to heart to be re-infused with more oxygen and recirculated again.

Cholesterol is also a vital necessity for us to live, albeit in a less immediate sense. Half of the dry weight of our brains are cholesterol. Our joints are lubricated by cholesterol. All our sex hormones (estrogens, progesterone, testosterone) are synthesized from cholesterol. Cholesterol is used to make bile, which is necessary to break down fats. Cholesterol is necessary to help synthesize Vitamin D. Cholesterol helps maintain the structural integrity of cellular membranes. I could summarize this entire paragraph by saying cholesterol is exceptionally important in order for the body to function properly on many levels. So why do we demonize it? Why would this necessary building block of life also be the very same culprit responsible for blocking blood flow?

This is one of the chapters of this book where I'm going to call a spade a spade and be categorically and directly antagonistic to what our allopathic friends believe and have been taught. Friends, you've been lied to. Cholesterol is not bad for you. It's necessary to survive.

Statin drugs on the other hand are toxic poison and should be avoided at all costs. How's that for blunt?

Statin drugs have over 300 *known* side effects, including muscle pain, weakness, damage, and atrophy. They can cause elevated liver enzymes, liver damage, and liver inflammation. Statins predispose people to type 2 diabetes, increase the risk of acute kidney injury by 34% (a condition that can be fatal), impair cognitive function/cause memory loss, increase the risk of ALS, Alzheimer's, Parkinson's, hair loss, birth defects, gastro-intestinal distress, the inability to deal with stress, they cause neurological side effects, decreased levels of vitamin E, weight gain, acidosis, anemia, pancreatic dysfunction, immune system suppression, sexual dysfunction, neuropathy, an increased cancer risk, they inhibit the synthesis of vitamin K, they inhibit your ability to manufacture vitamin D from sunlight, and dangerously interfere with your production of CoEnzyme-Q10, which is ironically vital for heart function. (Premature aging and DNA damage also result from having too little CoQ10.) It should have been considered a criminal act in 2012 when the FDA removed the long-time recommendation that patients on these drugs needed routine liver enzyme monitoring.

Are you scared yet? You should be. These aren't my opinions; these are clinically documented side effects. You can find most of them in the monograph pamphlet that comes with the drug.

The tone of this book is not meant to be divisive, it's meant to be illuminating, integrative, productive, and inclusive. But this is one topic where there simply is no gray area and where the mainstream has got it dead wrong. The only highly scientific term I can even come up with to describe statin drugs is that they are pure, unadulterated *bullshit*. Perhaps 'quackery' if you need a second qualifier. There are people with sky-high cholesterol that are at almost no risk of a heart attack or a coronary event, whereas there are people out there with a total cholesterol of 80 who are about one good sneeze away from congestive heart failure. Yes, the HDL to LDL *ratio* is important, but as a whole, **Cholesterol does not cause**

heart disease. Calcified coronary plaque and inflammation do. According to a study in the journal *Atherosclerosis*, published on PubMed in 2012, *statin use is associated with a 52% increased likelihood and degree of calcified coronary plaque as opposed to non-users.* **Just as many people have heart attacks who have a cholesterol of less than 200mg/dl, as do people with a cholesterol over 300mg/dl.** The country of France has one of the highest averages for cholesterol (~250mg/dl), and yet they have the lowest incidence of heart disease in all of Europe. Percentage-wise, they have approximately half the heart attacks we currently experience here in the contiguous United States. Again, these are not my opinions here, they are easily researchable (non cherry-picked) facts.

According to Raymond Francis, a chemist, a graduate of MIT, and author of the 2002 book *Never Be Sick Again*:

> Atherosclerosis—the main cause of heart attacks and strokes—is the accumulation of fatty plaque inside the walls of major arteries. As the disease progresses, arteries become increasingly narrow, making it easier for a blood clot or piece of dislodged plaque to completely block blood flow, resulting in either a heart attack or stroke.
>
> When cholesterol was found to be a major component of arterial plaque, the "cholesterol theory of heart disease" was born, thinking that high cholesterol levels cause atherosclerosis. The truth, however, is not so simple. Cholesterol is an anti-oxidant, a repair and healing molecule. The body produces more of it in response to stress and tissue damage, when repair and healing are needed. Remove the cause of the body's distress, like inflammation and oxidation, and you lower cholesterol. **It turned out that blaming cholesterol for heart disease makes as much sense as blaming the Red Cross for the disasters it responds to.**

Drug companies responded to the cholesterol theory by investing millions in developing cholesterol-lowering drugs. Now, although unbiased science has disproved the cholesterol theory, these companies have an enormous vested interest in keeping the cholesterol myth alive and well, and they're doing an excellent job of just that.

Pfizer's Lipitor is the best-selling drug of all time. It brings in ten billion dollars a year and has quadrupled Pfizer's net income. Up to 80 million Americans have elevated cholesterol according to the new guidelines, make them eligible to receive statins. That's 80 million potential customers not yet taking statins! Pfizer and other drug giants are spending millions to convince them and their doctors that they need statins, which are taken for life. With insurance and government subsidies, we're all paying for these ineffective, unnecessary, toxic drugs.

I'm of the opinion that the only safe place for statin drugs is in the trash can. It certainly isn't safe to put them in the human body. The only good thing about statin drugs, is that unlike most drugs, there are no side effects of stopping them abruptly (other than being one day closer to a state of better health). There are no withdrawals. Once you stop taking them, the half-life of the drug is quite long, and they continue on in your bloodstream for about a week before your body finally flushes the rest of that crap out.

Ok so now that we know cholesterol is a good guy and statins aren't the answer, the next natural question in the progression is **"What *does* cause heart disease?"** The answer is *arterial scarring*, oxidation, and inflammation. This is pretty straight-forward. It's already well known that the metabolic poisons sugar, white flour/gluten/grain, alcohol, most dairy, and the saturated fats we consume on a daily basis all cause inflammation. (Smoking does this too; we can't forget smoking as a major causative factor. But in the year 2017, it's almost superfluous to mention that.) If you are reading this book, chances are you already knew that those things are bad for you and cause inflammation. But what specifically *causes arterial scaring*? It's been my research that there are three major culprits... 1) **artificial sweeteners**, i.e. Splenda, sucralose, aspartame, HFCS, etc, 2) **hydrogenated oils**, i.e. fried foods, vegetable oils, and 3) *homogenized/pasteurized* dairy. The molecular structure of these unnatural dietary components is such that they each scar and damage our arteries. This degenerative cycle of chronic inflammation *leads to the oxidation of otherwise harmless cholesterol*, with this newly oxidized cholesterol being one of the major constituents of the subsequent plaque build-up that then creates occlusions and blockages on these now-scarred arterial walls.

And therein lies the 'devil in the details'...that is real reason why there are many patients with 'normal' cholesterol levels who suffer adverse cardiac events whereas there are plenty of patients with 'high' cholesterol who lead perfectly healthy, unremarkable (from a coronary perspective) lives. The difference has nothing to do with cholesterol, and it doesn't matter what your cholesterol number is on a lab report. The difference has *everything* to do with the amount of chronic inflammation in a person's body and whether or not their cholesterol is becoming oxidized. (Genetics also factor into the resilience and resistance against coronary disease, but we are strictly addressing self-inflicted causative factors here.)

If you are a physician and you only rely on basic lab work, common sense (not to mention science) dictate that the combination of a C-reactive protein reading and a homocysteine level is a much better indicator of heart health and coronary risk than a lipid panel. Also, a high-tech laboratory technology has recently emerged known as the Corus CAD test, developed by CardioDX. (CardioDX.com) This test is a powerful new tool that uses a composite score of several different factors (including age, sex, gene expression) to determine risk of coronary artery disease. Combining this test with a read of arterial plaque build-up would most likely lead to an optimal outcome for patient diagnosis and care. (Full disclosure, I have no monetary interest in the Corus CAD test or the company CardioDX, but we do use their lab at our clinic(s) as a beneficial tool in tandem with other diagnostic measures to help give our patients the best care possible.)

Now that we've diagrammed and understand the cause behind arterial disease, how to diagnose it, and how *not* to treat it, what can we do to reverse arterial disease? What can we do to *improve* arterial and vascular health? I'm glad you asked!

To heal, to repair, to rebuild proper arterial health, we need to bring in the big guns if we want to save already compromised patients from heart attacks and quadruple bypass surgeries. We need to 1) remove the distractors—i.e. inflammatory diets, statin drugs, arterial plaque build-up, and environmental toxins, and 2) we need to restore arterial health and rebuild the nitric oxide metabolic pathway.

To remove arterial wall plaque build-up, we have amazingly safe and effective therapies like intravenous chelation, backed by nearly 70 years of clinical usage and studies. The two primary types of IV chelation used today are EDTA and Phosphatidyl Choline (which goes by the trade name PlaqueX). EDTA is a general chelator that not only helps dissolve arterial plaque, but also binds to heavy metals and environmental toxins and converts them into a readily (via the kidneys) excretable form. Phosphatidyl Choline is an essential phospholipid that can directly reduce arterial plaque build-up and actively works to restore arterial wall flexibility, elasticity, and proper viscosity. Together, these two forms of chelation form the dynamic duo of heavy hitters that directly address the issue of preventative coronary care. They can work together synergistically (in tandem with a proper anti-inflammatory plant-based diet loaded with good fats) to significantly improve arterial health and help the body reverse the ticking time bomb of heart disease. Hirudotherapy (explained in another chapter) has also been shown to be effective in treating cardiovascular disease by having a beneficial effect on vascular walls, improving micro-circulation, and releasing the bio-active substance hirudin, which thins out the blood and can ease hypertensive issues.

The other major component of circulatory health is the Nitric Oxide metabolic pathway. Nitric Oxide is probably the most studied molecule in the human body. It is at the core of every major signaling function of the cardiovascular and circulatory system and without it absolutely nothing works. N-O is synthesized from the amino acid L-arginine, maintains/signals the vasodilation function of blood vessels and sustains the oxygen/nutrient transport system. It is imperative for good cardiovascular, endothelial, and circulatory function that we support this system, but in order to preserve it, we must first understand it.

N-O production is influenced by three major factors: age, diet and exercise. Borrowed from the NeoGenesis Labs/HumanN company website humann.com:

Age:

We already know our bodies change as we age. This is true for Nitric Oxide levels in the body as well. By the time we reach 40, studies have shown that we only produce about half or less of the Nitric Oxide we did at age 20. And it continues to decline as we age. There's also a difference when it comes to gender: by 40, men produce about 50% of the N-O they did in their teens and twenties. And women only produce about 35% of what they did in their twenties at age 50. Yet, our ability to produce and generate N-O within the body is a key element of a healthy body. Which means having an effective strategy to maintain optimal levels is critical because it affects how every cell in our body communicates with each other.

Diet:

A diet rich in green, leafy vegetables is known to be cardio healthy. For decades, nutritionists and scientists thought these effects were from the anti-oxidants found in those foods. Now we know that it's due to the dietary nitrates found in green, leafy vegetables and beets. Nitrates are metabolized into Nitric Oxide in the human body by oral nitrate-reducing bacteria. If we don't consume enough high nitrate vegetables, then we become N-O deficient and our N-O levels begin to fall.

Additionally, people who use antiseptic mouthwash can destroy all the good bacteria in the mouth that are responsible for reducing dietary nitrate into nitrite and Nitric Oxide. As a result, even though these individuals may eat sufficient amounts of high nitrate vegetables, they may become N-O deficient because they don't have the right bacteria necessary for metabolizing dietary nitrate.

Exercise:

Physical exercise is the most potent stimulator of Nitric Oxide production and is considered one of the top strategies for supporting overall cardiovascular health. However, when we don't exercise, we lose that important signal that tells our body to make more N-O. As a result, the enzyme that makes N-O in response to exercise becomes dysfunctional. This usually leads to N-O insufficiency. Just as in the aging process, the problem is the inability to utilize L-arginine to make Nitric Oxide. The good news, however, is that we once begin to exercise we may regain the functionality of that enzyme and begin to stimulate more N-O production.

Adjunctively, we've found a very valuable supplement called Neo40, backed by clinical studies, which is utilized to help patients over the age of 40 actually rebuild the nitric oxide metabolic pathway, as well as help their bodies heal and reverse the conditions associated with N-O dysfunction such as hypertension.

(Full disclosure, I do not have any vested or monetary interest in the NeoGenesis Labs/HumanN company, however I do carry their line of products at my clinic and am thankful to be able to do so because of the tremendous benefit these scientifically developed, naturally sourced, practitioner-grade supplements provide. However, I'm not interested in selling you a product, I'm interested in you being made aware of the totality of how the N-O metabolic pathway works, the importance of it, and *all* of the necessary steps you need to take to maintain this pathway in the grand scope of optimal health. These supplements are not a panacea or a cure all; they are meant to be used as a *supplemental* tool (when appropriate) in tandem with proper diet and exercise to achieve an optimal outcome.)

Lastly, one remarkably helpful and simple method to maintain vascular/venous health is the **inversion table**. Veins are the blood vessels that return blood to the heart. The summary of how they are designed is a dual-flap, bicuspid system that creates a de facto backflow valve, so that blood can only go one way. When the heart contracts/pumps, the valves open and blood is pushed, and when the heart relaxes in between contractions, the valves close so that the blood doesn't go back in the wrong direction. Over time and in certain (usually sedentary) circumstances however, the veins and their backflow system become damaged by varicosis or thrombosis, in which case the valves fail to deploy properly and blood flows backwards, increasing the pressure on leg veins, and causing blood pooling in the lower extremities. Noticeable symptoms start with leg aching/discomfort, and eventually degenerate to edema (fluid build-up/swelling) around the ankles. Over the course of an individual's life, using an inversion table regularly, even if it's only for two 30 to 60 second sessions a day, makes a remarkable difference in the slowing, prevention, and sometimes reversal of this condition. Inverting yourself allows gravity to temporarily work with you instead of against you. Just a quick couple of sessions are enough of a momentary pressure relief on your venous backflow system to allow them to 'catch their breath' from the normal 24-hour-a-day cycle they are typically tasked with working. The benefits of this therapy cannot be overstated, and they harmonize quite nicely with the rest of the recommendations in this chapter. My favorite inversion table to date is the IronMan 4000. You can usually find one of these on Amazon.com for around $350.

CHAPTER 7

BIO-ELECTRIC MEDICINE

Bio-electric medicine was touched on in the earlier chapter on acupuncture, but that was in an ancient 'old-school' sense (and hey, sometimes old school is the best school!). But what can modern science add to it? What can we improve upon? It turns out there is a whole lot we can do to augment the ancient traditions.

I highly recommend that everyone interested in this topic read three very important books: *Healing is Voltage* by Dr. Jerry Tennant, *PEMF the 5th Element of Health* by Bryant A. Meyers, and *The Body Electric* by Dr. Robert Becker and Gary Selden. Each can be cheaply found on Amazon.com or other major book outlets. The preview summary of *Healing of Voltage* reads:

> Every cell in the body is designed to run at -20 to -25 millivolts. To heal, we must make new cells. To make new cells requires -50 millivolts. Chronic disease occurs when voltage drops below -20 and/or you cannot achieve -50 millivolts to make new cells. Thus, chronic disease is always defined by having low voltage. This book tells you how to measure your voltage in each organ, how to correct it, and how to determine why your voltage dropped enough to allow you to get sick.

That seems important right? *Sigh*...it's a shame they don't teach that in med school! But I digress!

In addition to the ancient methods (acupuncture, earthing, grounding, bio-magnets, etc.) to restore the bio-electric pathways, we now have new technology called PEMF, which is short for 'pulsed electromagnetic field' therapy. These devices are extremely powerful tools which, over the course of just 8 minutes, begin to restore that millivoltage charge to all the cells in your body, *simultaneously*. They send a very specific frequency and type of wave form through the entire body to jumpstart all of the meridians, cells, and bio-electric pathways in order to assist the body in healing itself. More blood-flow, more oxygen, more micro-circulation, more energy, more cellular efficiency/function, and more bio-electrical conductivity = a much happier, healthier human being.

What makes this technology more important now than ever is that our bodies are constantly being bombarded by harmful frequencies emitted by cell phones, cell phone towers, Wi-Fi, smart meters, and whole host of other damaging electromagnetic frequencies emitted into our local environments. More and more studies are beginning to show the disruptive effects these devices have on cell function, brain waves, bio and circadian rhythms, sleep cycles, and overall health—everything from the increased prevalence of cancerous tumors to cardiac events. As of this writing, the critical mass of awareness of bio-shielding and PEMF therapy within the consciousness of the public is only beginning to emerge... however, in the near future, the proposed roll out of "5G" cell-phone technology and the associated health concerns may very well make them common household items. To those who are interested, research the side effects they are reporting in the 'test' cities where 5G is being rolled out. If we as a society allow this technology to become widespread...then, as they say in Game of Thrones...*a storm is coming.*

We need something that can negate the negative impact of these inescapably harmful devices and restore proper bio-electric function. Fortunately, we do have some respite via the valuable shielding capabilities of laboratory-developed devices like the

Q-Link (shopqlink.com), but that's only a passive approach in the form of shielding. We need something to actively re-empower the cells and by proxy the entire body to return to an optimal state of bio-electric energy.

The PEMF device that we currently use and recommend at our clinic is the BEMER Pro (which is the new evolution and improvement over the old Bemer3000 technology). We've had tremendous patient success, and it never ceases to amaze us how many benefits it provides and how well it augments the efficacy of our other holistic treatments. Do a quick Youtube search for "Bemer Microcirculation" and "Bemer Chitvan Malik" to get a scientific understanding of how it all works. If it's something that interests you as a practitioner or for personal use and you just want to know more, you can check out 8minutemat.com for additional information.

Full disclosure, I actually *do* have a vested financial interest in this product as a distributor. But I am *not* a brand-loyalist, I believe in what works. Before we ever had the Bemer Pro in our clinic, we first used the competitors IMRS-2000 and the Curatron. While I believe both of these other devices can be beneficial to a certain extent in their own right, we simply never saw anywhere near the positive patient results and outcomes that we've gotten with Bemer, which is what led to us becoming a Bemer distributor. Bemer also appears to have much more clinical data, studies, and research behind it as a technology, as well as a recently signed agreement with N.A.S.A. to integrate their technology into future applications designed for astronaut use. When it comes to clinical application, more 'power' is not better... specific beneficial frequencies and waveforms are what's needed to produce results, and Bemer gets that right.

I eagerly await what future iterations of this technology may bring as we enter a new era of bio-electric and voltage-based medicine.

CHAPTER 8

BREATHING AND HYDRATION

Hydration. Breathing. Is it really worth dedicating a whole chapter to this? The answer is a resounding *yes*. We don't know *how* to breathe. We don't know *how* to keep ourselves hydrated.

I have patients come to the clinic frequently whom we have a slightly difficult time starting an IV on them because they are dehydrated (and often over-caffeinated). I ask them about this and they either readily admit that they 'haven't drank any water yet today' or they have the opposite reaction...shock, because they claim to have already drunk one to two liters before the IV was started. The problem being that you can drink a sizeable amount of water and still be clinically dehydrated. Most people aren't aware that water alone isn't enough to properly hydrate. We need the six major electrolytes--sodium, calcium, phosphorus, chloride, potassium, and magnesium—for the kidneys to properly regulate fluid balance. In our typical crappy western diets, we simply don't get the electrolytes we need. Sure, we get plenty of sodium, too much in fact, but we need to balance it out with those that are insufficient, most notably magnesium and potassium. We should also be drinking truly purified water which is balanced with the right minerals needed to optimally maintain metabolic function. This is a catch-22 because most reverse osmosis systems, which are ostensibly designed to remove impurities from the water, also remove the trace minerals. When you drink overly purified water you aren't actually getting the necessary electrolytes and minerals into your system. (Some people swear by distilled water as being part of a daily cleansing ritual, and I have no problem with that, but it is still quite important to supplant the necessary electrolytes throughout the day.) Furthermore, while reverse osmosis units do a lot as far as eliminating particulate matter, they don't remove the toxins like Fluoride, unless you add a special bone-char filter element capable of binding to and extracting it. Buy bottled water and you get exposed to the BPA/plastic toxin, especially if the bottles are left out in the heat in your car for a couple of hours or during transport before you even purchase them.

So what do we do? How do we get the right water, and the right amount of it to facilitate optimal health? Once again I'm glad you asked! The electrolyte and mineral issue is a simple fix…. I'm a big fan of the Power-Pak brand of electrolyte packets you can get on Amazon.com for about $14 (for a 1-month supply)…dirt cheap, they are non-gmo, taste great, and have all 6 major electrolytes and 72 ionic and trace minerals. Combine that with drinking the roughly 0.5 ounce of water per pound (~35ml per kilogram) of body weight and you've got basic hydration covered. What you don't want to do is drink a 'sports drink' like Powerade which has also sorts of toxic artificial ingredients in it. (Also, if you are a coffee/caffeine drinker, it's important to drink more than the 0.5 ounce (per lb of bodyweight) to compensate. Caffeine has a vasoconstriction effect, and also acts as a diuretic, essentially worsening the dehydration problem.)

Obtaining the clean healthy type of water we need on the other hand is a little bit more difficult of a task, at least here in western society. The water we generally have access to here is somewhere along the sliding scale of bad, worse, and terrible. At the most toxic end is municipal tap water (especially in places like Detroit or Flint), loaded with neuro- and excito-toxins like fluoride and chlorine, as well as a lead, anti-biotic residue, pesticides, and other miscellaneous environmental toxins. If you value your health, never drink this. Ever. Heavily filter it before even taking a shower in it if you can. On the other end of our spectrum is the water that is purified to an extent (R-O, UV light, etc), which is an improvement, but it is still leaching the plastic from its own container over time and more importantly, it's dead. In doesn't have the life-giving properties found in nature.

If you want the best, cleanest, healthiest, most life-giving water on earth, I would encourage you to go to johnellis.com. There are certainly some sensationalist claims/entertaining elements to the website that I *don't* necessarily subscribe to or stand behind, but the water itself is unlike anything else on the planet. I've skeptically tried it, I was impressed, and to be honest rather astounded at the effects it had (which are duplicable and well beyond the possibility of placebo effect). I'm not going to make any additional claims (and I have no vested interest in the product), I'm only going to suggest that there is something to what he discovered (an application of Faraday's 1st and 2nd laws of electrolysis with regard to 114-degree hydrogen bond angle), and that you should consider trying it once (from a skeptic's point of view of course) and see what you think.

If that's not an option, however, at the very least, drink plenty of properly purified (and de-fluoridated) water stored in glass containers and add in the electrolyte packets, and you will be doing better than the overwhelming majority of people in the western hemisphere. The difference in overall health, energy, and stamina will be immediately noticeable if you're currently in a state of chronic dehydration (which most of us are).

Breathing

The Eastern cultures of old have this one right. Here in western society, our lives are generally ruled by stress. There are always deadlines, conflicts, and the soul-crushing pressures of the rat race. When the body is stressed, the breathing is shallow and held in our chest. We don't breathe deeply and fully with our diaphragms expanded as we should. We don't draw life-giving breath all the way in like we should. We aren't in a state of peace, a place of zen, and we don't feel centered. Cellular respiration is diminished, and we do ourselves a huge disservice as the rest of our metabolic, mental, immune, and emotional functions suffer for it. We get more lactic acid build up, we get fatigued easier, agitated, and begin signaling the body to increase the rate at which it releases stress-coping molecules like norepinephrine and cortisol to deal with the extra strain on the body. Vicious cycles are begun and repeated ad infimum until an early death unless we consciously act to break them.

Whether or not you readily acknowledge the existence of chi/prana/essence/living breath, you still can benefit tremendously from deep breathing exercises, most notably during the practices of meditation and yoga. Science now readily admits that. A fascinating study done at Harvard Medical School, titled *Now and Zen: How Mindfulness Can Change Your Brain and Improve Your Health* was recently presented in the spring of 2016 by Dr. John Denninger, Dr. Sara Lazar, and Dr. David Vago, and I highly encourage you to read through it. Deeper breathing brings more oxygen and vitality into the body tissues. Doing this in a meditative and mindful state has been shown to lower stress, blood pressure, improve cognitive function and create a whole host of biochemical improvements within the human body. Yoga actively facilitates better blood flow and stress reduction as well and has long been known to be a valuable tool for rejuvenating and rebalancing the mind, body, and spirit.

Lastly, and most importantly, when you are ready to step just past the physical and perhaps slightly into the metaphysical/spiritual, I might suggest looking into the practice of "warrior breathing." This is a whole new level of active breathing technique(s). It's intense, it's a workout and it isn't for the faint of heart. It forces extra oxygen into the tissues and induces a state of mild hyperventilation...but man does it make you feel awake and alive! At the very least this electively induced and hyper-vigilante state offers a valuable data point as to what the opposite end of the spectrum looks like as compared to our typical shallow, inadequate breathing and to show what is possible for the human body to achieve with simple breath-work.

The pinnacle of breath work and how it allows us to push past the absolute limits of the human body is clearly demonstrated by a Dutch man named Wim Hof. Known as the "Iceman," he is world-renown for his ability (and teachable method) to do the outright impossible when it comes to withstanding the extreme elements of nature, most notably by immersing himself in sub-zero temperatures while maintaining his core body temperature. He can also drastically influence his immune system and autonomic functions like heart rate and adrenaline secretion, which was previously thought to be impossible by modern science. I highly recommend you watch a few of these super human inspirational videos at wimhofmethod.com. It will change your life, even if it's only your perspective.

CHAPTER 9

CANCER

It is almost difficult to choose a starting point on where to begin writing this chapter. Just about every other topic in this book has one or more books written about it. Within those books, the eventuality is that the disease state in question is what leads to cancer...and you know what? They are all correct. Stress leads to cancer, poor voltage/pH opens the door to cancer, root canals, poor diet, cell phone radiation, inflammation, viruses, heavy metals, environmental toxins, parasites...they *all* cause cancer. There have been countless books written on the countless different types of cancer. I don't feel the need, nor do I feel it would be productive to take 100 pages of this book to summarize the endless volumes of cancer information that we have at our disposal.

What I do feel inclined to do is to reconcile the fact that all causes of cancer and all types of cancer need *not* be so overly isolated as if they existed in a vacuum. It may work like that on paper in the soulless confines of Academia, but out here in the real world all those things are interrelated. In the real world a patient can develop cancer because of an amalgamation of origins. A single person can have a root canal, inflammation, low voltage/pH, Lyme disease, be drinking a diet Coke, have emotional stress, and be talking on a cell phone *simultaneously*. Is it really that big of a mystery why 1 in 2 people in the U.S. and the U.K. 'get' some form of cancer in their lifetimes? I should think not. It would be more logical to marvel at the testament to the strength of the human body that 1 in 2 people somehow manage to *not* get cancer in their lifetimes.

Every human being on the planet has cancer cells in their body. This is normal. The body has a cycle of facilitating cellular turnover in cancer cells the same as it does with any other cells, through a mechanism known as cellular apoptosis. This is another way of saying 'pre-programmed' cell death. A cell has finite life cycle, limited by the ever-shortening length of its telomeres, and once it has exhausted this cycle, it initiates a (highly controlled and regulated) self-destruct sequence. Somewhere between 50 to 70 billion cells die *each day* in the average human adult as more new cells are produced. When carcinogenic factors are introduced, this process gets disrupted, certain cells begin to mutate, and the over-taxed immune system is unable to successfully eliminate them all. Upon mutation, the process that initializes the regularly scheduled cell death gets derailed and the mechanism (apoptosis) gets deactivated, often leaving us with 'immortal' or 'zombie' cells. It is generally accepted that groups of these cells are what usually become a form of cancer or cancerous/malignant tumor. (There are of course exceptions to this in which the cancer cells are non-immortal, but regardless, the normal apoptosis process has been subverted and these cells have mutated to a malignant state.)

Ok great, so how does this pathology lesson help us in the long run? What is the proper preventative approach to drastically reduce the rate of cancer, and what are my best options if I'm currently battling cancer? The answer is **Synergy**. This is a foreign concept to many specialists who hang their hat on one particular treatment or modality. The answer is to address everything contained within this book (and the other books referenced herein), not just this chapter.

With that thought in mind, let me present to you some of the best, most powerful options on the planet. It would be foolhardy to claim to have all the answers or to throw around four-letter words like 'cure.' We certainly haven't done that. What we have done is help create a very powerful starting point that goes down a path leading to various modalities than can *help the body heal itself.* Let's begin…

Vitamin D3

Vitamin D3 isn't just a vitamin, it's a hormone. It is part of the very foundation of your immune system. It plays a critical role in your endocrine system. It is key in preventing depression, bone density loss, and most importantly, cancer. The reference range of Vitamin D in blood serum concentration is 30 to 100ng/ml, but the low end of that range is based on a sick population. We like to see our patients at a minimum of 90ng/ml. I keep my personal level at approximately 120ng/ml (deduce from my personal information what you wish). Taking 5,000 i.u. a day typically facilitates a 'maintenance' dose, whereas patients who are deficient can benefit from taking 10,000 i.u. a day to titrate those levels up over time. Vitamin D is fat soluble, so it will slowly build up in serum concentration over the course of several months of supplementation. For patients that are severely deficient, we do 50,000 i.u. intramuscular injections once a week at the clinic to bring them up a little quicker.

Intravenous Vitamin C / Meyer's Cocktail

This is probably the most common treatment we administer at our clinic, and it's also one of the most effective. It is physically impossible to get to a therapeutic dosage of vitamin C when it is consumed orally. This is due to a mechanical limit (in the gut) with regard to how the human body uptakes water soluble vitamins. You can drink a literal gallon of oral vitamin C and it practically utterly useless, only serving to act as an expensive laxative that produces explosive diarrhea. When we administer vitamin C intravenously however, it bypasses this mechanical limit and goes straight to work, elevating blood concentration levels to therapeutic values. Extensive studies, most notably conducted at the University of Kansas research hospital, have shown that IV doses exceeding somewhere between 10 to 20 grams (10,000 to 20,000mg) of Vitamin C cause it to switch from an anti-oxidant therapy to a pro-oxidative therapy (thus converting it to a form of peroxide in the blood-stream), which kills cancer cells.

For more information, research 'Myer's Cocktail.' Every integrative clinic has their own custom version of it, but you specifically only want to go to a clinic for this therapy if they use (non-GMO) tapioca/cassava-based Vitamin C. You do not want the (probably GMO) corn-based 'manufactured' version of IV-C. This stuff is garbage and can cause inflammation, but it's much cheaper and more readily available, so be extra sure you're getting the right stuff. Remember the devil is *always* in the details. You also want a fair amount of Methylcobalamin (B12), Magnesium, and Sodium Bicarbonate in the bag to get the full benefits of a well-rounded 'cocktail.' This is an essential tool in helping the body fight cancer. **Human beings** *are one of the only mammals (along with primates, guinea pigs, and fruit bats) that* **cannot naturally produce their own vitamin C during times of distress or illness.**

IV Glutathione

This treatment is described elsewhere in the book but it is the body's master anti-oxidant molecule and helps detox the body/liver during cancer therapy. It should not be performed on the same day as pro-oxidative therapy such as high-dose Vitamin C, Silver Hydrosol, or UVBI because the effects can negate each other.

UltraViolet Blood Irradiation

This has been around for over half a century, but the newest version of the technology is the **UVLrx**. I won't make any specific claims on this device, but go to UVLrx.com for more info.

Vitamin B17/Laetrile

This is a very powerful anti-cancer nutrient that is mostly non-existent in the North American diet. This one has been suppressed for decades. For more information, read the book *World Without*

Cancer: The Story of Vitamin B17. If you feel this treatment is right for you, it is available for purchase at tjsupply.com/vitamin-b17-injections.html.

DCA

DCA—Dichloroacetate is a very well tolerated, non-toxic, highly affordable, extremely effective cancer treatment that is used with great success in tandem with other therapies. Go to DCAwatch.com for more information and the fascinating history about DCA. If you feel this treatment is right for you, it can be found and purchased at PureDCA.com.

BloodRoot

This is used in both oral preparation as well as a topical salve. Well known in Native American medicine, TCM, and herbology to be extremely effective treatment for both skin cancer and prostate cancer. Studies on the active plant alkaloid *sanguinarine* show cell blockade and apoptosis of human prostate carcinoma cells. See study here: mct.aacrjournals.org/content/3/8/933.short.

Anecdotally, we've had several patients come through our clinic who were/are under the care of a DOM/AP (doctor of oriental medicine/acupuncturist) who had successfully treated their skin cancer with this item.

DMSO

This naturally occurring solvent that has been safely used intravenously as an anti-inflammatory, anti-viral, anti-fungal, anti-bacterial, and anti-cancer treatment for decades. It works quite powerfully on its own, but when combined with a Myer's cocktail or with Sodium Bicarbonate, it can be extra effective at penetrating and fighting cancer cells. I recommend picking up a copy of the book *DMSO: Nature's Healer* by Dr. Morton Walker for more information. Also, be sure to check http://www.cancertutor.com/dmso/ to learn about how it can work with chemo to make it drastically more effective and much safer.

Medical Marijuana

Literally endless amounts of data and scores of both international and domestic studies showing both safety and efficacy. Has been used for thousands of years both as palliative therapy and for the treatment of illness (including cancer.) There is entire metabolic pathway in human beings known as the **Endocannabinoid** system that seems to be custom made for and restored by the use of marijuana. (See marijuana chapter.) The science is there; it's finally getting legalized. Let us hope that Big Pharma/Monsanto doesn't come in and GMO the ever-loving shit out of it, which would turn it sterile, useless and probably toxic.

IPT

IPT is Insulin Potentiated Therapy. True holistic practitioners typically try to have their cancer patients avoid chemo and radiation at all costs (and for mostly good reason if you look at the non-cherry-picked actual mortality/success rates), but for those patients who are convinced they need to do chemo, IPT is the best option. Cancer cells consume more than *20 times* as much glucose/sugar than normal cells. When there is an insulin spike (which is typically what happens naturally when a person consumes carbohydrates/sugar/glucose), the cancer cells get excited and become more receptive/open up because they are expecting the incoming sugar.

Through the manipulation of this process by injecting a patient with exogenous insulin at the same time they are administered chemotherapy, it 'tricks' the cancer cells into thinking they are getting a big meal of sugar/glucose, and it makes them more readily uptake the chemotherapy. This allows a considerably more targeted and effective treatment, and also allows the usage of much less chemo, usually about *one-tenth* the standard dosage. This is way less toxic on the body and drastically increases the rate at which the patient's body will survive the chemo itself.

IV Cesium Chloride

This is another promising therapy that works by (simplifying it here) drastically raising the pH of cancer cells to an alkaline state (around 8), thereby impairing the ability of the cancer cell's enzyme systems and abilities to reproduce and survive. I personally do not have any clinical experience with this particular modality, but it has been used with noteworthy success in parts of Europe, and there are compounding pharmacies in the U.S. that make it upon a doctor's order for IV therapy. Go to CancerTutor.com/cesium-chloride/ for more information.

Dendritic Cell Therapy

This is the new frontier of customized immunotherapy. Patients who are already battling cancer can have a sample of their blood taken, which is then recombined into a targeted cell-signaling therapy aimed at potentiating their own immune response towards specific types of cancer. The sample is then re-injected into the patient with the hope of having a significantly improved ability to fight off the cancer.

Myomin/DIM/Calcium-D-Glucarate

These are 3 easily attainable supplements (all 3 can be found on Amazon.com and other common websites). All 3 of them have the powerful ability to block and purge excess estrogens from the body (which includes chemical, false, xeno-estrogens), and this can be very helpful support to anyone who is fighting cancer, as there are several types of cancer that proliferate in the presence of excess estrogen.

Poly MVA

This is a clinically formulated, highly unique treatment containing a proprietary blend of the mineral palladium bonded to alpha-lipoic acid, vitamins B1/B2/B12, formyl-methionine, N-acetyl cysteine, and trace amounts of molybdenum, rhodium, and ruthenium. For more information, go to Polymva.com. The *intravenous* version is only available for purchase by doctors, and the oral version able to be purchased online. I won't make any claims other than to say I've seen it in action and it can be very *ahem*, helpful. Per the website:

> This formulation is designed to provide energy for compromised body systems by changing the electrical potential of human cells and facilitating aerobic metabolism within the cell. A member of the Lipoic Acid Mineral Complexes (LAMC), Poly-MVA may assist in boosting immune response by replenishing key nutrients and supporting cellular metabolism. What makes Poly-MVA unique is the proprietary manufacturing process by which palladium is sequestered to lipoic acid. No other company produces a product similar to Poly-MVA because of the preparation and bonding process through which LAMC is manufactured. The proprietary formulation of LAMC with other vitamins, minerals, and amino acids provides considerable nutritional support, helping to enable optimum functioning of essential body systems.
>
> When lipoic acid, a powerful antioxidant with many biological functions, is connected to an electrically-charged mineral substrate, and associated with B vitamins, the resulting complex has enhanced solubility in both water and fat. It can easily and safely travel throughout the body, even crossing the blood-brain barrier. Its ability to cross the blood-brain barrier (impossible even for most drugs, let alone ordinary nutritional supplements) suggests that, as a nutritional supplement, Poly-MVA may hold great promise in cases where other means of supplementing cell nutrition are ineffective.
>
> The Poly-MVA dietary supplement has a unique action because healthy cells have oxygen radical pathways. Normally, oxygen radicals are formed when fatty acids

donate electrons to oxygen. These oxygen radicals have an unpaired electron charge and are unstable. Special proteins in the mitochondria convert the oxygen radicals into water and usable energy. Poly-MVA has shown to assist and facilitate this process.

Numerous articles, studies and in-depth information on Poly-MVA are available. Please contact AMARC Enterprises at 1-866-POLY-MVA (866-765-9682), search or visit the additional pages of this website.

Silver Hydrosol

There is only one version of this I recommend, and it is the practitioner grade *Argentyn23* by Natural Immunogenics. The *intravenous administration* isn't really discussed by the company. But what I can tell you is that Argentyn23 is an excellent anti-viral, anti-fungal, anti-microbial, anti-pathogen, etc, and I've seen incredible 'positive results' with what it can do. It is 100% safe, you could drink it, or spray it in your eyes/nose (all of which I've done myself) with no risk of adverse reactions. Per there website (natural-immunogenics.com/products/argentyn-23.html):

> Argentyn 23 is a professional grade of silver hydrosol which is available only through licensed health care practitioners. Like Sovereign Silver, it represents the ultimate refinement and most significant breakthrough in colloidal technology, having consistently produced the smallest particles ever seen in colloidal silver products, with the most unique charge attributes (98% positively charged). The manufacturing technique is proprietary but particle size and particle charge have been confirmed by third party laboratories and universities. Argentyn 23 does not use additives or stabilizers, nor does it contain salts or proteins (often used to keep silver in suspension, but which create silver compounds). It is pure, meaning it contains only 99.999% pure silver suspended in

pharmaceutical-grade purified water. No other manufacturer can make these claims and support them with evidence.

I have used Natural Immunogenics' professional Argentyn 23 silver hydrosol in immune-suppressed patients for many years. I have been very impressed with its positive effects in a series of applications, as well as its safety record, as the likelihood of a significant side-effect is almost non-existent. I have not found other so-called silver products to be nearly as effective.

—Kent Holtorf, M.D.,
Holtorf Medical Group Affiliate Centers

Over the past 10 years, I have used thousands of dosages of Argentyn 23 with the most consistent results. Having a nano particularized silver, with the ultimate dispersion and zeta potential, makes it a formidable tool for daily use in my practice. Extremely low, if any, side-effect potential, coupled with broad-based efficacy, has made Argentyn 23 my product of choice for countless immune cases.

—Mitch Ghen, D.O., Ph.D.

It is without hesitation that I support and applaud Natural Immunogenics for its safety and quality in making an excellent and pure silver hydrosol product for public use.

—Dana Flavin, M.D.
Founder and Executive Director
Foundation for Collaborative Medicine and Research;
Former science assistant to the Associate Bureau
Director Division of Toxicology, US FDA,
Washington, DC

GcMaf

This may very well be a more important discovery than all of the other treatments, *combined*. I would encourage you to download the

100% free copy online of *The GcMAF Book* by Tim Smith, MD., while it's still available at http://gcmaf.timsmithmd.com/book/book/4/. Without getting too far into conspiracy, this information is being heavily suppressed, and it would appear that several holistic practitioners known to be successfully treating patients with this modality (approaching 90 of them as of this writing) seem to have *unintentionally 'suicided' themselves or found themselves dead from freak accidents* in the past couple of years. We'll say no more on that other than where there's smoke, there is usually fire. (And I don't really care what the manipulated mainstream media and the obviously bought-and-paid-for shill Snopes.com have to say on the subject.)

Paraphrased per an excerpt of The GcMAF Book:

> As far as the treatment... GcMAF—Group-specific component Macrophage-Activating Factor is the [naturally occurring] protein your body makes to activate your anti-cancer immunity. Your immune system contains some very large cells called macrophages that, when activated, will track down, attack, devour, and kill viruses and cancer cells. GcMAF—an immune protein made by your lymphocytes—is what literally turns them on. Without GcMAF, your macrophages remain in a state of suspended animation—sort of like zombies...This is not a subtle slowdown, either. In terms of killing power, an activated macrophage is about 40 times more aggressive than a de-activated macrophage. Without GcMAF, they just go to sleep.
>
> Cancer cells (and certain viruses) 'know' that if they block the production of GcMAF, they can disable their archenemies, the macrophages, and get the upper hand. Without GcMAF to activate them, the macrophages don't have a chance.

Per VDBP online:

GcMAF is also known as a Vitamin D Binding protein, and facilitates the transport of vitamin D metabolites. It has a major role in maintaining the total levels of vitamin D in the body and in regulating the amounts of free (unbound) vitamin D available for specific tissues and cell types to utilize. Other functions of VDBP are to control bone development, binding of fatty acids, sequestration of actin and a range of less-defined roles in modulating immune and inflammatory responses. The actin removal is considered to be a very important role for VDBP, actins being toxic and released into the body following cell death.

Two amino acids on this protein chain have been shown to be very strongly associated with the activation of macrophages. In some publications, the vitamin D binding protein is shown to respond to enzymes released by inflammation and this is often referred to as MAF (Macrophage Activating Factor). Studies show that this isoform not only activates macrophages, it turns them off when no longer needed, so it is an immune system regulator.

Studies in laboratory cultures have shown that Calcitriol (Vitamin D bound with VDBP) can significantly increase the number of dopamine neurons.

Vitamin D Binding Protein is otherwise known as:
- VDBP
- Gc-Protein
- Glycoprotein
- Transport protein
- Gc-Globulin
- GcMAF

Cancer cells block GcMAF production by making a protein called Nagalase. *Nagalase levels are always directly proportional to* *the levels of cancer in your body*, even if it is yet too early to see any sort of tumor/lump/mass on an ultrasound, MRI, or CT/PET scan. Whether cancer has reached conventionally detectable levels or not, as practitioners we can run one of the many available nagalase labs (it's easy to find found four or five here in the U.S. after 30 seconds of a simple Google search) and establish a baseline on a patient. If you are more conventionally/allopathically minded and aren't quite convinced, think of this as being similar (only better) to traditional CEA/CA 19-9/CA 125 cancer markers...i.e. you don't have to use them as diagnostic, but you can use them as reference markers to track a baseline and show a progression.

Here is the twist that circles briefly back into the shadows for the moment...it would appear that we now know from the **research** of several concerned doctors and scientists (some of whom are now deceased like Dr. James Jeffrey Bradstreet) **that the culprit cancer protein *nagalase* is included (free of charge!) in almost all of our childhood vaccines, flu shots, pneumovax/zostavax, etc.. Pharmaceutical companies do not deny this.**

They simply cry foul and say 'nagalase cannot cause cancer!' And *technically*, they are correct, it doesn't *cause* cancer. Every human being on the planet *already has cancer cells*. What they neglect to mention is what nagalase *does* do is *block the body's ability to fight cancer* via preventing macrophages from being activated, and by blocking the absorption, transport, and utilization of Vitamin D, thus allowing cancer to proliferate unimpeded. Whether or not this is intentional is for you to decide, but it is almost irrelevant at this point. The nagalase in these vaccines is a 'slow-kill' for everyone. When children are young, their stem cells are healthy and their bodies are little power-houses of energy, and they often manage to get by a full schedule of childhood vaccines with no immediately apparent side effects. But as we age (especially past 40), the strength of our stem cells deteriorates, and metabolic pathways begin to break down, we rely increasingly more on our immune systems, Vitamin D, and our ability to fight off cancer to survive. This becomes increasingly difficult with a crippled/impaired immune system.

As a side note the big Pharma crowd also claim that nagalase (in the form alpha-N-acetylgalactosaminidase) is naturally occurring and necessary for humans to not develop the *exceedingly rare* (less than 1 in 200,000 according to tracking/reporting which first began in the late 1980's) liposomal storage disorder known as 'Schindler disease' or 'Kanzaki disease.'

This is a ridiculously wet-toilet-paper thin argument on all fronts, and more specifically, the disease mentioned has to do with an isolated deficiency due to mutations in the NAGA gene on chromosome 22. **This very low, naturally occurring level of this enzyme** *cannot be in anyway logically construed to even be in the same ballpark as the massive quantities of synthetically derived nagalase included in the never ending schedules of childhood vaccines, boosters, flu shots, etc.*

If you would like to get more of a taste for why there is such a controversy brewing here, go to:
naturalnews.com/050582_nagalase_GcMAF_cancer_industry_prof its.html.

Friends, patients, practitioners, we have a very real solution that is being violently suppressed by a $100 billion dollar a year cancer *industry*. The science behind GcMaf is very real, it is very clear, it is easily duplicated, and it is already a core element of the body's innate ability to fight of cancer. Drug companies will *never* produce the funding and put it through the process of becoming a prescription item because it falls under the FDA's classification of a naturally occurring molecule within the human body, and therefore it cannot be patented. Even if it could, it would wipe out a massive industry. As practitioners, we often want to maintain an altruistic mindset, and see the good in everyone. But to understand true good, you also must understand that there is true evil, true darkness, and true greed in the world. You are a fool if you believe otherwise. It is important to state again that it's time that we *raise our consciousness* to the very real threats around us. The science is there, it's time we change our philosophies and mindsets to match it.

Ok so we've discovered some awesome and powerful treatments...what about understanding and eliminating some of the causes? I'm glad you asked! Let's begin with a few clear examples of what we need to observe and eliminate.

Addition by Subtraction

When it comes to understanding medicine, health, biochemistry, disease, and the human body in general, we often run into one of two problems: gross oversimplification or needless complication. Let's give some examples of each:

Gross Oversimplification:

All stress is bad for the body. This once commonly held belief is now known to be untrue. There is eustress, which the good kind of stress you might get from an intense, but enjoyable workout, and there is distress, which is itself an over-simplified umbrella term that encompasses all 'bad' forms of stress. Consider this excerpt from world-renown author Anthony William:

> **The Many Blends of Adrenaline:**
>
> [Mainstream] medical science and research currently believe there is only one type of adrenaline produced by the adrenals, but this isn't true. It's not yet known that **there are actually 56 different blends of adrenaline** that are produced and change in response to different everyday emotions and situations, including dreaming, showering, exercising, falling in love, have a car accident, arguing, debating, singing, even listening.
>
> ...our adrenals have the wisdom to release any of the 56 hormone blends to power us through our immediate needs.

Needless Complication:

Thanks to the hundreds of millions of dollars being frittered away in needlessly specific, ultra-complex, and inherently myopic cancer research, lots of well-paid, bespectacled academicians (i.e. people who spend their entire lives sequestered in a lab instead of seeing actual patients in the real world) have come to the conclusion that the prevalence of breast cancer must have some complex genetic/hereditary origin that causes genes like *BRCA1*, *BRCA2*, and *PALB2* to mutate at an absurdly high rate relative to the general population.

Guess what, it's not. ***It's because of deodorant***. What? Let's say it again—it's because of the deodorants/anti-perspirants that most people use. At the risk of being called a quack or conspiracy theorist, let's dig a little deeper, provide some reasonable evidence, and look at the facts, shall we? Here are some of the main ingredients found in several brand name deodorants/anti-perspirants:

- **Propylene Glycol**—when they put this in your radiator, they call it 'anti-freeze.' Known to cause heart, liver, and nervous system damage. Probable carcinogen.

- **TEA** and **DEA**—Triethanolamine and Diethanolamine, readily absorbed into the skin and known to cause liver and/or kidney damage. Known carcinogens and already banned in Europe because of it (but not here in the U.S. for some reason).

- **Triclosan**—kills bacteria and is classified as a pesticide. When combined with water it has the potential to make the compound known as chloroform, which is a known carcinogen.

- **Phthalates**—disrupt androgen function, impairs reproductive ability in men, linked to impaired fetal development, lower IQ's, and higher rates of asthma. Probable carcinogen.

- **Parabens**—disrupts hormonal balance, acts as a xeno-estrogen, known to disturb the body's hormonal balance and promote both breast and prostate cancer.

- **Talc**—potential to contain asbestiform fibers, as in the well-known carcinogen *asbestos*. The quantity of asbestiform fibers in deodorants is heretofore unknown because it *isn't regulated* in cosmetic products.

- **Steareth-n**—derived from vegetable oil but reacted with ethylene oxide, a known carcinogen.

- **Aluminum Compounds**—main active ingredient (this is what temporarily clogs underarm pores to block sweating)—linked with Alzheimer's disease and other forms of cognitive/neurological degeneration. Exposure has now also been linked with both direct carcinogenic activity as well as interfering with estrogen levels, which can directly and indirectly stimulate the growth of breast tissue cancer. PubMed Studies anyone? Just for the sake of overkill (because I like killing a house-fly with a nuclear weapon), here are *five* that I found after a mere 30 seconds of looking. (There are probably more but I got bored of reading all of them):

  1) *Aluminum, Antiperspirants, and Breast Cancer*
     www.ncbi.nlm.nih.gov/pubmed/16045991

  2) *Aluminum and Breast Cancer: Sources of Exposure, Tissue Measurements, and Mechanisms of Toxicological Actions on Breast Biology*
     www.ncbi.nlm.nih.gov/pubmed/23899626

  3) *If exposure to aluminum in antiperspirants produces health risks, its content should be reduced*
     www.ncbi.nlm.nih.gov/pubmed/24418462

4) Aluminum and the human breast
   www.ncbi.nlm.nih.gov/pubmed/26997127

5) Aluminum chloride promotes tumorigenesis and metastasis in normal murine mammal gland epithelial cells
   http://www.ncbi.nlm.nih.gov/pubmed/27541736

And if that wasn't enough information to give you pause, consider that the majority of breast cancer tumors form in the upper outer quadrant of the breast, closest to where the deodorant/anti-perspirants are applied. Apply these deodorants one time, and you are probably ok. Apply them to your underarms (where there is also breast tissue and lymph nodes) every day for 40 years, and ask yourself how in the world you *don't* have breast cancer (assuming you don't already). Can genetics play a role in all this? Sure, they can, but it's more a matter of genetic *susceptibility* or genetic '*toughness*' with regard to *resisting* mutations that cause cancer when exposed to carcinogens, as opposed to the current model, which seems to indicate that the body arbitrarily attacks itself. Ask yourself which one makes more sense. The human body is a marvel of engineering, it's designed to maintain homeostasis and keep itself alive as best it can for as long as it can. Therefore, it would stand to reason that we would not have such a ridiculously high incidence of things like breast cancer relative to the general population. What we have are people who are genetically not strong enough to resist 40 or 50 years of bastardized combinations of carcinogens being applied directly to their lymph nodes and breast tissue. Even this of course, occurs within the vacuum of not considering the addition of all the other carcinogens, environmental toxins, heavy metals, pesticides, stresses, etc. one might experience over the course of a lifetime. We are literally just talking about deodorant thus far...which is why it can be infuriating to see stuff like this:

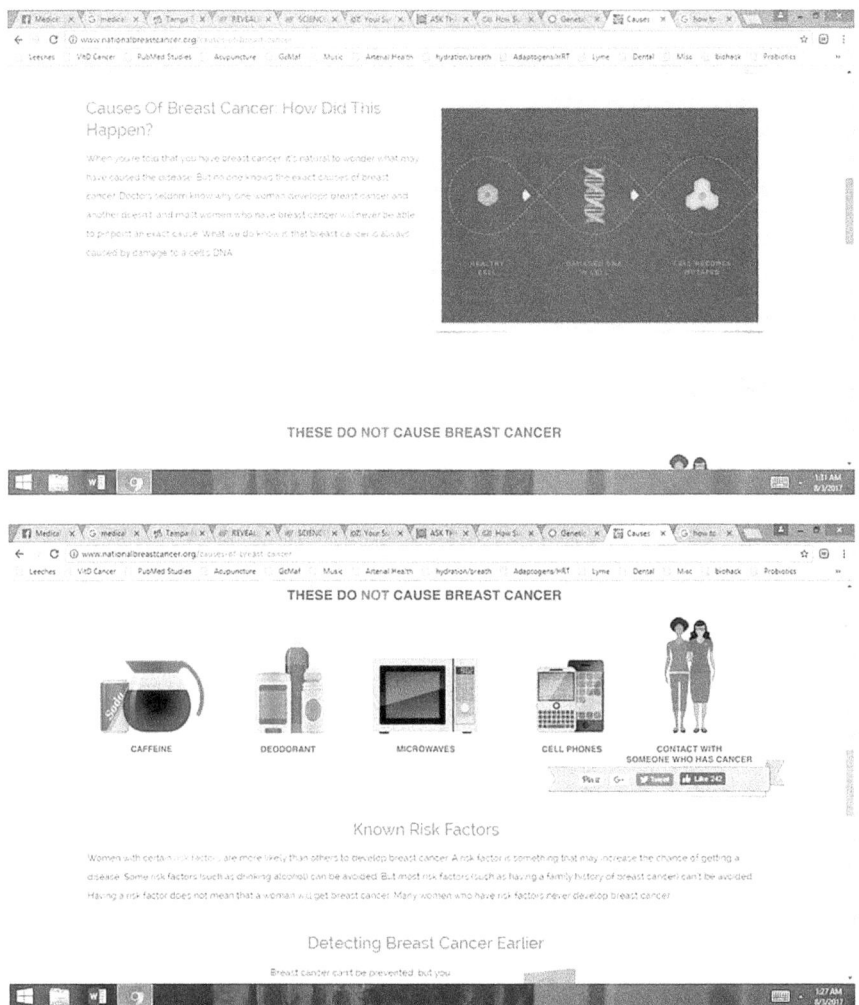

THESE DO NOT CAUSE BREAST CANCER

Folks, the 'information' in this second screen shot is *felony stupidity*. If we didn't know better, we might think this type of ass-hattery was from the satire news site *The Onion*. But sadly, it's not. It's from nationalbreastcancer.org/causes-of-breast-cancer. The *first four of the five items on their list are major causes of cancer*. The fifth item is still up for scientific debate given the current meta-data available, but with it now being known that certain viruses (which can be transmitted via bodily fluids) play a critical role in the development of certain cancers, I think it's safe to say that #5 is a strong candidate to play a role as well. Now let's look back to the first screen shot, where we have a grossly oversimplified version of how breast cancer might occur. They have a progression made for kindergarteners that says:

> "Healthy Cell → Damaged DNA in Cell → Cell Becomes Mutated."

Hmm...ok well how did the DNA get damaged and the cell become mutated? It certainly can't be any of these 5 items listed below like carcinogen-laden deodorant or cell phone radiation, that's for damn sure! Because if that *was* the case, then what *the hell* do you need us for and why the hell would you go to the massive section of our website dedicated to donations, fundraising, corporate partnering, getting signed up for the Art of Hope Gala, purchasing hats/t-shirts/coffee mugs from the NBCF gift shop, or getting your very own Fundraising Tool-kit?? One day, on the 12th of Nevertober we'll find the 'cure,' but in the mean time we've got to do everything we can to distract people from the *root cause* and sell plenty of merchandise.

The tone here is not meant to sound callous or flippant, but it is meant to sound incredulous with a hint of outrage. Support groups and fellowship are extremely important for sufferers, survivors, and family members of breast cancer. But go to the TheTruthAboutCancer.com/susan-g-komen-pink-ribbon-façade and educate yourself on the shameful scams out there that masquerade as true charities.

As a side note, the first iPhone was released on June 29th, 2007. To me this was the dawn of the 'smart-phone era.' Now, over 10 years later, smartphone use is ubiquitous, and we know from overwhelming anecdotal evidence as well as several ongoing studies that cell phone radiation disrupts cellular function, brain-wave function and has drastically increased the rate of brain tumors, most specifically on the same side of the head that the user typically holds the phone to. I suspect that there is a high percentage (somewhere around 100%) that cell-phones being carried around in woman's bra (a common storage location) now directly competes with anti-perspirant as the main cause of breast cancer. But hey, they also aren't mutually exclusive (perhaps on paper, not in the real world). Cell phones and deodorant don't have to compete. They exacerbate—i.e. it's probably a safe bet (though there is admittedly no data to support this) that most people (men included) that store a cell phone in either a shirt pocket or a bra probably also wear deodorant.

Let's look at the data from a 2013 multi-focal breast cancer study with regard to cell-phone proximity to breast tissue (skip past it if you just want the summary) and see what it has to say:

Case Report

Multifocal Breast Cancer in Young Women with Prolonged Contact between Their Breasts and Their Cellular Phones

John G. West[1], Nimmi S. Kapoor[1], Shu-Yuan Liao[2], June W. Chen[3], Lisa Bailey[4], and Robert A. Nagourney[5]

[1] Breastlink, Department of Surgery, 230 S. Main Street, Suite 100, Orange, CA 92868, USA
[2] Department of Pathology, St. Joseph Hospital, University of California Irvine, 1100 West Stewart Drive, Orange, CA 92868-5600, USA
[3] Breastlink, Department of Radiology, 230 S. Main Street, Suite 100, Orange, CA 92868, USA
[4] Bay Area Breast Surgeons, Inc., Department of Surgery, 3300 Webster Street, Suite 212, Oakland, CA 94609, USA
[5] Department of Obstetrics and Gynecology, Rational Therapeutics, University of California Irvine, Long Beach, CA, USA

Received 30 July 2013; Accepted 19 August 2013

Academic Editor: Hans-Joachim Mentzel

Abstract

Breast cancer occurring in women under the age of 40 is uncommon in the absence of family history or genetic predisposition, and prompts the exploration of other possible exposures or environmental risks. We report a case series of four young women—ages from 21 to 39—with multifocal invasive breast cancer that raises the concern of a possible association with nonionizing radiation of electromagnetic field exposures from cellular phones. All patients regularly carried their smartphones directly against their breasts in their brassieres for up to 10 hours a day, for several years, and developed tumors in areas of their breasts immediately underlying the phones. All patients had no family history of breast cancer, tested negative for BRCA1 and BRCA2, and had no other known breast cancer risks. Their breast imaging is reviewed, showing clustering of multiple tumor foci in the breast directly under the area of phone contact. Pathology of all four cases shows striking similarity; all tumors are hormone-positive, low-intermediate grade, having an extensive intraductal component, and all tumors have near identical morphology. These cases raise awareness to the lack of safety data of prolonged direct contact with cellular phones.

1. Case Reports

1.1. Case 1

A 21-year-old female presented with left spontaneous bloody nipple discharge. Her history was notable for keeping her cellular phone tucked into her bra on the left side for several hours each day. Her mammogram showed extensive pleomorphic calcifications and densities from the retroareolar region to the chest wall spanning a length of 12 cm. A magnetic resonance image (MRI) showed extensive abnormal nonmass enhancement in a segmental distribution corresponding to changes seen on her mammogram (Figures 1(a)–1(c)). She was treated with mastectomy and pathology revealed extensive ductal carcinoma in situ (DCIS) with multifocal microinvasion. Sentinel lymph nodes were negative for metastatic disease.

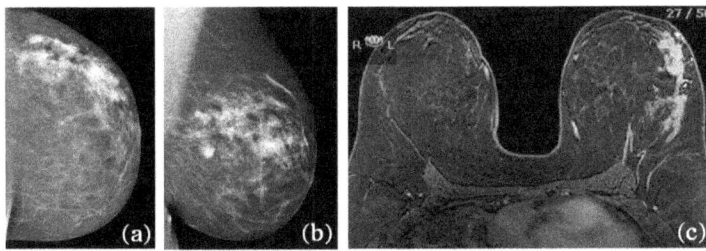

Figure 1: Representative imaging of patient in Case 1. Left mammogram showing clustered calcification corresponding to multiple sites of disease in craniocaudal (a) and mediolateral-oblique (b) projections. MRI showing extensive nonmass enhancement in the lateral hemisphere of the left breast in segmental distribution (c).

1.2. Case 2

A 21-year-old female presented with a palpable breast mass in the area where her cellular phone was kept in direct contact with her left breast. She had been placing her cellular device in her bra for eight hours a day or longer for the past six years. Breast MRI demonstrated four distinct separate lesions ranging from 15 to 18 mm in diameter involving an extensive area of the upper hemisphere of the left breast. Pathology of her mastectomy showed multifocal invasive cancer with extensive DCIS. Two of nine axillary lymph nodes were positive for metastatic disease. Later studies found metastasis to the bone.

1.3. Case 3

A 33-year-old female presented with two palpable masses in the upper outer quadrant of her right breast directly underneath where her cellular phone was placed against her breast in her bra. She had been placing her cellular phone in her bra intermittently for eight years. In the two years prior to diagnosis she would routinely place her phone in her bra while jogging 3-4 times per week. During this time period she would use a global positioning system (GPS) application on her cellular phone to determine her location while jogging. MRI demonstrated at least six suspicious lesions spanning a length of 8 cm in the upper outer quadrant of the right breast. Mastectomy specimen showed extensive DCIS with multifocal invasion. A 5 mm metastasis was found in one sentinel lymph node.

1.4. Case 4

A 39-year-old female presented with three palpable breast masses in the area of cellular phone contact with her right breast. She had been placing her cellular phone in her bra while commuting and using a Bluetooth device to talk for hours each day for the past ten years. MRI demonstrated multiple mass-like and tubular areas of enhancement essentially involving the entire upper right breast from the 11 to 1 o'clock position. Mastectomy showed four separate invasive ductal carcinomas ranging from 1 to 3 cm in size with 10 cm of DCIS. Two of nine lymph nodes were positive for metastatic disease. Pathology of the insitu and invasive ductal carcinomas observed in all four cases shows striking similarity, and the representative histological figures are illustrated in Figure 2.

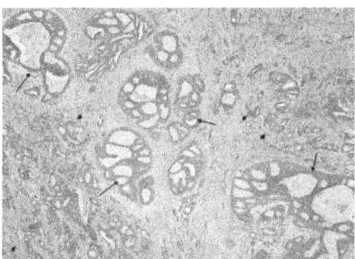

Figure 2: Representative histology of all four cases. There is extensive DCIS with cribriform configuration (arrow). The multiple foci of invasion (arrowhead) occur in between the DCIS (magnification ×100).

2. Discussion

The majority of breast cancer occurs sporadically in postmenopausal women with no family history of the disease. Breast cancer occurring in women in their 20s and 30s is uncommon, accounting for fewer than 5% of all breast cancer cases, and is often associated with a genetic predisposition [1]. These four cases of young women with sporadic, multifocal breast cancer bring forth the possibility of a relationship between prolonged direct skin contact with cellular phones and the development of breast cancer. To date there is insufficient laboratory or clinical evidence to establish a definite relationship between exposures to the electromagnetic radiation (EMR) emitted from cellular devices and the risk of developing cancer. Some studies have suggested that such a relationship exists, but larger and more robust studies have not been confirmatory [2–6]. Nonetheless, the International Agency for Research on Cancer has classified radiofrequency waves of the electromagnetic spectrum, the form of EMR that cellular devices emit, as a possible human carcinogen [7].

Cellular phones emit EMR in the microwave spectrum and produce both a thermal and nonthermal effect. The EMR emitted from cellular phones has insufficient energy to ionize molecules and is not capable of producing direct DNA damage as occurs with diagnostic and therapeutic radiation [2]. The primary thermal effect from cellular phones is the heating of tissue, which has controversial clinical significance [2, 8–10]. EMR emitted from cellular devices couples with the body to create currents within the tissue, potentially having an effect on cellular microenvironments [9]. A recent study using fluoro-deoxyglucose injections and positron emission tomography concluded that exposure to radiofrequency waves within parts of the brain closest to the cellular phone antenna resulted in increased levels of glucosemetabolism, but the clinical significance of these findings is unknown [11].

One of the first clinical reports of a possible carcinogenic effect of exposure to EMR from cellular phones suggested that cellular phone users were at increased risk of developing brain cancers [5]. The largest and longest study of cellular phone use to date is the INTERPHONE study which included data from 13 countries [6]. This retrospective study could not identify a significant increase in risk of gliomas or meningiomas with the use of cellular phones. There were, however, indications of an increased risk of glioma at the highest exposure levels, but biases and error prevent a causal interpretation. The INTERPHONE study concluded that the possible effects of long-term, heavy use of mobile phones require further investigation. A more recent meta-analysis showed an association between gliomas and acoustic neuromas in ipsilateral users (using the phone on one side of the head most often or always) who were also heavy users of cellular phones, compared to nonusers [3]. Moreover, the risk of cancer was found highest in people with longest exposure and exposure that began before the age of 20.

The issue of cellular phone exposure on male fertility has also been reported [12]. Both laboratory and clinical studies have demonstrated alterations in fertility, motility, and morphology in sperm exposed to EMR from cell phones. Similar reports of clinical responses resulting from exposure to cellular phone EMR have been made for changes in the blood brain barrier and cognition, but attempts to confirm these findings have been inconsistent [13–15].

The data collected from the majority of the aforementioned cellular phone studies was from the early 2000s. Since that time, cellular phone usage has continued to increase, with over 303 million subscribers to cellular phone service in the United States alone in 2011 and almost six billion subscribers worldwide [16]. This is triple the number of reported users in 2000. Children and young adults are now more likely to be using mobile devices and are among some of the heaviest users [17]. This group is potentially at greatest risk of harm from EMR, as dividing tissue, such as that occurring in prepubertal breast buds, is more prone to the adverse effects of radiation [18].

Current cellular phone safety regulations were established in the United States by the Federal Communication Commission (FCC) in 1996 [19]. The regulations were based on studies which measured the level of EMR penetrating the plexiglass head of a simulated 200 pound man. The studies were designed to measure the specific absorption rate (SAR) which is a measure of the rate at which energy is absorbed by the body when exposed to cellular phone EMR. The FCC set an exposure limit of 1.6 watts per kilogram of tissue. Any cellular phone functioning below this limit is considered to be safe. The duration of exposure during a SAR test is only 30 minutes and does not reflect the total amount of EMR exposure consumers experience with more prolonged exposure. Furthermore, FCC guidelines do not address the issue of risks associated with direct skin contact with cellularphones. This is a critical issue, as the long-term consequence of the direct thermal effect of EMR on developing breast tissue for extended duration has not been documented. In addition, unlike older cellular devices, smartphones have the ability to regularly transmit information, sending and receiving an intermittent signal even when the user of the device is not actively handling it. The accumulation of this passive exposure to EMR is also not well studied.

Although the FCC has not addressed the issue of skin contact, cellular phone manufacturers typically place a warning in their manuals stating that direct contact with the skin should be avoided. For example, the iPhone 4 user manual advises to keep the phone 1.5 cm or more away from the body [20]. Similarly, the safety manual for the BlackBerry Bold Smartphone recommends using an approved holster to carry the phone and to keep the phone 15 mm away from the body when the device is transmitting [21].

This series of four young women with cellular phone-related breast cancer is noteworthy, but caution must be exercised in drawing any conclusion from our small sample. Millions of women are using cellular devices, and it is predictable that rare events will occur. From this small case series, one cannot infer causality but can only consider association. Additionally, no data is available on the number of women who place their cellular phones in contact with their breast and do not develop breast cancer. Finally, the duration of exposure and the location of placement of the cell phone in direct contact with the breast are subject to recall bias.

However, the unusual pattern of multifocal cancers and extensive DCIS occurring in areas of direct cell phone contact on the breast is noteworthy. Each patient had multifocal cancer, but the tumors were all clustered within the area of breast tissue directly underlying the cellular device, and nowhere else. Furthermore, from a pathological point of view, the morphological features of insitu and invasive ductal carcinomas are interesting. All of the carcinomas exhibited similar, if not identical, histology characterized by a mixture of tubular and solid patterns with identical nuclear morphology and grade. All were estrogen and progesterone positive but Her2 negative, luminal-type carcinomas. The ductal and lobular units away from the areas of cellular phone contact showed no significant histological changes. While the cancers appear to be centralized to the region of the breast exposed to the cellular devices, they still possess the ability to metastasize as evidenced by three patients in this series with lymph node metastasis and one with bone metastasis (Case 2). Although the numbers of reported cases here are too small to have a scientific conclusion, the findings are intriguing and support the notion that direct cellular phone contact may be associated with the development of breast carcinoma.

There are fundamental differences between the available literature on cellular devices associated with cancer development and the four cases presented here. First and foremost, unlike the brain which is protected by the skull as well as a spatial distance from the cellular device, each patient here had direct contact between their device and their breast. The effect of EMR on tissues is directly related to the distance between the body and the source [2]. No study has yet to evaluate this direct effect. Second, the period of exposure was prolonged, over many years. Patients from earlier studies in general had a shorter duration of exposure to cellular EMR compared to those in our series. Lastly, it has been demonstrated that the effect of EMR on children can be several times higher than that of adults [22]. It is possible that the growing, dividing breast tissue that occurs during puberty may be particularly vulnerable to cellular phone EMR, accounting in part for at least two of the cases reported here (Cases 1 and 2).

Cellular phone use continues to expand rapidly, especially among young adults. Until more data becomes available, efforts should be made to encourage cellular phone users to follow the recommendations of mobile device manufacturers and to avoid skin contact. Further research is urgently needed in this area. In our practice, we have started to incorporate frequency of cellular phone use and placement location into part of our routine patient-history documentation. Physicians should document this behavior and also inform their patients that, until sufficient safety data becomes available, prolonged skin contact with cellular devices should be avoided.

[1] American Cancer Society, Breast Cancer Facts and Figures 2011-2012, American Cancer Society, Atlanta, Ga, USA, 2011.

[2] R. Baan, Y. Grosse, B. Lauby-Secretan et al., "Carcinogenicity of radiofrequency electromagnetic fields,"

The Lancet Oncology, vol. 12, no. 7, pp. 624–626, 2011. View at Google Scholar • View at Scopus

[3] L. Hardell, M. Carlberg, and K. Hansson Mild, "Use of mobile phones and cordless phones is associated with increased risk for glioma and acoustic neuroma," Pathophysiology, vol. 20, no. 2, pp. 85–110, 2013.View at Publisher • View at Google Scholar • View at Scopus

[4] J. Schüz, R. Jacobsen, J. H. Olsen, J. D. Boice Jr., J. K. McLaughlin, and C. Johansen, "Cellular telephone use and cancer risk: update of a nationwide Danish cohort," Journal of the National Cancer Institute, vol. 98, no. 23, pp. 1707–1713, 2006. View at Publisher • View at Google Scholar • View at Scopus

[5] L. Hardell, M. Carlberg, and K. Hansson Mild, "Pooled analysis of case-control studies on malignant brain tumours and the use of mobile and cordless phones including living and deceased subjects," International Journal of Oncology, vol. 38, no. 5, pp. 1465–1474, 2011. View at Publisher • View at Google Scholar • View at Scopus

[6] E. Cardis, "Brain tumour risk in relation to mobile telephone use: results of the INTERPHONE international case-control study," International Journal of Epidemiology, vol. 39, no. 3, Article ID dyq079, pp. 675–694, 2010. View at Publisher • View at Google Scholar • View at Scopus

[7] IARC Monographs on the Evaluation of Carcinogenic Risks to Humans, Non-Ionizing Radiation, Part II: Radiofrequency Electromagnetic, vol. 102, IARC Press, Lyon, France, 2011.

[8] H. Bartsch, C. Bartsch, E. Seebald et al., "Chronic exposure to a GSM-like signal (mobile phone) does not stimulate the development of DMBA-induced mammary tumors in rats: results of three consecutive studies," Radiation Research, vol. 157, no. 2, pp. 183–190, 2002. View at Google Scholar • View at Scopus

[9] D. J. Brenner, R. Doll, D. T. Goodhead et al., "Cancer risks attributable to low doses of ionizing radiation: assessing what we really know," Proceedings of the National Academy of Sciences of the United States of America, vol. 100, no. 2, pp. 13761–13766, 2003. View at Publisher • View at Google Scholar • View at Scopus

[10] G. O. Acar, H. M. Yener, F. K. Savrun, T. Kalkan, I. Bayrak, and O. Enver, "Thermal effects of mobile phones on facial nerves and surrounding soft tissue," Laryngoscope, vol. 119, no. 3, pp. 559–562, 2009.View at Publisher • View at Google Scholar • View at Scopus

ADAPTOGENETIC MEDICINE

[11] N. D. Volkow, D. Tomasi, G.-J. Wang et al., "Effects of cell phone radiofrequency signal exposure on brain glucose metabolism," Journal of the American Medical Association, vol. 305, no. 8, pp. 808–813, 2011. View at Publisher • View at Google Scholar • View at Scopus

[12] A. Agarwal, F. Deepinder, R. K. Sharma, G. Ranga, and J. Li, "Effect of cell phone usage on semen analysis in men attending infertility clinic: an observational study," Fertility and Sterility, vol. 89, no. 1, pp. 124–128, 2008. View at Publisher • View at Google Scholar • View at Scopus

[13] A. Agarwal, A. Singh, A. Hamada, and K. Kesari, "Cell phones and male infertility: a review of recent innovations in technology and consequences," International Brazilian Journal of Urology, vol. 37, no. 4, pp. 432–454, 2011. View at Publisher • View at Google Scholar • View at Scopus

[14] H. Nittby, A. Brun, J. Eberhardt, L. Malmgren, B. R. R. Persson, and L. G. Salford, "Increased blood-brain barrier permeability in mammalian brain 7 days after exposure to the radiation from a GSM-900 mobile phone," Pathophysiology, vol. 16, no. 2-3, pp. 103–112, 2009. View at Publisher • View at Google Scholar •View at Scopus

[15] R. Luria, I. Eliyahu, R. Hareuveny, M. Margaliot, and N. Meiran, "Cognitive effects of radiation emitted by cellular phones: the influence of exposure side and time," Bioelectromagnetics, vol. 30, no. 3, pp. 198–204, 2009. View at Publisher • View at Google Scholar • View at Scopus

[16] The World in 2011, "ICT facts and figures," June 6th, 2013, http://www.itu.int/ITU-D/ict/facts/2011/material/ICTFactsFigures2011.pdf.

[17] F. Söderqvist, L. Hardell, M. Carlberg, and K. Hansson Mild, "Ownership and use of wireless telephones: a population-based study of Swedish children aged 7–14 years," BMC Public Health, vol. 7, article 105, 2007. View at Publisher • View at Google Scholar • View at Scopus

[18] A. K. Ng and L. B. Travis, "Radiation therapy and breast cancer risk," Journal of the National Comprehensive Cancer Network, vol. 7, pp. 1121–1128, 2009. View at Google Scholar

[19] "Radio frequency safety," June 7th, 2013, http://www.fcc.gov/encyclopedia/radio-frequency-safety.

[20] "iPhone 4 important product information guide," June 7th, 2013, http://manuals.info.apple.com/en_US/iphone_4_important_product_information_guide.pdf.

[21] "Safety and product information. Blackberry Bold 9900/9930 Smartphones," June 7th, 2013, http://docs.blackberry.com/en/smartphone_users/deliverables/32435/BlackBerry_Bold_9900-9930_Smartphones-Safety_and_Product_Information–1334716-0615045228-001-US.pdf.

[22] O. P. Gandhi, L. L. Morgan, A. A. De Salles, Y.-Y. Han, R. B. Herberman, and D. L. Davis, "Exposure limits: the underestimation of absorbed cell phone radiation, especially in children," Electromagnetic Biology and Medicine, vol. 31, no. 1, pp. 34–51, 2012. View at Publisher • View at Google Scholar • View at Scopus

—

If that whole study was a TL:DR (too long: didn't read) moment, let's summarize it: storing a radiation-damaging, frequency-emitting device next to your breast tissue for several hours a day and for years on end, will probably give you an excellent chance of getting breast cancer. This study was completed four years ago as of this writing, and frankly, even without the study, one could probably extrapolate the same conclusion/results with common sense and deductive reasoning...the deodorant studies were conducted between 2005 and 2016, and yet that utter nonsense from nationalbreastcancer.org is still up on their website, well...*now*. As we enter into the newer "5G" era of cell phone technology, we as a population will most likely begin to suffer even greater effects from this phenomenon.

If you would like an even better summary of the cancer-causing effects of cellphones, got to TheTruthAboutCancer.com/mobile-phone-radiation/.

If you're still reading this chapter, it's assumed you are still interested in knowing more about this type of stuff and haven't skipped to the next one. So let's keep going down the rabbit hole! Next up we have the cancer causing substance known as 'sunscreen.' Let's hear what Dr. Arthur W. Perry, MD, FACS, board certified plastic surgeon, and adjunct professor at Columbia University has to say on the subject in this article posted on doctoroz.com:

Your Sunscreen Might Be Poisoning You

By <u>Arthur W. Perry, MD, FACS</u> Dr. Perry is a board certified plastic surgeon, an Adjunct Associate Professor at Columbia University, and a member of the Medical Advisory Board for The Dr. Oz Show.

Posted on 5/07/2013 | By Arthur Perry, MD, FACS

Sunscreens have been around for nearly 100 years. The goal was to block ultraviolet (UV) light, the harmful rays of the sun. Sunscreens started out with pasty zinc oxide that no one would use. So scientists created sunscreens with clear chemicals that absorbed UV light. In 1944, Coppertone® became the first mass marketed sunscreen. Fast forward to now, when about a billion dollars worth of sunscreen are sold each year in the United States.

UV light causes skin cancer and prematurely ages the skin, and so it's very important to protect our skin with sunscreen. We don't want to block sunshine completely – about 20 minutes each day is good for us – it boosts our vitamin D and improves our mood. Beyond 20 minutes, however, and our <u>immune system suffers</u>. We either need to spend the rest of the day inside or protect our skin with sunscreen.

There are 17 individual sunscreen ingredients that are FDA approved: 15 of these are clear chemicals that absorb UV light and two are made of minerals that reflect UV light. Of these 15, nine are known endocrine disruptors. To be effective, chemical sunscreens need to be rubbed into their skin 20 minutes before sun exposure. They do a pretty good job at blocking UV light, but they actually get used up as the sun shines on them. In fact, some sunscreens lose as much as 90% of their effectiveness in just an hour, so they need to be reapplied often. This is not the case with zinc oxide and titanium dioxide, the two mineral, or physical, sunscreens. These two work very differently – they sit on the surface of the skin and physically block UV light.

Chemical sunscreens don't sit on the surface of the skin – they soak into it and quickly find their way into the bloodstream. They scatter all over the body without being detoxified by the liver and can be detected in blood, urine, and breast milk for up to two days after a single application. That would be just fine if they were uniformly safe – but they're not.

As I mentioned, nine of the 15 chemical sunscreens are considered endocrine disruptors. Those are chemicals that interfere with the normal function of hormones. The hormones most commonly disturbed are estrogen, progesterone, testosterone, and thyroid. Endocrine disruptors, like some ingredients in chemical sunscreens, can cause abnormal development of fetuses and growing children. They cause early puberty and premature breast development in girls, and small and undescended testicles in boys. They cause low sperm counts and infertility. Endocrine disruptors that act like estrogen can contribute to the development of breast and ovarian cancers in women, and other endocrine disruptors may increase the chance of prostate cancer in men.

Sounds pretty unsettling, doesn't it? But there's more. As I said earlier, chemical sunscreens function by absorbing UV light. In the process, some may get used up and mutate. Some generate DNA-damaging chemicals called "free radicals." These may lead to cancers.

I'm pretty negative about chemical sunscreens, and while I do have to tell you that I believe they are not proven to cause cancer, as I said on The Dr. Oz Show, "Where there's smoke, there's fire."

Poisoning that takes place over decades is difficult to study. Chemicals like arsenic and botulism make us sick very quickly, and so it was easy to figure out that they are toxins. Lead is a toxin that takes longer to cause illness, so it was many years before the government listened to scientists and restricted its use. And chemical sunscreens are even harder to study since their effects are subtle and take a long time to appear.

As you read this, you might be saying, "Why is this guy – a plastic surgeon – saying something I've never heard about before?" This information isn't new for me. My patients know I've been talking about sunscreen and other cosmetic toxicity for about 15 years. But I'm just an interpreter of science. And experts agree with me.

R. Thomas Zoeller, MS, PhD, is a Professor of Biology at the University of Massachusetts. He's an author of the Endocrine Society's scientific statement about endocrine disrupting chemicals and their official representative. He said, "Dr. Perry makes an important point that sunscreens are applied to skin in a formulation that serves as a drug delivery system and that some sunscreens are known to interfere with hormone action. The way in which these chemicals can interact with hormone systems could plausibly increase the risk of various cancers as well as other endocrine disorders."

If there were no good alternatives, we'd be in a pickle – we'd have to make some hard decisions whether or not to use sunscreen. But, fortunately, we have great alternatives.

Zinc oxide and titanium dioxide are rocks that are ground down to a fine consistency. They do a great job at blocking both UVA and UVB light. Zinc is less whitening on the skin and blocks nearly all dangerous UV light. Inexpensive versions of these sunscreens are gooey and while you might put them on your kid's skin, most people don't like them. But newer zinc oxide sunscreens contain particles so small that they are transparent. These sunscreens are called micronized and do a great job at protecting against UV radiation. Even newer sunscreens use rocks that are ground into smaller bits called nanoparticles. Nanoparticles have their own issues, and some people don't consider them to be uniformly safe.

Some people may call me "self-serving" because I have my own skin care company and I produce a SPF 20 sunscreen with micronized zinc oxide. But I created this product because of my attitude toward sunscreens. I really do feel that people are poisoning themselves by putting ounce-quantities of chemical sunscreens on their bodies, and I cringe when I see women, particularly pregnant or breastfeeding women, and small children slathering that stuff on their skin.

Bottom line? Use a micronized zinc oxide containing SPF 15 broad-spectrum sunscreen every day of the year and an SPF 30 when you're on the beach or working in the garden. How much should you use? An ounce spread over your whole body should do it. And reapply it every 2 hours or so. For more information, I've posted scientific references on the toxicity of sunscreens and cosmetics on PerryPlasticSurgery.com.

Article written by Arthur Perry, MD, FACS
Dr. Perry is a board certified plastic surgeon, an Adjunct Associate Professor at Columbia University, and a member of the...

—

Interesting at the very least! Ok here's one more from author Arjun Walia:

HOW SUNSCREEN COULD BE
CAUSING SKIN CANCER, NOT THE SUN

Arjun Walia February 13, 2017

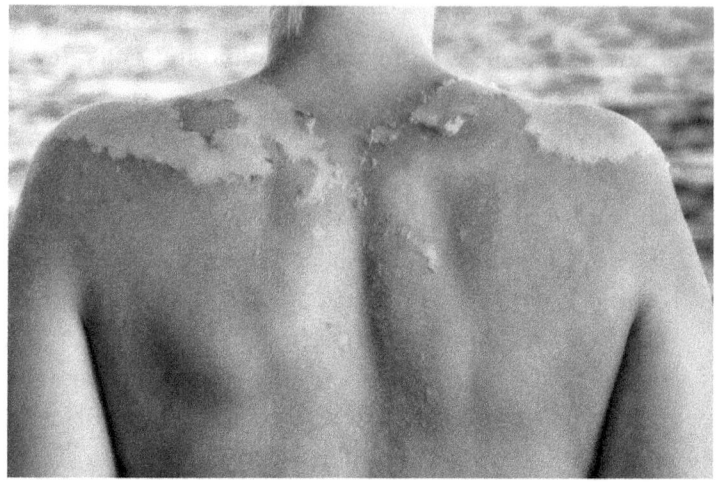

Summer may be a long way off, but it's never too early to start thinking about protecting your skin. For most people, this means covering themselves in sunscreen, which corporate marketing campaigns encourage at every turn. Yet, while we do indeed need protection to prevent sunburns, blocking out the sun entirely is not ideal. Rich in vitamin D, it offers a number of other health benefits, including, oddly enough, cancer prevention. We've been made to fear the sun, and, as a result, adults and children are choosing to drench themselves in a bath of toxic, hormone-disrupting chemicals.

Science has long shown that what we put on our skin ends up in our bodies, and quickly. Multiple studies from across the world have examined sunscreen in particular, evaluating its ingredients and how it penetrates and absorbs into the skin after application. One study, conducted at the Faculty of Pharmacy at the University of

Manitoba, Canada, sought to develop a method for quantifying common sunscreen agents. Results demonstrated a significant penetration of all sunscreen agents into the skin, meaning all of these chemicals are entering multiple tissues within the body. (source)

Conversely, a study published in Environmental Health Perspectives showed a significant drop in hormone-disrupting chemicals that are commonly found in personal care products after participants switched to 'cleaner' products. These chemicals include oxybenzone, triclosan, parabens, phthalates, and more. You can read more about that and access the study here. All of these ingredients are found within most popular sunscreens.

So, the next question becomes, are the ingredients used to make sunscreen, which are entering into our bloodstream, something to be concerned about? The science given to us by the corporations who profit from the sale of sunscreen says no, but I think by now we have established how trustworthy such corporately-funded 'science' is. It wasn't long ago that Johnson & Johnson, for example, was found guilty of knowingly putting a cancer-causing baby powder on the market. You can read more about that here.

This is precisely why we wanted to bring attention to an article published by the Huffington Post titled "Excuse Me While I Lather My Child In This Toxic Death Cream." In it, mother Sarah Kallies shares how exhausted she feels trying to navigate today's world and do the best for her children when everything, everywhere, seems to be killing us. For every purchase she makes for her children, there is science telling her it's great on the one hand and toxic on the other, and so she highlights how confusing the consumer marketplace has become. We are dished a wealth of information that differs from source to source, on a variety of different topics, making it difficult to make even the simplest of choices without second-guessing ourselves.

Yet we know the various chemicals found within sunscreens are toxic, and we know that our skin absorbs whatever we put onto it. Below are a few examples of these chemicals:

Oxybenzone

This could in fact be the most troublesome ingredient found in the majority of popular sunscreens. Used because it effectively absorbs ultraviolet light, it's also believed to cause hormone disruption and cell damage, which could promote cancer.

According to the Environmental Working Group:

Commonly used in sunscreens, the chemical oxybenzone penetrates the skin, gets into the bloodstream and acts like estrogen in the body. It can trigger allergic reactions. Data are preliminary, but studies have found a link between higher concentrations of oxybenzone and health harms. One study has linked oxybenzone to endometriosis in older women; another found that women with higher levels of oxybenzone during pregnancy had lower birth weight daughters. (source)

There are many other studies out there on this chemical. For example, one study done by the Department of Clinical and Experimental Endocrinology at the University of Gottingen in Germany observed regulatory effects on receptor expression for oxybenzone that indicate endocrine (hormone) disruption.

A study out of the Institute of Pharmacology and Toxicology from the University of Zurich determined that oxybenzone may also mimic the effects of estrogen in the body and promote the growth of cancer cells.

Prompted by multiple studies, a study out of the Queensland Cancer Fund Laboratories at the Queensland Institute of Medical Research in Australia recognized the significance of systemic absorption of sunscreens. Researchers discovered that oxybenzone inhibited cell growth and DNA synthesis and retarded cycle progression in the first of the four phases of the cell cycle. They determined that sunscreen causes mitochondrial stress and changes in drug uptake in certain cell lines.

Journal of Health Science by the National Institute of Health Sciences in Japan examined UV stabilizers used in food packages as plastic additives. They found that some UV stabilizers in sunscreen products have estrogenicity in an MCF-7 breast cancer cell assay as well as an immature rat uterotrophic assay. They tested a total of 11 UV stabilizers. 20 kinds of benzophenones were tested using the same assay to demonstrate their estrogenic activity.

The list goes on and on.

Retinyl Palmitate (Vitamin A palmitate)

A study conducted by U.S. government scientists suggests that retinyl palmitate, a form of vitamin A, may speed the development of skin tumors and lesions when applied to the skin in the presence of sunlight (NTP 2012). "Retinyl palmitate was selected by the Center for Food Safety and Applied Nutrition for photo- toxicity and photocarcinogenicity testing based on the increasingly widespread use of this compound in cosmetic retail products for use on sun-exposed skin," reads an October 2000 report by the National Toxicology Program.

As Dr. Joseph Merocla explains, this suggests that sunscreen products could actually increase the speed at which malignant cells develop and spread skin cancer, because they contain vitamin A and its derivates, retinol, and retinyl palmitate.

Fragrance

Fragrance refers to a host of harmful hormone-disrupting chemicals mentioned earlier, like parabens, phthalates, and synthetic musks.

Sun Exposure Can Protect You From Cancer

The sun isn't as bad as it's marketed to be, however. Corporations are concerned with profit, not people, and telling us that sun exposure can actually protect against cancer isn't going to get us to buy sunscreen. Yet several studies have made this connection, confirming that the appropriate amount of sun exposure can actually protect us against skin cancer.

As many of you probably already know, humans require sunlight exposure for vitamin D. Sunburns are indeed a concern, and there are many studies that link sunburns to melanoma, but due to a wide range of factors, such as cultural changes and marketing campaigns, our skin has become less resistant to sun exposure. If you spend a large portion of your time in the sun, your skin adapts to build a natural immunity. We are naturally built to receive sunlight, and we have gone backwards in this regard. There are alternative ways to protect yourself from sunburns. You can buy natural sunscreens without harmful chemicals. Questioning big name advertisements is crucial to our health in these times of information awareness.

Only 10% of all cancer cases are attributed to all forms of radiation, and UV is a very small part of that. When we think of skin cancer we automatically want to blame the sun, but what about other causes of skin cancer that are out there? Arsenic, found in a number of things we ingest or work around, pesticides, and leather preservatives are all causes for concern.

Sunscreens are a huge contributor to toxins in the body, being absorbed within seconds of application. Is it not important to know what you are putting into your body? We now live in a culture where we fear the sun, which is ironic considering it has created all life on Earth. It's important to remember that fear eventually manifests as reality. The sun has many health benefits, so using natural products will ensure that you receive these benefits while keeping your skin safe.

Healthier Alternatives

When shopping for sunscreens, be sure to read the labels and avoid buying sunscreens containing toxic chemicals. They may be tough to find, but a trip to a natural health store can often do the trick. Look for sunscreens that contain **zinc** and **titanium minerals** as opposed to the active ingredients listed above. Remember, the best sun protection is shade and clothing. It is not necessary to wear sunscreen every time you are out in the sun. Sunscreen does NOT allow the body to absorb any vitamin D from sunlight. So if you plan on being outside for a short period of time, skip the sunscreen and feed your body the vitamin D that will keep it healthy.

Coconut oil has been shown to provide an SPF of about 8 when it comes to sun protection. This means that, although it's protection isn't very high, it can help. If you were to apply it often, it would not only offer sun protection, but it would also hydrate the skin, making it less susceptible to burning. You may also want to try combining natural sunscreens with coconut oil for protection. To do this, at the beginning of your long day out in the sun, use natural sunscreen, and after a few hours, try applying coconut oil to supplement the natural sunscreen and hydrate the skin.

—

Summary: Cancer is bad, we've got some amazingly effective treatment options, and more importantly we can take significant steps to prevent it. Let's continue.

Here is one last article on why we should *never*, (emphasis on 'never') use a microwave. Some people (even those in the holistic field) have a hard time with this one, they don't seem to understand why it can be *that* harmful. The reason may not be what you think…sure the radiation is bad, but you get more radiation exposure from taking a quick flight from Dallas to Tampa on an airplane than you do from having one meal out of the microwave. The real issue is that putting food in the microwave deforms and *denatures* it on a molecular and enzymatic level. The nutritionists scream that the nutrient content is technically the same, the caloric, protein, fat, and carbohydrate content is the same, and that is *technically* accurate. But the *life force* of the food is either damaged our outright destroyed. This can actually be seen via a method called **Kirlian Photography** which has the ability to photograph the bioelectric energy field of any living thing. So if you take a picture of an apple, it will have a smooth looking healthy field around it. Microwave that apple, and then use Kirlian Photography to look at it again, and the field will be very rough, darker, and jagged looking.

But let's imagine for just a moment, and for the sake of argument, that all that sounds like a bunch of nutter-butter nonsense and you don't buy it. You're skeptical. Hey, no one could blame you, none of what was just written is accepted science and this book could just be making some of that up. Fair enough, **what if it could be proven to you that the microwave was harmful in a very cheap, easy, unbiased experiment that you can perform yourself?** Got your attention? Do this: Go to Lowe's or Home Depot and buy 6 common house plants of the same species. They can be something like Azelea's, Philodendron,

Hydrangea's, etc. Make sure they are cheap because three of them are going to die. The experiment is simple, divide the plants into two groups of three. Give all six of them the normal amount of sunlight that is recommended for whichever particular species you purchased. Give all six of the plants the exact same amount of spring water from the same source, *but microwave the water that you give to three of the plants first*, and don't microwave the water you give to the other three plants. Now *obviously*, wait until the water cools off and returns to room temperature from the microwave before you give it to the plants, we aren't trying to burn them to death.

In this experiment, the three plants that receive the regular spring water are the 'control' group. The plants that receive the microwaved water are the experimental group. Keep the two groups of plants separated so that you don't get them mixed up, and keep up this watering schedule every other day (or whatever the appropriate watering cycle is for that particular plant, we don't want to overwater them). After 3 to 6 weeks, evaluate and critically analyze the results. (Spoiler Alert: 3 of the plants will be dead or dying, you may speculate as to which 3). You can also perform this same experiment with goldfish or guppies in an aquarium and the fish whose tank you added microwaved water to would die, but that's kind of cruel and I don't advocate that. (Just to clarify, I don't mean adding hot microwaved water to a fish tank, I mean after you've microwaved it and let it return to room temperature.) You could repeat these experiments a thousand times, and you would get the same, or nearly the same result *every* time. Let's learn a little more:

Are Microwaves Safe?
(Must Read if You Use a Microwave Oven)
by Lloyd Burrell

Where would you be without your microwave oven? Aren't they just a huge time-saver? You can cook a meal in seconds. Even frozen food can be defrosted and ready to eat in a matter of minutes.

But **have you ever wondered... are microwaves safe? Are there any dangers to using them?** How could there be any dangers? If there were, the government would have taken microwave ovens off the market, right? These are the questions we're going to explore in this article.

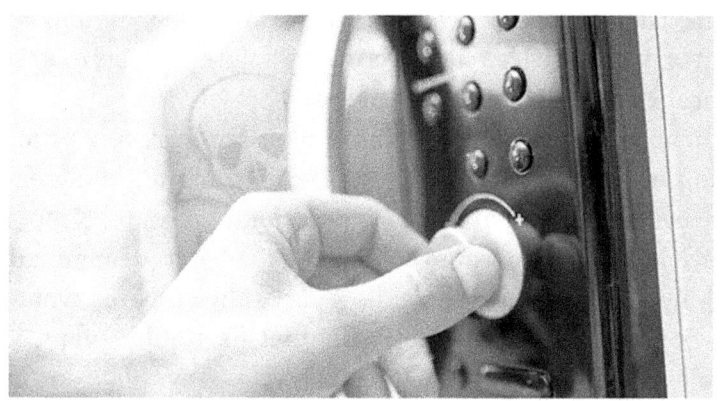

Microwave Ovens Use Microwaves – a Form of EMF

As the name suggests, "microwave ovens" use microwaves. These microwaves, which are a form of electromagnetic field (EMF) generated by a magnetron, vibrate at a speed of 2.4 billion times per second. This causes the water molecules in the food to resonate at very high frequencies and generate heat.

Conventional heating of food is a different, much gentler process altogether. Heat is transferred by convection from the outside to the inside.

Cooking with microwaves begins in the cells and molecules where water is present. This energy is transformed into frictional heat. These are called thermic effects. Added to this are athermic effects which are not currently measurable but are thought to deform the structures of molecules and have qualitative consequences.

Microwave Ovens Microwave Your Home

Few people realize that when you use a microwave oven, *the microwaves do not stay within the confines of the oven.*

Microwave ovens have to meet safety standards set by the FDA. These standards "limit the amount of microwaves that can leak from an oven throughout its lifetime to 5 milliwatts (mW) of microwave radiation per square centimeter at approximately 2 inches from the oven surface." This might sound quite rigorous, but it's not.

My tests with an EMF meter show that *even brand new microwave ovens emit significant levels of microwave energy*, otherwise known as radio frequency radiation.

What this means is that when you switch your microwave oven on these EMFs permeate into your home... traveling through walls, ceilings, and you. These EMFs, though being in the non-ionizing range of the EMF spectrum, are not negligible.

In May 2011 the World Health Organization officially classified this type of EMF exposure as a class 2B possible carcinogen.

Added to this, a microwave ovens' cables and motor also give off high magnetic fields, often over 10 milligauss. *Exposures of just 4 milligauss have been firmly linked to leukemia.* Not surprisingly these magnetic fields have also been categorized as carcinogenic.

Over 70 Years of German and Russian Research Point to Microwave Dangers

Twenty years of Russian research, and German studies dating back to 1942 in Berlin, make a strong case against the safety of microwave cooking.

The Nazis are thought to have invented the first microwave ovens to provide mobile food support to their troops during their invasion of the Soviet Union in World War II. After the war the United States War Department was given the task of researching the safety of microwave ovens. But it's the Russians who are credited with having performed the most thorough research.

After the war the Russians set about researching the biological effects of microwave ovens. *This led to microwave ovens being banned in Russia in 1976.* The ban was later lifted during Perestroika to promote free trade with the west.

Their findings led the Russian government to issue an international warning about possible biological and environmental damage associated with the use of microwave ovens and other similar frequency electronic devices such as cell phones.

Are Microwaves Safe? What the Research Tells Us

The research on microwave ovens reveals the following…

- Microwaving prepared meats to ensure sanitary ingestion was found to provoke the formation of
- d-Nitrosodienthanolamines, a well-known carcinogen.
- Microwaving milk and cereal grains was found to convert some of their amino acids into carcinogenic substances.
- Swiss clinical trials have found that microwaving food increases cholesterol levels. It was also found to decrease red and white blood cell counts while decreasing hemoglobin and producing radiolytic compounds.

- Thawing frozen fruits was found to convert their glucoside and galactoside containing fractions into carcinogens.
- Even very short exposure of raw, cooked, or frozen vegetables to microwaves was found to convert their plant alkaloids into carcinogens.
- Russian and Japanese studies have shown how food can lose nearly 60% to 90% of its food value when cooked or heated in a microwave oven. Significant portions of Vitamins B, C, E, and essential minerals have been found to be lost.
- Food cooked in a microwave oven with a little water can lose up to 97% of its beneficial antioxidants.
- Another issue with microwave ovens is that many people cook food in plastic and paper containers. Carcinogenic toxins can leach out of this packaging into your food. Studies have shown that chemicals such as polyethylene terpthalate (PET), benzene, toluene, and xylene can leach from the packaging of common microwavable foods such as pizzas, fries, and popcorn.

5 Tips to Break Free From Your Microwave Oven

In the light of the above I take a firm line with microwave ovens. I cleared my microwave oven out of my kitchen a long time ago.

Here's how to survive without a microwave oven:

1. Invest in a turbo oven or steamer instead. These are much healthier alternatives to microwaving.
2. Plan your meals. Take your dinner out of the freezer that morning or the night before so you don't end up having to speed-defrost food.

3. Frozen soups and stews can be taken out the freezer an hour before mealtime and partially defrosted in a sink of water then when sufficiently thawed put in a pan to heat on the stove.

4. If you do insist on keeping your microwave oven, don't allow children, pregnant women, and people with low immunity in your kitchen (or in the adjacent rooms) when your microwave oven is on.

5. Keep as far away as you can from your microwave oven when it is working. Your risk of EMF exposure will be reduced significantly.

Your Quality of Food = Your Quality of Life

There's no doubt the food we eat affects our health. But already the foods we eat contain more toxins and are nutritionally poorer than they were only a few decades ago. If you use a microwave oven, not only are you diminishing the nutritional value of food which is already less nutritional than it was previously, you are also exposing yourself to potential harmful electromagnetic fields which are known carcinogens.

Are microwaves safe? The resounding answer is NO. Do yourself and your family a favor and remove them from your home and take steps to limit your exposure at work and other areas where they're used.

Please share this important information about microwave oven safety with friends and family. *It could save someone's life!*

Article Summary

• Have you ever wondered… are microwaves safe? But how could there be any dangers? If there were, the government would have taken microwave ovens off the market, right? Not necessarily…

- As the name suggests, "microwave ovens" use microwaves. These microwaves are a form of electromagnetic field (EMF). When you use a microwave oven, the microwaves do not stay within the confines of the oven.
- When a microwave oven is turned on these EMFs permeate into your home... traveling through walls, ceilings, and you. In May 2011 the World Health Organization officially classified this type of EMF exposure as a class 2B possible carcinogen.
- A microwave ovens' cables and motor also give off high magnetic fields, often over 10 milligauss. Exposures of just 4 milligauss have been firmly linked to leukemia. These magnetic fields have also been categorized as carcinogenic.
- Research on microwave ovens reveals the following...
  - Microwaving prepared meats to ensure sanitary ingestion was found to provoke the formation of
  - d-Nitrosodienthanolamines, a well-known carcinogen.
  - Microwaving milk and cereal grains was found to convert some of their amino acids into carcinogenic substances.
  - Microwaving food increases cholesterol levels. It was also found to decrease red and white blood cell counts while decreasing hemoglobin and producing radiolytic compounds.
  - Thawing frozen fruits was found to convert their glucoside and galactoside containing fractions into carcinogens.
  - Even very short exposure of raw, cooked, or frozen vegetables to microwaves was found to convert their plant alkaloids into carcinogens.

- Russian and Japanese studies have shown how food can lose nearly 60% to 90% of its food value when cooked or heated in a microwave oven.
- Food cooked in a microwave oven with a little water can lose up to 97% of its beneficial antioxidants.
- Many people cook food in plastic and paper containers in microwaves which can cause carcinogenic toxins to leach out of this packaging into your food.

—

But wait, there's more! Let's consider the role that GMO foods play. To clarify, I don't mean natural hybridization of similar sub-species of plants, for instance the tangelo, which is offshoot of breeding tangerines with either pomelos or grapefruits. This has been done by farmers for thousands of years. I'm talking about the franken-food (and I used the term 'food' loosely) that is genetically spliced, mutated, and bastardized, into a human-gene-altering, synthetically engineered carcinogenic product that the body cannot properly digest or detoxify from.

If you've ever seen the 1997 movie *Alien: Resurrection* and remember the gruesome scene where Ripley (Sigourney Weaver) walks into the part of the ship where there are horribly disfigured and mutated clones of herself, and one of them chillingly looks over at her and hoarsely whispers "Kill.....me" before Ripley puts it out of its misery with a flame-thrower, then you kind of get a version of the image that should go through your head when Monsanto/GMO foods come up. The only problem is that the horribly disfigured/mutated part is within the genes (i.e. genotype) of the food, even though the way they look on the outside (i.e. the phenotype) looks perfectly normal. The more important point to take away is that any studies proving how toxic things like GMO corn are often get violently suppressed, and/or dismissed on a technicality. To give example, one study involving rats that had a high percentage cancer development from eating GMO foods was completely disregarded *because the rats most notably developed cancer in their forestomachs*, an organ which human beings don't have. Really? Yes, really.

We would encourage you to do your own research on this, eat locally grown organic whenever possible, and avoid Monsanto/GMO products (including their glyphosate weed killer Round Up if you don't want your dog to get cancer from playing out in the yard). Go to thetruthaboutcancer.com/eating-gmo-foods/ and/or thetruthabo utcancer.com/implication-of-gmo-foods/ for more information and watch the quick 2-minute videos (also available on Youtube) from Mike Adams and Jeffrey Smith on GMO foods. Here is another informative article from cancertutor.com/the-truth-about-cancer-and-gmos/:

> In an increasingly processed and packaged world, most of us have a decent understanding of what is "real food" and what is not. We avoid the nitrates, the additives, and the mile-long list of chemicals that manufacturers try to pass off as ingredients.
>
> When we first begin attending to our health, it can be a victory simply to stick to the perimeter of the grocery store, avoiding the boxed carcinogens that lie deep within the store's aisles. Unfortunately, even the produce section, where the food looks like food and you gather your own — real — ingredients, can be deceptive and even dangerous. GMOs are to thank for that, and their connection to cancer cannot be understated.
>
> Even more unfortunate is the lobby behind GMOs, carrying untold amounts of cash and a vested interest in protecting their practices. As a result, a good bit of misinformation, shady marketing, and biased lawmaking have ensued, leading to health problems and lawsuits – not to mention the damage that is yet to be seen as an entire

generation grows up on Frankenfoods. Arm yourself with information before GMOs become the norm.

Misleading Claims about GMOs

GMOs, genetically modified organisms, really began to come into their own in the last three to four decades. Instantly, agribusiness saw potential in soy and corn crops – two of the most widely used crops in the world. What the original scientists had in mind when pursuing this technology, we may never truly know, but it didn't take long for seeds of GMO plants to make it to industrialized farms, allowing indiscriminate pesticide use without killing the plant.

If we're looking to the root of the problem, it's probably there – that we have giant farms who need to spray heavily in order to more easily produce mass amounts of "food," much of which will be processed into empty calories anyway. Yet, here we are, and until consumers vote with their dollars and refuse to support such practices, they will carry on.

In justifying the use of GMOs, much has been said — and many have been misleading. Without combing research or knowing someone directly impacted, consumers are left with a "he said, she said" situation about many hot-button issues and GMOs are not exempt. Some of the top claims about GMOs that mislead consumers include:

- That GMOs have always been around
- That GMOs increase yield
- That long term human studies aren't needed

Each of these reasons for justification is flawed in their own way, without addressing or negating very serious concerns with substances to be distributed as food throughout the world.

GMOs have not always been around

To soften the idea of altering seed DNA, proponents like to say that this isn't a new practice – that, to some extent, farmers have always made modifications to their crops' gene structure. This is not only an overstatement but completely misleading.

The practice of selective breeding and hybridization has been in place for hundreds of years – if not thousands – this much is true. Farmers would (and do) identify specific plants that resisted disease well, produced a solid harvest, or handled environmental conditions favorable, and use them to create new varieties of plants. If you've ever planted a vegetable garden, you know how many varieties are out there and how important it is to select varieties that do well in your region.

Genetic modification, as practiced in labs in our era, is not only different than hybridization, but it's also very new. The USDA reports that the upswing in use of GMO seeds only began in the late 1990s. In less than a generation, we've moved from hardly any GMOs to half of our farmland consumed with genetically altered seeds. (1)

The practice of genetic modification is obviously different from hybridization, but it's the reason for modification that endangers our health: the USDA report also noted that the primary reason for choosing GMO seeds is overwhelming to resist herbicides and pesticides. In other words, half of our farmland can be doused with even more chemicals thanks to GMOs – chemicals that can poison the air and leave residue on our food.

GMOs do not increase yield

So many of our decisions in this world must boil down to a risk vs benefit analysis. Even when there are risks to a given choice, sometimes the benefits are greater and it's still worth pursuing. Pro-GMO arguments often include higher crop yields as a benefit meant to outweigh concerns about GMO safety.

Setting aside the fact that higher yields would still not likely improve our outlook on GMOs, this isn't even an accurate statement at all.

In a summary of a detailed, long-term evaluation of crop production, the Union of Concerned Scientists had this to say:

This report is the first to evaluate in detail the overall, or aggregate, yield effect of GE after more than 20 years of research and 13 years of commercialization in the United States. Based on that record, we conclude that [genetic engineering] has done little to increase overall crop yields. (2)

While it may be simpler on paper to produce a similar annual crop with the help of uninhibited sprays for every obstacle, the big picture tells a different story. Crop yields have little to do with GMO justification.

Long-term safety studies are needed

In spite of the heavy and increasing use of GMOs — and the subsequent pervasive use of chemicals that follows — long term evaluations ensuring human safety are nowhere to be found.

The counter to this concern typically points to studies that utilize animals, pointing to results and claiming them as the be all, end all. The pro-GMO Genetic Literacy Project claims this rebuttal in one of their articles on the topic, pointing to long-term studies that were all conducted on animals. Yet they admit that "there have not been human clinical trials on GMOs." (3)

While researchers have gleaned countless leads and untold knowledge from animal studies, it's important to remember where they fall in the grand scheme of things. Animal studies tell us a lot about a substance or process, but they don't tell us exactly how it will translate to the human body.

Until we have confirmation, in the human body, that long term effects of GMOs and our current farming practices are safe, the current research is nothing more than a hint. Of course, if we're being honest, few of us would sign up for a trial like that, since there actually is evidence of harm even in short term and pieced together evidence.

Isn't that telling? An entire generation of our country, effectively acting as an experiment, giving our consent with every trip to the grocery store.

How GMOs risk our health

From the environment to our dinner tables to the very cells of our bodies, GMOs are invading our lives more and more each year. What exactly are they doing to our bodies? If the mainstream claims about them are untrue, then what actually is true – and how does it relate to cancer?

The risks that GMOs pose are very real and affect us even when we don't directly consume them. The pesticide-laden farming practices that GMO seeds enable further poison our air and water. GMO seeds are more than a farming practice; they are shaping our entire way of life.

Understanding these risks can help us to be better stewards — even activists — for our land, air, and bodies, helping to create a cleaner world where seeds are simply seeds and cancer isn't a household term.

We risk genetic transfer

Even before we acknowledge that GMOs do damage our bodies, we can't deny that their impact reaches far beyond meals or incidental exposure. Researchers are finding that modified seeds change more than growing patterns – their modified produce may change our DNA, as well.

One study, published in 2013, summarizes this risk in disturbing clarity:

Here, based on the analysis of over 1000 human samples from four independent studies, we report evidence that meal-derived DNA fragments which are large enough to carry complete genes can avoid degradation and through an unknown mechanism enter the human circulation system. (4)

They went on to note that some blood samples actually included more plant DNA than human. What does that mean practically? It means that the practice of genetic modification itself cannot be waived off as only about the way plants grow.

Those altered genes can make it into our bodies. And not just ours – there is also evidence that the toxic residue and altered DNA that GMOs leave behind are transferred from maternal blood to the growing baby. (5)

This is about more than growing plants. It's about our health, our children, and our very DNA.

We risk internal health

Who hasn't snidely quipped about the sudden increase in gluten sensitivity, often the butt of jokes about imaginary illness? Chances are, however, that it's not our paranoia that has driven the gluten-free trend but a generation of young adults raised on gut-damaging GMOs.

This connection is not, as some suppose because wheat is genetically modified. In fact, you may be surprised to learn that wheat itself is not a GMO crop. The wheat we have today has changed over the centuries, but not because of lab technicians.

Instead, the Institute of Responsible Technology proposes that it's the exposure to all of the other GMO crops in our diet that damages the gut and keeps it from properly processing gluten. (6)

We risk cancer

Here's where it all culminates: Our circulating DNA affected. Our digestive system broken. Our children beginning their lives in utero exposed to toxins. And cancer around every turn.

The risk factors don't stand alone, you see. It's not like you can say it's okay to pursue and consume GMOs because one or the other may not be so bad – it's a package deal! Years of chipping away at our internal systems lead to chronic illness. People with chronic illness were found to have "significantly higher" herbicide residue in their urine than healthy individuals, as evaluated by German scientists in 2014. (7)

Perhaps these risks are most poignantly demonstrated in people who have the misfortune of working directly with GMOs and the corresponding herbicide and pesticide loads. In recent years, an uptick in lawsuits against Monsanto shares a common theme: farm workers are using their chemical sprays and then finding that they have cancer.

A write-up in Reuters walks through some of the most prominent lawsuits that are active: bone cancer, leukemia, with the World Health Organization countering the US declaration that glyphosate is non-carcinogenic. (8)

This tempered statement on the common herbicide is disappointing but hardly surprising; it's no secret that Monsanto has a heavy lobbying wing and is interwoven with the US government. It's up to consumers, it seems, to stick up for ourselves where our government will not.

The World Health Organization, on the other hand, tells us that popular herbicides and pesticides are "probably carcinogenic," citing links between glyphosate and animal tumors as well as genetic damage in humans after glyphosate exposure. (9)

The truth about GMOs and cancer is that the further we move away from the original design for creation, the more acutely we will feel the effects of this broken world. Not only are altered genes a departure from nature itself, but the fact that we are doing so in order to douse our food with toxins is telling.

In the US at least, the tide will not begin to turn until consumers make it so. Whether that simply means intentionally choosing non-GMO products (a must) or sharing information with our friends and neighbors (a plus) or activism on a larger scale (a calling), we have a responsibility to do something with the information we have been given.

As researchers continue to detail exactly how GMOs affect our bodies and how increased sprays affect our environment and our health, there's more than enough evidence for us to know that it's a dangerous practice, from conception to growth to harvest to table.

Article Information

(1) https://www.ers.usda.gov/amber-waves/2014/march/adoption-of-genetically-engineered-crops-by-us-farmers-has-increased-steadily-for-over-15-years/K

(2) http://www.ucsusa.org/sites/default/files/legacy/assets/documents/food_and_agriculture/failure-to-yield.pdf

(3) http://www.geneticliteracyproject.org/2015/09/23/myth-busting-anti-gmo-activist-claims-no-long-term-safety-studies-demolished/

(4) http://journals.plos.org/plosone/article?id=10.1371/journal.pone.0069805

(5) https://www.uclm.es/Actividades/repositorio/pdf/doc_3721_4666.pdf

(6) http://responsibletechnology.org/media/images/content/Press_Release_Gluten_11_25.pdf

(7) http://www.omicsonline.org/open-access/detection-of-glyphosate-residues-in-animals-and-humans-2161-0525.1000210.pdf

(8) http://www.reuters.com/article/2015/09/29/us-monsanto-lawsuit-idUSKCN0RT2L220150929

(9) http://www.iarc.fr/en/media-centre/iarcnews/pdf/MonographVolume112.pdf

—

To conclude this chapter, it is imperative to do your own critical analysis and make decisions on the *preventative* side of things, instead of simply reacting to a disease state and wondering how it came to be.

We've got to use more common sense to our approach. Let's mention one last example:

It would be wise to cook your food in ceramic or cast-iron pans, Teflon is toxic, and the fumes emitted are carcinogenic. If you have a pet bird sitting on your shoulder when you cook with Teflon, that bird has an excellent chance of sudden death. Hundreds of pet birds die from this every year. This is well known and not debated. If this can quickly kill a smaller animal, the intelligent mind would wonder if the human body is being harmed as well.

If we as a society begin to apply this logic, reasoning, and critical thinking to everything around us, even the small things like deodorant and cookware, we can begin to evolve past a needlessly rampant scourge like cancer.

CHAPTER 10
CHIROPRACTIC AND SPORTS MEDICINE

The world of sports medicine and rehabilitation has come a long way in the last 15 years. Stem Cell/PRP therapy is now becoming mainstream. We understand physiology and body mechanics so much better now (though there is still a lot to learn). Chiropractors have been integrated into our mainstream care system and have made a tremendous difference in the realm of healing, repairing, and optimally rehabilitating injuries from sports or auto accidents. They've perfected newer, highly specific techniques like Atlas Orthogonal. But what these guys are really good at is healing the spine/central nervous system, and getting different parts of the body and brain to communicate with each other again. My good buddy David Snellgrove, DC in Pensacola, Florida was a God-send when I was recovering from both minor sports injuries and a car wreck when at age 19, and we've been friends ever since. Through the mastery of spinal manipulations and proper realignment techniques, I was almost immediately able to get back on the field and not have to worry about any residual nagging injuries thanks to him. He was one of the early influences in my life with regard to 'alternative' (or as I call it, 'normal') approaches to medicine.

Another friend of mine in Tampa, Richard Shaker, DC has worked with many professional and amateur athletes, drastically accelerating their bodies' ability to heal/repair/recover from major injuries like torn ACL's and reducing down time. He is one of the early adopters of **Trigenics** (<u>trigenics.com</u>), the field of myo-nerual medicine. It is a state-of-the-art neuro-kinetic sensorimotor assessment, treatment, and training system, which instantly relieves a significant amount of pain and increases strength and movement.

If you have back nagging back injuries or sports-related injuries, there is a whole new world of options that can heal and restore optimal function. There is no longer a reason to suffer from repairable 'mechanical' injuries indefinitely anymore, nor is there reason to simply relegate yourself to living on Ibuprofen.

(Full disclosure, I have no vested or financial interest in Trigenics, but I've met and know many of the professional athletes that swear by it and have seen the dramatic improvement in their injuries during rehabilitation. More importantly, I've seen their injuries healing *properly*. I've also personally been worked on to address minor sports injuries and am very impressed with the technique.)

Athletic Performance

For the ultimate guide in athletic performance, there is no need for me to write a chapter or a book on what it takes to get the absolute very best out of an athlete. Why not? Because someone already beat me to it, and his name is Tom Brady. He is the single greatest NFL quarterback of all time and has won many Super Bowls with the New England Patriots. Even though he isn't the most athletically gifted player to ever play the game (far from it in fact), his method of preparation is second to none. The reader is encouraged to pick up a copy of his book, *The TB12 Method*, and see for yourself why he has rewritten the rules on longevity, health, and athletic performance, most notably with an emphasis on nutrition, flexibility/pliability, and whole-body maintenance. This valuable guide is by no means football-specific, it applies to everyone at every stage of the game.

CHAPTER 11

COGNITIVE FUNCTION AND LONGEVITY

The human mind, and its physical housing (the brain), is an unbounded marvel of engineering. We haven't even come close to understanding the complete nature and complexities of it, and despite our increasingly advanced diagnostic technologies, there are properties of human consciousness—the will, the sentience of self-awareness, the *spirit*, that shall always transcend our ability to completely quantify and qualify the true essence of what composes and *animates* us as human beings. Without delving too far into the metaphysical, existential, or philosophical, it would be fair to say that true consciousness is indubitably more than the sum of its parts.

So let us speak further on that which we *do* understand about the mind/brain connection, and how to avoid certain known habit/diet patterns that are now well-established to be causative factors in the role of cognitive decline.

A great starting point is to pick up a copy of the book *Brain Grain* by world-renowned neurologist David Perlmutter, MD, which details the 'silent killers' of the brain— wheat/gluten and sugar, and how these distractors create a cascade reaction directly attributed to the onset of conditions like dementia, ADHD, anxiety, chronic headaches, depression, and many others. He follows this with his second book *Brain Maker: The Power of Gut Microbes to Heal and Protect Your Brain—for Life*, which goes into extraordinary depth on how to dietarily replenish the state of the microbiome in your gut (the importance of which we previously touched on in the 'probiotic' chapter). The brain-gut connection is one of the key pillars of optimal health and as practitioners we can no longer compartmentalize and artificially isolate these two organs as being separate or unrelated entities. You cannot affect one without influencing the other, therefore you cannot truly heal one without healing the other.

In line with this understanding is the concept of properly addressing **Neurotransmitter** imbalances. The major neuro-transmitters (some of which also function as hormones) that we currently address are *dopamine, serotonin, GABA, glutamate, acetylcholine, norepinephrine, histamine, epinephrine, melatonin, adenosine, nitric oxide, glycine, endorphins, cannabinoids, oxytocin, orexin/hypocretin, and corticotropin.* (There are several others, but they are not as critical and have more obscure functions.)

As we alluded to earlier, neurotransmitters are mostly formed in the gut, and are at the core of our brain chemistry. Neuro-transmitters compose a large component of the very makeup of our dynamic emotional states, primal/limbic urges (eating, sleeping, sex drive, stimulus reaction, self-preservation, pain avoidance), how we handle stress, our natural predispositions, and constitute a balance which allows us to function and interact with other human beings.

It's when this delicate balance of neurotransmitters gets improperly altered that an individual may struggle to 'fit-in' with society, may become reclusive, show signs of self-harm, may display violent tendencies, irrational fears, paranoia, insomnia, hyper-vigilance, depression, anxiety, and an indefinite list of what we can easily identify as deleterious/self-destructive behavioral traits. The truly sad thing with respect to these relatively common imbalances is that modern psychiatry has only one answer: mind-numbing, soul-stealing drugs.

Friends, it's important to be blunt here: SSRI's are *not* the answer. Zoloft and Prozac and Abilify and Seroquel are *not* a viable solution, they are merely a modern day, less bloody version of the surgical lobotomy of the early 1940's. They are the equivalent of throwing a hammer in the dark and hoping a problem goes away. Surely we can do better than that for our patients...

Perhaps we already are? Enter the brave new world of **Neurotransmitter Testing**. In decades past, if we wanted to measure someone's neurotransmitters, we would have either had to collect a sample of cerebrospinal fluid (which is highly impractical and invasive) or performed a brain biopsy (which is extremely impractical and dangerously invasive). Therefore, psychiatrists, while mostly well-meaning, have been essentially limited to doing evaluations of symptomology/behavioral patterns, and prescribing psychiatric drugs to compensate. This model barely functions as a band-aid, and often times makes the underlying problem worse in the long run. But what if we could get to the *root cause*?

For a few years now, we have had access to a state-of-the-art lab known as the HPA-T Axis neurotransmitter assay. We now have the technology to take a look at the neuro-analytes from a combination of urine and saliva collection, and we use the amalgamation of those two sets of data to determine the composition/balance of a patient's neurotransmitter levels. This is groundbreaking, this is beyond exciting, this is a whole new world of being able to give patients proper mental health care. The science is there, the clinical data is there, it's simply a waiting game and an uphill battle to get this into the mainstream.

Fortunately, for the patients who seek this out, it's readily available to them in the field of holistic medicine/psychiatry. Once the lab is administered and the results are received approximately 2 weeks later, we are able to custom tailor the appropriate therapy for the individual patient, using the exact practitioner-grade neutraceutical supplements the patient needs, and in very specific doses. We mostly deal with the primary axis neurotransmitters, and start rebuilding/rebalancing the **inhibitory** side of things *first*, which we exclusively address during the first 3 weeks of therapy. This typically means boosting/supporting/rebuilding Serotonin and

GABA. (The inhibitory side of neurochemistry is typically what constitutes peacefulness, zen, focus, tranquility, being able to relax, get restful sleep, etc.) Once we've seen some initial improvement, we then begin addressing the **excitatory** side, most notably by assisting the production of Dopamine. (The excitatory side of neurochemistry is generally what constitutes motivation, enthusiasm, will-power, happy feelings, and zest for life, but we also must be very careful to manage this appropriately, because over-correction here can lead to psychosis.) The formulas we use are powerful, practitioner-grade, clinically studied nutraceuticals that are only prescribed in the unique combination that the patient (based on their neuro-lab results) needs. These formulas do *not* mask symptoms the way SSRI's do. These formulas very specifically give the body what it needs to actually *rebuild its own neurotransmitters* to a state of optimal balance, which then becomes *self-sustaining*. These supplements are in no way addicting, they are in no way habit forming. Once they've done their job, the patient is typically able to discontinue the supplements altogether around the 4 to 6-month point of therapy, at which point we do follow-up neurotransmitter testing (in tandem with symptomology evaluation) to confirm that optimal balance has been achieved. Fellow practitioners, this is an example of a true solution. Please *let it not be lost upon you that the optimal number of drugs for a patient to be on is **zero***.

Ok, so all that sounds amazing and wonderful (and it *is*). But surely that can't be all there is to it (it's *not*). Nothing is that simple, human beings are definitely not that simple. It bears reiteration that we humans are more than the sum of our parts. We are a combination of mind, body, and spirit, and soul. A true physician, a true *healer* must be able to address all four, not just figure out a formula or write a prescription. Repairing neurotransmitters is a huge step in the right direction, but it doesn't fix the whole person, nor does it necessarily resolve their underlying trauma. How did they get a neurotransmitter imbalance in the first place? Wait, wait, wait...aren't we overstepping our bounds here? Are we getting out of our lane? Isn't that a *personal* problem? Sure it is, and they've come to you to for help. At the very least, point them in the right direction on their journey. As a wearer of the white coat, and as a taker of the Hippocratic Oath, I would humbly suggest you make *damn* sure you know how to do that, even if that aspect of patient care isn't taught in med school (*hint: it isn't*).

One of the most common types of patient that walk through the door looking for psychiatric help are war veterans with PTSD. My heart goes out to them. They served our country honorably, they represent the very best and bravest of us, and they've witnessed horrors the likes of which would prevent most of us from ever being able to sleep again. They've seen their buddies get blown up and die in their arms, they put their lives on the line to defend our freedoms, and they've endured a level of pain and suffering that no human should ever have to face. But then they have to deal with the even greater torment of a health-care system that fails them, loads them up with toxic psychiatric drugs, and hangs them out to dry, all while the sheer inertia of government bureaucracies like the VA forces them to languish in agony. They almost never get the adequate treatment that they were promised, that they deserve, and that they paid for in blood, sweat, and tears. We've had the honor and privilege of first, thanking these brave men and women for their service, and second, helping them undo the trauma of the abject horrors they experienced. We do that by rebalancing, rebuilding, and restoring their neurotransmitters. But this is where the 'holistic' element of philosophy comes in. We very specifically tell our PTSD patients that this isn't just a physical or neuro-chemical injury...this is a **spiritual injury**. (Yeah, as a reader, let that sink in for a moment, it's heavy.) So what does all this mean and where are we going with this?

Our intent is this...to make the treatment and the healing more human to human, not just doctor to patient. We tell our PTSD patients that they are still going to need to find their own version of solace, forgiveness, wholeness, and peace by whatever means they find appropriate whether it's prayer, meditation, group therapy, yoga, etc.

The awesome part of all this though is that when you fix or remove the physical component (i.e. the neurotransmitter imbalance), you've effectively removed what we refer to as the *'distractor,'* and it makes healing the spiritual/emotional component 90% easier. When you've removed hyper-vigilance, anxiety, fight-or-flight response, insomnia, sky-high cortisol/norepinephrine, and any other *physical* imbalances, all of the sudden it becomes much more of an attainable goal for the patient to find healing for their own *spiritual and emotional* injuries.

I wonder how long it's going to take before they teach this in med school…

For practitioner reference, we use the *HPA Neurotransmitter Lab* by Sanesco Labs. (www.SanescoHealth.com) We like this one because it includes an Adrenal Stress Index (ASI) test that gives us a 4-point cortisol (stress hormone) read in addition to the neurotransmitters. There are a few other similar labs that some of our sister clinics like to use including the *NeuroScreen Expanded (9123)* by Pharmasan Labs, and/or the *NeuroEndocrine Profile* by NeuroScience Labs (www.integrativepsychiatry.net)

Some of our most well utilized products for rebalancing neurotransmitters are **Serotone** by Apex Energetics, **GABA** by Pure Encapsulations, **Kavinace Ultra PM** by NeuroScience, (soy-free) **Phosphatidyl Serine** by Integrative Therapeutics, **DopaTropic Powder** by Biotics Research, and **L-Theanine** by Pure Encapsulations.

Shifting to another element of mental health is the field of cognitive and/or neurological degeneration. We again reference world-renowned neurologist Dr. David Perlmutter. The reader is highly encouraged to go to YouTube and take a few minutes to watch the quick 3-minute videos of Dr. Perlmutter and the success he has in real time treating a Parkinson's patient with **intravenous glutathione**. In the videos an elderly Vietnam veteran goes from severe stuttering and shakily walking to speaking and moving normally within minutes immediately following an IV administration of (3000mg) glutathione. We now have access to these amazing treatments, most notably IV glutathione, IV stem cell therapy, and IV glycero-phosphatidylcholine which can drastically improve patient outcomes for conditions like Parkinson's, ALS, Alzheimer's, and Dementia, and Autistic Spectrum Disorders. More on these treatments later in the book!

Bio/Body Hacking

A huge trend in health in the past few years has been the emergence of the concept and culture of "Bio-Hacking." This ideology is predicated on bending/pushing past the rules and limits of normal human abilities to reach super-human thresholds of strength, focus, stamina, mental/cognitive ability, sexual prowess, etc. It's all about taking self-improvement to the extreme.

One of the pioneers of the movement is Dave Asprey, CEO and Founder of the *Bulletproof* brand, most famous for its "bulletproof" coffee recipe which combines MCT/Coconut oil and grass-fed butter with gourmet coffee. This formula provides the brain with some seriously 'high-octane' fuel in the form of slow-burning healthy fats, and it gets an additional kick from the caffeine. Even though we are not a fan of caffeine/stimulants, this formula is admittedly a very effective method for achieving razor sharp focus, concentration, and optimal mental efficiency for several hours. So if you're going to drink coffee, at least drink it this way.

Dave helped coin the term, the movement, and the definition as articulated on blog.bulletproof.com:

> **Biohacking** (verb, noun): (v): changing your environment from the inside-out so you have full control of your biology; using your body as your personal laboratory, finding the exact hacks that work for you.
>
> (n): The art and science of becoming superhuman.

A couple more firebrands in the genre are Wim Hof, the famous 'iceman' who can resist extreme temperatures and control his autonomic body functions (www.WimHofmethod.com) and Timothy Ferriss, author of *The 4-Hour Body*, which introduces radical methods of achieving things like rapid fat loss, 15-minute orgasms, polyphasic sleeping, and tapping into new levels of psychological perseverance in order to achieve a goal. I highly recommend you look at both, if only to spark a new conversation with yourself and introduce a different perspective of what you are truly capable of as a human being.

Another big component of this movement is the sudden resurgence of interest in the class of drugs known as *Nootropics*, which have sustained a newfound celebrity-status among the private sector tech industry as well as in the public eye thanks to Hollywood movie productions like the Bradley Cooper film *Limitless*. These substances are known as 'smart' drugs, recognized for their abilities to improve cognitive function, focus, memory, creativity, mental clarity, and motivation. The final verdict is still out with regard to long term effects, however, the decades-long ongoing clinical studies seem to support a dramatic improvement in cognitive function with only the potential for very minimal side effects (i.e. mild headache, temporary insomnia).

It is essential to clearly point out that there are two 'types' of nootropics. Some of them are drugs (mostly within the *'racetam'* family), but there are also natural substances which produce various elements of enhanced mental acuity/cognitive ability. Some formulas combine one or more of the 'racetam' drugs with the natural enhancers for a synergistic effect, which is categorized as 'stacking.'

The oldest and most well-known of the nootropic drugs is Piracetam, a cyclic derivative of GABA synthesized in 1964 by (Romanian chemist and psychologist) Corneliu E. Giurgea. He is credited for coining the term 'nootropic' in 1972. Piracetam and the entire 'racetam' family of nootropic drugs have, for decades, been shown to be exceedingly safe with a profile of extremely low toxicity rates, and have been used to not only improve cognitive abilities in patients with degenerative conditions like Alzheimer's, but in healthy adults as well.

Natural brain boosters have presently garnered an equal amount of recent notoriety, and a significant number of clinical studies are validating the safety and efficacy of substances like Vinpocetine, Huperzine-A, Bacopa, Acetyl-L-Carnitine, Ginko Biloba, Phosphatidyl Serine, Alpha GPC, L-Theanine, and more.

At our clinic, we have three favorite nootropic supplements that, at the present moment, we believe to be of the highest grade, the safest, and the most effective. The first one is **Nootroo**, which has an alternating schedule of noopept, and phenylpiracetam combined with choline, and l-theanine. This stuff is potent, powerful, and the clinical studies/data are readily available on the company website (*nootroo.com*) for those who wish to see the research. We've personally tried it at the clinic and believe it to be a very effective product. I personally wouldn't want that much of a 'charge' everyday, so I only take it occasionally when I need a little boost to complete a mentally intensive project, but then again I'm not a morning coffee drinker either, so this might be a better, more effective option for the roughly 64% or so of Americans who do drink coffee every day.

The second supplement we recommend is a practitioner-grade product called **MemorAll** by Xymogen. There are no drugs (racetams) in this formula, it's non-stimulatory, and it has more of an aggregate effect on improved cognitive ability over time. It contains methyl-lated B vitamins as well as most of the 'natural brain boosters' mentioned two paragraphs ago. It is a very effective option for natural brain support and is an integral part of the therapy we offer for our patients suffering from early stage Alzheimer's, dementia, and other forms of cognitive decline. There are also newer promising supplements continuing to surface on the market like Qualia Mind and Alpha Brain which anecdotally appear to produce solid results as well.

We are entering the generation of the super-human mind, hopefully we can practice due diligence and guide it in a healthy direction.

CHAPTER 12

COLON HYDROPTHERAPY

This is perhaps an unpleasant, but highly necessary chapter. The average middle-aged American has somewhere between 10 to 20 *pounds* (~5 to 10 kilograms) of impacted fecal matter in their gastrointestinal tract. This is due to the indigestibility of all the processed foods we eat and chemicals/toxins they contain. Richard Anderson, ND, NMD coined the term *Mucoid Plaque* to describe this condition, and if you have a strong stomach and wish to see what it looks like, you can Google Image search that term. The N.I.H. estimates that at least 70 million Americans experience poor digestive health. It's not hard to imagine that number is significantly understated.

The major problem we have with this putrefying mucoid plaque build-up is that the level of build-up directly correlates to how clean your bloodstream is. Dietary nutrients are absorbed into the bloodstream through the walls of the small intestine, but so are toxins. People with high levels of mucoid build up often suffer from poor nutrient absorption. It can also produce a sluggish liver which struggles to process and turn over those toxins, leading to physical symptoms such as food intolerance, over active seasonal allergies, skin rashes, irritability, insomnia, weight gain, IBS, fatigue, and several others. The length of the colon (also known as large intestine) is roughly equivalent to a person's standing height. Each foot can store roughly 5 to 10 pounds of feces, which means a 6-foot-tall male has the theoretical capacity to carry 60 pounds of poop. Now obviously that theoretical capacity is only on paper/in a vacuum and would be highly uncommon, but there have been many autopsies done in which the deceased patient's colon was distended and contained *over 40 pounds* of mucoid plaque, which resembles some sort of disgusting rubbery beef jerky/rawhide combined with encrusted glue. Yeah, that's fun.

One of the most helpful tools we have at our disposal (in addition to eating a proper diet) is the ability to preempt and reverse this impacted condition via the modality of Colon Hydrotherapy. A colon hydrotherapist is able to use a highly specialized set of state-of-the-art machinery with properly (and minimally) pressurized sterile water to go in the 'back way' and cleanse the bowels of harmful mucous, toxins, and excess bad bacteria, and to stimulate/exercise/strengthen the colon muscle so that it works more efficiently thereafter. I speak from personal experience and from the experiences of my friends/family/patients that this is a tremendously beneficial therapy. Following the colon hydrotherapy, a great additional modality to employ is a coffee enema. The type of coffee used is not the same type of coffee that you drink, and you definitely wouldn't want to taste it! It's much more bitter and potent than regular coffee. When prepared in solution and administered rectally, it helps further clean out the GI tract, but more importantly stimulates the liver to purge remaining toxins.

It's important to note that colon hydrotherapy does pose certain risks in the hands of a poorly trained practitioner (such as colon wall perforation), and it's imperative to find a good one before venturing down this avenue to assist in the healing process. If you happen to be in the Tampa Bay area, I recommend Bonnie Barrett, LMT/CT. She's a personal friend of mine and has been a licensed colon hydrotherapist for over 25 years. Her website is **Renewlifefla.com** (full disclosure, I have no vested or financial interest in promoting Bonnie or her practice, she is just an excellent and trusted practitioner within my network and I routinely refer patients to her who end up benefiting immensely from her therapies).

Another helpful method of G.I. detox is something called the "**Master Cleanse**." This formula has been around since the 1940's and consists of only four ingredients: Maple Syrup, Cayenne Pepper, Fresh Lemon Juice, and Pure Water. Anyone who is need of weight loss or is suffering the symptoms of G.I. toxicity should consider looking into this cleanse. The book to read is *The Master Cleanser: With Special Needs and Problems* by Stanley Burroughs. (You can a copy of either the e-book or paperback on Amazon.com for less than $4.)

Done properly (by easing onto it and off of it *slowly*), this cleanse permits the digestive system to get some much-needed rest and allows the body to reallocate the energy/resources normally required for digestion into healing itself, naturally. We do recommend that this cleanse is done under the supervision of a licensed health care practitioner. During the cleanse, it is an optimal time for other healing modalities, like lymphatic drainage massage, to be utilized. This type of massage loosens and releases toxins into the blood stream to be removed by liver. Since a cleanse is already in progress, it's significantly easier for the body to then eliminate this remaining detritus.

pH

One of the other major purposes of doing these types cleanses/detoxes is to restore pH of your body and its acid/alkaline balance. When the body is at an optimal pH and in a slightly alkaline state (about a 7.2 on the traditional litmus test), it virtually cannot get sick, and can heal significantly easier. When we have terrible diets, the body tends to get more acidic, even to the point where it falls into the condition known as Acidosis. Being overly acidic puts us into a compromised immune state, allowing us to become significantly more predisposed to conditions like cancer and diabetes.

The restoration of *balance* is the key factor here though; the intent is not to go in a radical direction chasing alkalinity, and there is a fair amount of pseudoscience on this subject, including a billion-dollar sales industry dedicated to selling snake-oil products which promise to make you alkaline. If we were extremely alkaline, that would be harmful too. There are certain places in the body like the stomach, which need to remain acidic. Adding in basic/alkaline substances here and raising the pH (which is what proton pump inhibitor medications do) can be a bad thing, and opens the body up to opportunistic infections like H. pylori. Conversely, ingesting alkali-forming foods like dark green vegetables, sprouts, legumes, and good essential fats from avocadoes and fish is a good thing, and those foods take on differing levels of acidic and alkaline properties as they pass through the various sections of the gastrointestinal tract. This is way the system is *supposed* to work.

There are no shortage of books and health regimens founded upon the topic of pH, however I believe improper pH is often the symptom, not the cause of disease states. When we cleanse the body of excess toxins, clean up our sugary/processed/artificial diets, and restore our emotional health/stress balance, then the body should have no problem very easily and effortlessly bringing its overall pH into balance, and maintaining the appropriate acid/alkaline ratios in different organs/body systems.

CHAPTER 13

DENTAL HEALTH

Everyone loves going to see the dentist…in some weird alternate parallel universe, definitely *not* in this one! We are all so busy in our day to day lives that we often don't spend enough time taking care of our teeth, and we suffer for it and end up at the dentist. But what if even those of us who *do* spend plenty of time on our teeth have been given very poor information on *how* to properly care for our teeth? What if the outdated or outright wrong information we had on dental care not only led to oral health issues, but to other health issues like cancer? What if that which is thought to help us is actually causing us harm? Sadly, that very well may be the case. A starting point for sage wisdom on this subject is the book *Whole Body Dentistry* by Mark A. Breiner, DDS. This book should be required reading in the first year of dental school and is a foundational piece/critical reading to understanding treating dental issues from a whole body perspective.

The past few years I've had the privilege to spend many hours of thought-provoking dialogue with my good friend Carlo Litano, DMD. Dr. Litano owns and runs *Natural Smiles of Tampa Bay*, a state-of-the- art biological dentistry practice that specializes in neuromuscular restorative dentistry. They are about 15 years ahead of the industry standard and are 100% metal-free and root-canal free. They perform extractions without discomfort through the use of the patient's own harvested stem cells (via platelet rich fibrin), localized ozone therapy, and bio-compatible mineral bone grafts. If you are experiencing any significant dental issues, I highly recommend you seek out an experienced biological dentist like him!

On to the story...let's go piece by piece into the dangers of *not* using a natural/biological dentist, i.e. the health hazards of being subjected to the draconian procedures of old.

> **Mercury Amalgams/Fillings—** Mercury is a known carcinogen and health hazard (in both methyl and ethyl form). It is also known to have adverse neurological side effects (neurotoxicity) and is considered a biohazardous material. It has been clinically linked to suppressing the immune system, causing chronic fatigue, migraines, anxiety, tremors, mood disorders, and memory loss. Apparently the only safe place then to store it would be in the human mouth. Wait, what? That can't be right! The old "silver" fillings consist of an amalgamation of mercury, tin, silver, and copper, which are supposedly stable and do not off-gas mercury. That's what was taught in dental school for nearly a hundred and fifty years. We now know that that could not be further from the truth. Every time you chew food, every time you brush your teeth, every time you drink a carbonated beverage, etc., mercury is being off-gassed at a rate that the EPA considers extremely toxic. Compounding matters is that the mercury is located in your mouth, and directly crossing into the blood/brain barrier. Over time the resultant health effects are often exacerbated and intensified as the amalgams corrode and become galvanized.
>
> Galvanization occurs when a metal takes on an ionic charge. With the saliva in your mouth acting as an electrolyte, you've essentially created a battery in your head. I've attached an excerpt written by Michael G. Rehme, DDS, NMD at the end of this chapter that further explains this process.

Also, *I highly recommend* you go to Youtube and watch the 2-part series that Dr. Oz did on the "Dangers of Mercury Fillings" with natural dentist Dr. Gerry Curatola. The videos are approximately 5 minutes each, clearly demonstrating in real time the off-gassing of mercury amalgams, and the docs further expound upon the associated health risks.

Root Canals— A root canal in your mouth is a permanent infection in your body, period. When a root canal is performed, it is initially sterilized and then sealed with a substance called gutta-percha. However, in very short order, anaerobic bacteria (bacteria that don't need oxygen to survive) begin to proliferate and fester. There is no way blood flow, oxygen, or even anti-biotics can get in to clean up this cordoned off infection, and it can lead to a cascade of very serious health complications. We also now know that teeth are very important end points for meridians/bio-electric pathways, so a permanently infected tooth means a compromised/blocked bio-electrical energy field as well. This correlates directly with chronic illnesses (one of which is the proliferation of oral spirochetes, a component of Lyme disease). At the end of this chapter is an attached article from Dr. Joseph Mercola which goes into more detail about the dangers of root canals. You can also go to bigdiastema.com/apps/toothchart to view an interactive meridian tooth chart which diagrams the direct relationship from individual teeth to certain body systems.

But amidst all this there is hope. At biological dental practices around the country (like Dr. Litano's office), mercury amalgams and root canals are a thing of the past (and they also specialize in removal/ proper restoration of both). All filings are done with the tooth-colored 'composite' materials which are completely inert and actually strengthen what is left of the tooth. More importantly, instead of performing a root canal, a biological dentist will make sure the dead tooth, all of its roots, and any cavitations are completely removed/cleaned-up and sterilized with O3 (Ozone) gas, and an amazingly innovative and organic procedure is done in its place:

A phlebotomist comes and takes several vials of blood from the patient. Those vials are spun at a specific rpm in a centrifuge until the **Platelet Rich Fibrin** (and plasma) are separated from the blood. PRF is then condensed and harvested in the form of a semi-solid bio-jelly. This substance is then sutured into the open socket where the extracted tooth was formerly rooted. Since PRF contains the patient's own stem-cells and healing co-factors, it actually begins to *regrow* the patient's jaw-bone. After a couple of months of healing, the bone fusion and accompanying gum regrowth are complete, and it looks as though there was never a tooth there to begin with. At this point, a zirconium implant can be drilled and anchored into the *brand new* section of jaw bone. Zirconium is inert, chemically unreactive and is very well tolerated by the body. It is the generation of technology beyond stainless steel or titanium implants. After the implant has had a chance to anchor and the surrounding jaw-bone has healed around it, the porcelain crown (the part that looks like the actual tooth) is custom made and secured to the implant, giving the patient restored chewing function. This entire approach is *vastly* superior to having a root canal done, and it lands on the exact opposite end of the spectrum with regard to overall patient health. After all I've seen and learned over the years, I am firmly of the opinion that *you absolutely cannot be in a state of optimal health with a root canal (and/or mercury amalgams) in your mouth.* It is simply imperative to get this stuff cleaned up. Dental health is a core component of and inextricably linked to total body health.

Ok so what else do we need to firmly update our approach on with regard to dental health?

> **Fluoride**. It's a neurotoxin. It's a common ingredient in several rat/roach poisons. It's a waste by-product of the

fertilizer industry. It's been clinically linked to lowered IQ in children and to causing developmental disabilities. The brain-numbing, soul-stealing SSRI/drug Prozac (fluoxetine) is a hybridized form of fluoride. Fluoride is actually harmful for your teeth, causing fluorosis, technically hardening enamel, but in a non-beneficial way that makes the enamel more brittle. A report in March of 2014 from the world's oldest and most prestigious medical journal, *The Lancet*, has officially classified fluoride as neurotoxin and/or a developmental neurotoxicant. The study, published by Philippe Grandjean MD, and Philip J. Landrigan, MD, titled *Neurobehavioural Effects of Developmental Toxicity*, very clearly linked early-life exposure to neurotoxins (including fluoride and several others like lead, methylmercury, polychlorinated biphenyls (PCBs), arsenic, and toluene) to neurobiological disease and degenerative changes during the early brain development and functional maturation phases of life, but also noted *that the wide range of adverse effects on the brain could manifest as functional impairments or disease at any point in the human lifespan, from early infancy to old age.*

You have to ask yourself, if fluoride really was that beneficial, why has there been such a violent backlash for decades and a struggle against it? Why is there resistance worldwide within the collective consciousness of the human population, including countless educated medical professionals? It's funny, we don't seem to have the same level of aversion to things that are actually healthy, like say magnesium. According to *Wikipedia*:

> *"When voted upon, the outcomes tend to be 'negative,' and thus fluoridation has had a history of gaining through **administrative orders** in North America."*

If fluoride was so critical for health, then why do they have to force us to take it at gunpoint? Why not just let an individual decide if they wanted to use fluoride toothpaste or not instead of drugging the water supply?

Fluoride was not only discontinued based on the overwhelming scientific evidence of being harmful, it was completely banned in a significant number of civilized European nations. Germany, Sweden, the Netherlands, the Czech Republic (formerly Czechoslovakia), Russia (formerly USSR), and Finland have all discontinued the use of water fluoridation (most of this was stopped between the early 1970's to the late 1980's. (The Asian country of Japan also stopped water fluoridation in 1972.) It has been linked many times (although not categorically proven) to the Communist and Nazi regimes as a means of prisoner/enemy subjugation via a form of slow tranquilization.

It's time we removed this injurious contaminant from our day to day lives and from our water supply. You can purchase any number of brands of fluoride-free toothpaste online or at your local health-food store (but make sure they are free of sulfates as well). You can also purchase multi-stage water filtration systems for your home to filter your shower/sink water, but it needs to have a 'bone-char' elemental filament layer in it to remove fluoride. Most simple R.O. units do not have this layer.

As far as fluoride detoxification for the body, the best way to accomplish this from our current research is supplementally. Regular use of practitioner grade **Curcumin/Turmeric** is number one, as the active alkaloids protect the brain and kidneys from fluoride toxicity, as well as prevent damage to the DNA from fluoride present in human lymphocytes. **Tamarind** extract, and getting plenty of **iodine** have also proven quite useful with regard to fluoride elimination from the body.

Oral Pro-biotics/ Mouthwash— Here is a very overlooked but critical component of dental care that has just now come to the forefront of emerging dental practice. We over-sterilize our mouths with alcohol-based mouthwashes like Listerine. Sure, they can be helpful at killing off the bad bacteria, but they also kill off the *good* bacteria in our mouths, which creates an unnatural condition that is both harmful to dental health, and to the entire digestive tract. We have disrupted the very first stage of digestion. We no longer have the 'first responders' of proper mouth bacteria that begin the nitrate/nitrite conversion process that is supposed to occur before the food ever even reaches the stomach. We need to maintain this healthy eco-culture and conversion process in our mouths as well as our guts in order from proper nutrient absorption to occur. So for those of us who used Listerine their whole lives (like me), what do we do now? Glad you asked!

1) We can begin a regimen of oral probiotics, at least temporarily, to jump start the re-population of good bacteria in the mouth. The most prominent on the market, and the one my dentist friends recommend is **EvoraPro/Evora Plus**. These can be found on Amazon.com and a few other retailers.

2) We can switch our alcohol-based mouthwashes out for something way healthier. There is a product called **Tooth and Gums Tonic**, made by the Dental Herb Company, which is an essential oil based mouth wash, developed by a dentist (Dr. Bernard Schecter) with a background in microbiology and herbology. It's been clinically shown (study at the University of Rochester) at being even more effective at the killing of certain bacteriological profiles than prescription strength chlorhexidine gluconate, and yet it is also more hospitable to the mouth's natural flora.

3) A cheaper but equally effective option is the ancient Ayurvedic practice of **oil pulling**. This consists of swishing roughly 1 tablespoon of either coconut or extra virgin olive oil around in your mouth for 20 minutes and then spitting it out. While the oil is in your mouth it draws out toxins and helps rebalance the bacteriological profile, as well as providing several other health benefits.

It is the intent of this chapter to open the eyes of the reader once more to the very real dichotomy between what's been accepted as standard for the last 100 years vs. what the newer proven scientific data shows us is actually beneficial for us (with regard to dentistry in the scope of the *whole body*). Once again, the real controversy does *not* lie in the science, the science is there. Nor does it lie in studies or funding, we already have those as well. The real issue is always getting past obstructionist philosophy, reaching a critical mass with regard to teaching new information, and convincing certain stalwart/stubborn practitioners and bodies of medicine (in this case the A.D.A.) that it's time to rid ourselves of draconian and barbaric practices in order to maintain the Hippocratic Oath of first doing no harm and moving onward in the progression of our abilities to truly heal patients.

What the Future Holds

There are revolutionary new procedures on the event horizon of regenerative dentistry. As this book is being written in 2017, there are not one, but *three* new pioneering methods of completely *regrowing* teeth. The first involves using a collagen-derived biomaterial to deliver stem cells to help regenerate dental pulp-like tissue. The second method is a type of low power laser therapy being developed at Harvard University to coax stem cells into reforming dentin. The results have been published in the journal *Science Translational Medicine*. The third method is being studied at King's College London (KCL) in which they combine the Alzheimer's drug Tideglusib (which works by stimulating dormant stem cells) with a substance called glycogen synthase kinase and apply it to the damaged tooth with a biodegradable sponge made from collagen. There has also been significant progress at Queen Mary University (London) on a project that found a protein capable of re-mineralizing tooth enamel.

There isn't a question 'if' these new procedures will emerge, but 'when.' The real question is 'how long will these procedures be violently resisted, suppressed and fought against before we allow them to replace dentistry as we know it?'. I for one, say we combine the laser, the stem cells, the protein, and the Tideglusib into one treatment, re-allocate funding to it from one of the many other places it's being squandered, and begin tests on it this week! If that isn't feasible, let's at least allow ourselves to have that discussion, and get into that type of innovative mindset where new science and discovery is encouraged and fast tracked into the modern world.

(Full disclosure, I have no vested interest in Natural Smiles Dentistry or any of the products in this chapter that I've spoken about. I do highly recommend Dr. Litano as superb biological dentist if you happen to be in the Tampa/Clearwater area.)

CHAPTER 13A

DENTISTRY ARTICLES
(Dr. Michael Rehme, DDS, CCN)

Is There A Battery In Your Mouth?

By Dr. Michael Rehme, DDS, CCN
on January 27, 2013 in *Heavy Metals*, Mouth-Body Health
reprinted with permission

That's a strange question to ask or is it? Did you know that most metals found in your mouth have the ability to create an electrical charge? This charge can be responsible for numerous side effects that are rarely associated with the dental work found in your mouth.

Galvanic current is a term that has been used in dentistry for over 100 years. It is a condition created by the presence of dissimilar metals in the oral cavity of the teeth and gums, with saliva serving as the electrolyte. Have you ever felt a "shock" to your teeth caused by a piece of tin foil or a spoon that touches a sliver or mercury filling in your mouth? If you answer yes to this question, you've experienced a galvanic event.

There are several different types of galvanism: 1) A silver/mercury filling is placed in opposition or adjacent to a tooth restored with gold. These dissimilar metals in conjunction with saliva and body fluids constitute an electric cell. When brought into contact, the circuit is shorted, the flow of electrical current passes through the pulp, and the patient experiences pain. 2) Dissimilar metals coming into contact when the upper and lower teeth come together and touch each other. 3) Two adjacent teeth are restored with dissimilar metals. The current flows from metal to metal through the dentine, bone and tissue fluids of both teeth resulting in discomfort and tooth sensitivity.

We learned about the galvanic current in dental school. We've read about it in dental journals. However, how often do dentists follow the protocols that are necessary to avoid this condition from occurring? The dental profession needs to be more aware of the negative effects that are caused by galvanic currents and be committed to prevent the unwanted, and often harmful, electrical charges or imbalances from occurring.

Other than tooth sensitivity, galvanism can cause a metallic or salty taste in the mouth, increase salivary secretion, and burning or tingling sensation of the tongue. Other systemic complications may include headaches, chronic fatigue, memory loss, sleep deprivation and even irritability due to its effects to the central nervous system.

The brain operates on 7 to 9 nano-amps which is 1000 times weaker than the currents resulting from non-precious metals found in the oral cavity. That is the difference between touching a 9 volt battery and sticking your finger in the light socket as far as the brain is concerned. Since the upper teeth are less than 2 inches from the brain, it is of concern that adding this much excess electrical activity has the potential of creating mis-directed impulses in the brain.

How can you tell if you have a galvanic current occurring in your mouth? The good news is that it can be measured. An electrical potential meter known as the Rita Meter can be used to measure electrical charges on fillings, crowns and metallic appliances. (Normal readings range from +2/-2 micro-amps.)

Healthy gold crowns or composite resins (tooth colored fillings) most often register a positive charge. When they register a negative charge greater than -2, it usually indicates either decay under an old filling or there's an amalgam/mercury filling under a crown.

If these symptoms sound familiar or if you've had 4 or 5 different dentists caring for your dental needs over the years, chances are much greater that there are several dissimilar metals to be found in your mouth.

Metals will not necessarily always cause the galvanic effect in the mouth. It depends on the specific metal and alloy being used along with quantity and placement in the mouth. However, knowing that some of the above symptoms could be dental related may provide you with an opportunity to evaluate your mouth from a different perspective and discover once and for all if there is a galvanic current present in one or multiple sites in your mouth.

Solution? Remove the offending material(s) connected with that particular tooth or teeth in order to reduce this unwanted electrical charge and create a balanced condition. Biological dentistry views galvanism as an obstacle to achieving overall health and wellness. Keep it simple, keep it safe. A balanced body is a healthy body.

Tooth Organ Charts

Borrowed from Michael G. Rehme
with permission – ToothBody.com)

Is it possible that your teeth have a biological effect on other parts of your body? In order to understand this concept, let's consider the therapeutic effects of Chinese acupuncture.

Chinese acupuncture believes there is a universal life energy called Chi (also spelled "Qi") present in every living creature. This energy is said to circulate throughout the body along specific pathways that are called meridians. As long as this energy flows freely throughout the meridians one's health is maintained. However, once the flow of energy is blocked, the system is disrupted, and pain or illness will occur.

Imagine rivers that flood and cause disasters or an electrical grid short-circuiting that causes blackouts. Acupuncture works to "re-program" and restore normal functions by stimulating certain points on the meridians in order to free up the Chi energy.

How does this theory apply to dentistry? Years ago, I was first introduced to the Tooth/Organ chart which lists each tooth in the mouth and describes its relationship to other major organ systems in the body.

I must admit that I was a bit skeptical when this information was first presented to me. However, after years of observations, clinical experience, and patient testimonials, it's quite apparent that our teeth are connected to these energetic pathways called meridians and the relationship to other body parts is quite real.

If a tooth is compromised by infection or contains a high galvanic current, an imbalanced condition will develop, and the natural flow of energy is blocked. When this occurs, any organ system connected to the tooth's meridian pathway can be affected in a negative way and eventually diminish your overall health and wellness.

Biological dentistry teaches us how to address these dental problems by eliminating the imbalances and restoring or "re-programming" the oral cavity back to its balanced energetic condition. Changes in systemic conditions, e.g. digestive problems, joint pains, fatigue, headaches, sinus infections and even heart palpitations, can correct themselves after correcting the dental concerns.

It continues to amaze me how often I witness the positive results that dental interventions have on the rest of the body. In the last 10 years, I've recorded hundreds of testimonials that support this theory of energetic pathways and meridians. Two accounts are listed below.

Patient testimonial 1: "I had an infected, cracked molar which had been affecting both my thyroid and my heart. My heart had been pounding for months. Within minutes after the tooth was removed my heart returned to normal and I felt better than I had in months."

Patient testimonial 2: "I had a great deal of swelling in my lower right jaw adjacent to the infected tooth. I also had a lot of pain in the upper left quadrant which was relieved immediately after the infected tooth was removed. My fatigue has lifted, and the heart palpitations are finally gone."

Let us not forget, holistic health care includes the entire body and the oral cavity should always be part of a complete medical evaluation. Education is the key ingredient for your continued success with biological dentistry. Application of this information can provide major breakthroughs for patients searching for the missing link to improve their health.

DENTISTRY ARTICLE
(Dr. Joseph Mercola)

The Role of Dental Health in Chronic Disease

by Dr. Joseph Mercola

Do you have a chronic degenerative disease? If so, have you been told, "It's all in your head?" Well, that might not be that far from the truth… The root cause of your illness may be in your mouth. There is a common dental procedure that nearly every dentist will tell you is completely safe, despite the fact that scientists have been warning of its dangers for more than 100 years. Every day in the United States alone, 41,000 of these dental procedures are performed on patients who believe they are safely and permanently fixing their problem. What is this dental procedure? The root canal. More than 25 million root canals are performed every year in this country. Root-canaled teeth are essentially "dead" teeth that can become silent incubators for highly toxic anaerobic bacteria that can, under certain conditions, make their way into your bloodstream to cause a number of serious medical conditions—many not appearing until decades later. Most of these toxic teeth feel and look fine for many years, which make their role in systemic disease even harder to trace back. Sadly, the vast majority of dentists are oblivious to the serious potential health risks they are exposing their patients to, risks that persist for the rest of their patients' lives. The American Dental Association claims root canals have been proven safe, but they have NO published data or actual research to substantiate this claim. Fortunately, I had some early mentors like Dr. Tom Stone and Dr. Douglas Cook, who educated me on this issue nearly 20 years ago. Were it not for a brilliant pioneering dentist who, more than a century ago, made the connection between root-canaled teeth and disease, this underlying cause of disease may have remained hidden to this day. The dentist's name was Weston Price—regarded by many as the greatest dentist of all time.

Most dentists would be doing an enormous service to public health if they familiarized themselves with the work of Dr. Weston Price. Unfortunately, his work continues to be discounted and suppressed by medical and dental professionals alike. Dr. Price was a dentist and researcher who traveled the world to study the teeth, bones, and diets of native populations living without the "benefit" of modern food. Around the year 1900, Price had been treating persistent root canal infections and became suspicious that root-canaled teeth always remained infected, in spite of treatments. Then one day, he recommended to a woman, wheelchair bound for six years, to have her root canal tooth extracted, even though it appeared to be fine. She agreed, so he extracted her tooth and then implanted it under the skin of a rabbit. The rabbit amazingly developed the same crippling arthritis as the woman and died from the infection 10 days later. But the woman, now free of the toxic tooth, immediately recovered from her arthritis and could now walk without even the assistance of a cane. Price discovered that it's mechanically impossible to sterilize a root-canaled (e.g. root-filled) tooth. He then went on to show that many chronic degenerative diseases originate from root-filled teeth—the most frequent being heart and circulatory diseases. He actually found 16 different causative bacterial agents for these conditions. But there were also strong correlations between root-filled teeth and diseases of the joints, brain and nervous system.

Dr. Price went on to write two groundbreaking books in 1922 detailing his research into the link between dental pathology and chronic illness. Unfortunately, his work was deliberately buried for 70 years, until finally one endodontist named George Meinig recognized the importance of Price's work and sought to expose the truth. Dr. Meinig, a native of Chicago, was a captain in the U.S. Army during World War II before moving to Hollywood to become a dentist to the stars. He eventually became one of the founding members of the American Association of Endodontists (root canal specialists). In the 1990s, he spent 18 months immersed in Dr. Price's research. In June of 1993, Dr. Meinig published the book *Root Canal CoverUp*, which continues to be the most comprehensive reference on this topic today. You can order your copy directly from the PricePottenger Foundation.

In the middle of each tooth is the pulp chamber, a soft living inner structure that houses blood vessels and nerves. Surrounding the pulp chamber is the dentin, which is made of living cells that secrete a hard mineral substance. The outermost and hardest layer of your tooth is the white enamel, which encases the dentin. The roots of each tooth descend into your jawbone and are held in place by the periodontal ligament. In dental school, dentists are taught that each tooth has one to four major canals. However, there are accessory canals that are never mentioned. Literally miles of them! Just as your body has large blood vessels that branch down into very small capillaries, each of your teeth has a maze of very tiny tubules that, if stretched out, would extend for three miles.

Weston Price identified as many as 75 separate accessory canals in a single central incisor (front tooth). Microscopic organisms regularly move in and around these tubules, like gophers in underground tunnels. When a dentist performs a root canal, he or she hollows out the tooth, then fills the hollow chamber with a substance called gutta percha, which cuts off the tooth from its blood supply, so fluid can no longer circulate through the tooth. But the maze of tiny tubules remains. And bacteria, cut off from their food supply, hide out in these tunnels where they are remarkably safe from antibiotics and your own body's immune defenses. These formerly friendly organisms morph into stronger, more virulent anaerobes that produce a variety of potent toxins. What were once ordinary, friendly oral bacteria mutate into highly toxic pathogens lurking in the tubules of the dead tooth, just awaiting an opportunity to spread. No amount of sterilization has been found effective in reaching these tubules—and just about every single root-canaled tooth has been found colonized by these bacteria, especially around the apex and in the periodontal ligament. Oftentimes, the infection extends down into the jawbone where it creates cavitations—areas of necrotic tissue in the jawbone itself. Cavitations are areas of unhealed bone, often accompanied by pockets of infected tissue and gangrene. Sometimes they form after a tooth extraction (such as a wisdom tooth extraction), but they can also follow a root canal. According to Weston Price Foundation, in the records of 5,000 surgical cavitation cleanings, only two were found healed. And all of this occurs with few, if any, accompanying symptoms. So you may have an abscessed dead tooth and not know it. This focal infection in the immediate area of the root-canaled tooth is bad enough, but the damage doesn't stop there.

As long as your immune system remains strong, any bacteria that stray away from the infected tooth are captured and destroyed. But once your immune system is weakened by something like an accident or illness or other trauma, your immune system may be unable to keep the infection in check. These bacteria can migrate out into surrounding tissues by hitching a ride into your blood stream, where they are transported to new locations to set up camp. The new location can be any organ or gland or tissue. Dr. Price was able to transfer diseases harbored by humans to rabbits, by implanting fragments of root-canaled teeth, as mentioned above. He found that root canal fragments from a person who had suffered a heart attack, when implanted into a rabbit, would cause a heart attack in the rabbit within a few weeks. He discovered he could transfer heart disease to the rabbit 100 percent of the time! Other diseases were more than 80 percent transferable by this method. Nearly every chronic degenerative disease has been linked with root canals, including: Heart disease, Kidney disease, arthritis, joint and rheumatic diseases, Neurological diseases (including ALS and MS), Autoimmune diseases (Lupus and more).

There may also be a cancer connection. Dr. Robert Jones, a researcher of the relationship between root canals and breast cancer, found an extremely high correlation between root canals and breast cancer. He claims to have found the following correlations in a five-year study of 300 breast cancer cases:

- 93 percent of women with breast cancer had root canals

- 7 percent had other oral pathology tumors—of which the majority of cases occurred on the same side of the body as the root canal(s) or other oral pathology.

Dr. Jones claims that toxins from the bacteria in an infected tooth or jawbone are able to inhibit the proteins that suppress tumor development. A German physician reported similar findings. Dr. Josef Issels reported that, in his 40 years of treating "terminal" cancer patients, 97 percent of his cancer patients had root canals. If these physicians are correct, the cure for cancer may be as simple as having a tooth pulled, then rebuilding your immune system.

How are these mutant oral bacteria connected with heart disease or arthritis? The ADA and the AAE claim it's a "myth" that the bacteria found in and around root-canaled teeth can cause disease. But they base that on the misguided assumption that the bacteria in these diseased teeth are the SAME as normal bacteria in your mouth—and that's clearly not the case. Today, bacteria can be identified using DNA analysis, whether they're dead or alive, from their telltale DNA signatures. In a continuation of Dr. Price's work, the Toxic Element Research Foundation (TERF) used DNA analysis to examine root-canaled teeth, and they found bacterial contamination in 100 percent of the samples tested. They identified

42 different species of anaerobic bacteria in 43 root canal samples. In cavitations, 67 different bacteria were identified among the 85 samples tested, with individual samples housing between 19 and 53 types of bacteria each. The bacteria they found included the following types: Capnocytophagaochracea, Fusobacteriumnucleatum, Gemellamorbillorum, Leptotrichiabuccalis, Porphyromonasgingivalis.

Are these just benign, ordinary mouth bugs? Absolutely not. Four can affect your heart, three can affect your nerves, two can affect your kidneys, two can affect your brain, and one can infect your sinus cavities... so they are anything BUT friendly! (If you want see just how unfriendly they can be, I invite you to investigate the footnotes.)

Approximately 400 percent more bacteria were found in the blood surrounding the root canal tooth than were found in the tooth itself, suggesting the tooth is the incubator and the periodontal ligament is the food supply. The bone surrounding root-canaled teeth was found even HIGHER in bacterial count... not surprising, since bone is virtual buffet of bacterial nutrients.

Since when is Leaving a dead body part *in* your body a good idea? There is no other medical procedure that involves allowing a dead body part to remain in your body. When your appendix dies, it's removed. If you get frostbite or gangrene on a finger or toe, it is amputated. If a baby dies in utero, the body typically initiates a miscarriage. Your immune system doesn't care for dead substances, and just the presence of dead tissue can cause your system to launch an attack, which is another reason to avoid root canals—they leave behind a dead tooth. Infection, plus the autoimmune rejection reaction, causes more bacteria to collect around the dead tissue. In the case of a root canal, bacteria are given the opportunity to flush into your blood stream every time you bite down.

The ADA rejects Dr. Price's evidence, claiming root canals are safe, yet they offer no published data or actual research to substantiate their claim. American Heart Association recommends a dose of antibiotics before many routine dental procedures to prevent infective endocarditis (IE) if you have certain heart conditions that predispose you to this type of infection. So, on the one hand, the ADA acknowledges oral bacteria can make their way from your mouth to your heart and cause a life-threatening infection. But at the same time, the industry vehemently denies any possibility that these same bacteria—toxic strains KNOWN to be pathogenic to humans—can hide out in your dead root-canaled tooth to be released into your blood stream every time you chew, where they can damage your health in a multitude of ways. Is this really that large of a leap? Could there be another reason so many dentists, as well as the ADA and the AAE, refuse to admit root canals are dangerous? Well, yes, as a matter of fact, there is. Root canals are the most profitable procedure in dentistry.

I strongly recommend never getting a root canal. Risking your health to preserve a tooth simply doesn't make sense. Unfortunately, there are many people who've already have one. If you have, you should seriously consider having the tooth removed, even if it looks and feels fine. Remember, as soon as your immune system is compromised, your risk of developing a serious medical problem increases—and assaults on your immune system are far too frequent in today's world. If you have a tooth removed, there are a few options available to you:

- Partial denture: This is a removable denture, often just called a "partial." It's the simplest and least expensive option.

- Bridge: This is a more permanent fixture resembling a real tooth but is a bit more involved and expensive to build.

- Implant: This is a permanent artificial tooth, typically titanium in the past implanted in your gums and jaw. There are some problems with these due to reactions to the metals used. Zirconium is a newer implant material that shows promise for fewer complications. But just pulling the tooth and inserting some sort of artificial replacement isn't enough.

Dentists are taught to remove the tooth but leave your periodontal ligament. But as you now know, this ligament can serve as a breeding ground for deadly bacteria. Most experts who've studied this recommend removing the ligament, along with one millimeter of the bony socket, in order to drastically reduce your risk of developing an infection from the bacterially infected tissues left behind.

I strongly recommend consulting a biological dentist because they are uniquely trained to do these extractions properly and safely, as well as being adept at removing mercury fillings, if necessary. Their approach to dental care is far more holistic and considers the impact on your entire body—not JUST your mouth. If you need to find a biological dentist in your area, I recommend visiting toxicteeth.org, a resource sponsored by Consumers for Dental Choice. This organization, championed by Charlie Brown, is a highly reputable organization that has fought to protect and educate consumers so that they can make better-informed decisions about their dental care. The organization also heads up the Campaign for Mercury-Free Dentistry.

Sources and References:
  i.   Weston A. Price Foundation
 ii.   Price-Pottenger Foundation
iii.   Weston A. Price Foundation June 25, 2010
 iv.   Quantum Cancer Management
  v.   American Association of Endodontists
 vi.   Journal of Clinical Microbiology February 2007
vii.   Journal of Clinical Microbiology July 2003
viii.   Clinical Infectious Diseases June 1996
 ix.   Science Daily January 4, 2011
  x.   The Wealthy Dentist July 12, 2011
 xi.   ToxicTeeth.org

CHAPTER 14

WEIGHT LOSS/DETOXIFICATION

They say if you want to get rich that you should write a book on weight loss. Does that mean I can get kinda rich if I write a chapter on it? That's sarcasm coming through, but it's aimed at the ridiculous number of fad diets, yo-yo diets, and outright snake oil that people tout and sell promising massive weight loss. The biggest obstacle that seems to elude and riddle the general population is that *there is no magic bullet*. But fortunately there is an *entire arsenal*. The true solution to weight loss is knowing two things:

1) You have to treat *all the underlying issues of the body* (including toxins and illness), not just the *symptom* of weight gain, or else you will never achieve the results you're looking for and 2) if you are significantly overweight, you can't oversimplify, compartmentalize and distill the concept of fat loss down to one little tonic (i.e. the 'magic bullet'). It requires a comprehensive understanding of *how you got there in the first place*. In other words, if you skipped straight to this chapter, then it's imperative to read the rest of the book.

With that being said we can transition to stating that the problem with generalized weight-loss programs is that they don't work for everybody. Human beings each have an amazingly complex and completely unique biochemistry, therefore you have to find what is going to work for *you*. Humans also generally fall into one of 3 body types: *endomorphs*—those who readily store more body fat, *mesomorphs*—those who typically have a well-developed musculature, and *ectomorphs*—those distinguished by having a lack of both fat and muscle tissue. Completely different types of exercise and fitness training are required to optimize these body types, as well as differing diets. What makes one person lose weight will make another gain weight. "Keto" works great for some people and it's terribly unhealthy for other people. With respect to the biochemistry aspect, we also have different blood types, sub-types, and antigens. There is a book called *Eat Right for Your Type*. I definitely don't think it's absolute gospel by any means, but it's worth skimming through and does present some good information, points, and theories.

What you can see here is that in just two paragraphs, we've already highly differentiated people into very specific categories. Within that single basic (9th-grade-biology level) 'punnet square' of cross-referencing, [3 body types x 8 major blood types], we've just created 24 combinations of a 'type' of person...and they all respond vastly differently to exercise(s) and diet(s). This is, of course, a gross oversimplification itself considering there are hundreds of thousands of variables and components in biochemistry and genetic make-up, not just two. So where the heck do we even start? Glad you asked.

Detoxing

Yes, my allopathic friends, these enigmatic, nebulous toxins <u>*do*</u> exist, whether you want them to or not, and no the body can't always easily rid itself of a lot of them, especially the synthetic ones that haven't existed for most of human history. Read the whole rest of the book to get a handle on them, but for the sake of having a concise list in one place, let me list certain *distractors* to weight loss...i.e. we need to remove these things first if we want our body to have an easier time losing, and not storing fat:

- Removal of Heavy Metals (lead, mercury, aluminum) via IV Chelation

- Discontinue Unnecessary Pharmaceutical Drugs
- Discontinue Fluoride toothpaste, detox fluoride with Turmeric
- Dental Issue Clean-up (removing root canals, removing mercury fillings, which allows for better endocrine/metabolic function)
- Discontinuing the consumption of GMO's, processed foods
- Discontinuing the consumption of any product with artificial sweeteners or the word 'diet' on it (i.e. Diet Coke)
- Discontinuing (at least temporarily) the 'big 4'—sugar, dairy, gluten, and alcohol
- Removal of impacted fecal matter via Colon Hydrotherapy
- Removal of Candida/Parasites via Parasite Cleanse
- Removal of dietary components which cause food intolerance and histamine response
- Removal of Clogged Liver and restoring function to sulfation pathways via Intravenous Glutathione
- Improvement of sluggish micro-circulatory system with Bemer/PEMF
- Gallbladder Cleanse (i.e. the organ that processes fat)
- Removal of excess and artificial (xeno-) estrogens via Myomin, DIM, and Calcium-D-Glucarate (excess estrogen signals fat storage)
- Removal of continual cycles of anti-biotics and re-establishing pro-biotic colonies/micro-biome
- Lowering of Cortisol (stress hormone)
- Toning of Bio-Electric Pathways via Acupuncture
- Daily (at least 5 days a week) consumption of 16 to 20oz of raw, organic celery juice
- **Removal of toxic belief systems, negative emotions, and stress**

Suffice to say that list is a great starting point for now. If we even begin to work our way down that list, drastic improvement should soon follow. Noticed how we haven't even introduced some snappy new exercise program yet? More importantly, did you notice how the last item on the list is highlighted in bold letters? Did you notice how it is perhaps a little bit different from all of the other things on the list? Mainstream medical science may not acknowledge this for another half a century, but let us be clear: *the mind, emotions, and spirit have a direct influence on the vessel (your body) and the complex mechanisms of biochemistry within it. We know this scientifically...now.* **Your emotions and beliefs take up physical resonance in every single one of the trillions of cells in your body.**

If you jumped straight to this chapter desperately looking for answers on fat loss and you feel like nothing has worked, I want you to forget everything else on that list for a moment and say this three times out loud:

> "It is **impossible** to effectively lose weight if I continue to harbor negative emotions like anger, hatred, resentment, grief, sorrow, anxiety, self-loathing and resentment."

That concept absolutely must *resonate* within you if you ever want to completely reclaim your life, your health, and lose the weight. Let's repeat, those negative emotions take up an actual physical residence within the bio-electric pathways, tissues, organs, and cells within your body, *there is no separation,* and you must find the solace, the harmony, the grace, the mercy, the forgiveness, the love, and an absolute peace that passes all understanding if you ever want to be truly healthy on all levels. One single negative thought begins to create a cascade reaction of elevated cortisol, norepinephrine, and all sorts of compensatory stress molecules in the body that are downright *corrosive* when they remain elevated in a sustained, unhealthy fashion. All the negative emotions you've swallowed and held on to over the years *no longer serve you,* and it is time to let them go.

Take a moment to digest that, let it sink into the core of your being, stop suppressing those negative emotions, feel them fully for a few moments, let out a good cry if you have to, thank them for the lessons they've taught you, and then begin to *let them go*.

Take a few minutes if you need them but willing to make that *decision* to actively move forward...

When you are ready to truly begin the next chapter of your life (and close the last one), I want you to be open to an entirely new concept and paradigm...a new way of thinking altogether. All the time you've spent here on this planet, you've been busy convincing yourself that you've had this huge void in your life, that you've been incomplete, that you somehow weren't good enough, or perhaps that you were underserving or unworthy of love or happiness. (And perhaps you've tried to self-medicate some of those painful or negative emotions with low-quality/high quantity food, alcohol, and other self-destructive behaviors). If that's the case, I want you to admit that to yourself right now. Be completely honest about it with yourself. If I'm honest I'm going to admit that right along with you.

We'll take a few more minutes if you need them...

Now, be open to the idea...that you were *always* good enough, you were *always smart* enough, you were *always* whole, and you were *always* deserving of **love and happiness and joy**. You really *are deserving of* all those things!

If you are physically able to, I want you to stand up from the couch or wherever you're sitting right now, and repeat that out loud at least three times loudly:

> "I was _always_ good enough, I was _always_ smart enough, I
> was _always_ whole inside, I was _always_ deserving of love
> and happiness and peace and joy, and I _deserve_ the very
> best that life has to offer!"

149

If you said that out loud and you meant it, you've begun to change your belief system.

Take a full deep breath in through your nose right now, hold it for 4 seconds, and breathe it out through your mouth slowly over four or five seconds.... as your belief system begins to change, you can shift your perspective and your focus to a positive one. If you are doing that, then *as we speak* right now, the stress hormone cortisol is beginning to lower within you...slowly, but surely. Your adrenals are beginning to calm, and your histamines, cytokines, C-reactive protein, homocysteine, and other inflammation markers are beginning to lessen, lower, and cool off *as you read this*. That's how powerful the mind/body/spirit connection is, it begins to work in real time. Set your intention to make this change permanent, and maintenance it on a daily basis, *and it will be so.*

If you're still reading I'm assuming you've come back to this chapter at some later point after removing those *distractors*, emotional blocks, and belief systems, and now you're ready to rock and roll. Awesome! As I previously mentioned, everyone (due to the sheer level of bio-diversity within the human species) needs to find what works for them. But here are a few powerful/helpful modalities that you can try out to see if they benefit you:

- **Master Cleanse and Colon Hydrotherapy, Celery Juice and Probiotics**—This really is square one. Buy the $2.99 Kindle-edition copy of the book (or splurge and get the paperback for $6.00) *The Master Cleanser*, find a good colon hydro-therapist, blend up 6 to 8 sticks of organic celery daily, and get some heavy duty probiotics going (Primal Defense Ultra and ProbioMax DF--100 billion are both great ones). The first 15 pounds (7kg) of weight loss are easy here.

- **Intermittent Fasting/Fasting One Day a Week**—Work up to this one, it can be difficult at first, but it can help completely reset your insulin resistance and glucose metabolism over time.

- **Ketosis/Ketogenic Diets**—Helpful option for some. Should be done under the supervision of a physician. Don't do the 'Atkins' version where you can eat 5lbs of bacon but not a single apple. Keto powder supplements that more easily induce ketosis may be appropriate jump starters (very short term) for some patients, but not everyone. Keto/Paleo *should be done short term, not long term or permanently.* The body is not meant to permanently have to deal with large amounts of saturated animal fats on a never-ending basis.

- **Anti-Histamine Therapy**—If you've suddenly removed a lot of the distractors (from the large list earlier in this article, you might be dealing with a mild type of a 'herxheimer' or detox reaction to where you feel lots of mucous build up, runny nose, allergy symptoms, etc. We try to use pharmaceuticals as sparingly as possible, but if you are experiencing these symptoms, consider alternating Zyrtec and Allegra every 12 hours, **but only for a total of 3 days**. This kind of mini-anti-histamine therapy is an old trick a several old-school doctors use to calm down the runaway histamine response, which results in better body homeostasis and dropping a few pounds of excess weight.

- **Pescatarian Diet**—This is the one I personally have had the most success on, but it is also specific to my body type. It's basically vegetarian, but includes things like organic egg whites, and quality fish protein (mahi-mahi, wild salmon, swordfish, Chilean Sea Bass), etc. It's also heavy on good fats from organic avocadoes and hummus. If I occasionally have red meat, I'll save it for special occasions at a steak restaurant where it's going to be grass-fed, aged kobe or wagyu beef. Stay away from the nitrate-filled red meat and the arsenic-filled blue chicken at Walmart at all costs. Watch the documentaries *"Supersize Me" and "What the Health is Going On?"* (although take that latter 'documentary' with a grain of salt, you don't have to completely drink the propaganda kool-aid and cut out meat altogether, just keep it to grass fed/free range-organic when you do eat it.)

- **Hydration**—Start the day with a class of lemon water and an electrolyte packet, reference the hydration chapter of this book, this is key for any weight loss program.

- **Apple Cider Vinegar and/or Digestive Enzyme** after any heavy meal. Drastically improves digestion, nutrient uptake, and absorption

- **L-Carnitine**—very important for the metabolism for fat. Can be taken supplementally

- **Hot Yoga**—simply amazing, spiritual and physical workout at the same time

- **Power Plate PRO5 sessions**—one of the hardest workouts you'll ever have and it is probably the best core workout on the planet

- **HCG Diet/Injections**—this should be limited to one cycle per year. Very powerful in tandem with right dietary constraints.

- **De Vany Training**—Dr. Arthur De Vany came up with a concept called 'Evolutionary Fitness.' It works for a lot of people and I'm including an article on it at the end of this chapter (13a).

- **Cool Sculpting**— can be safely used under the guidance of a licensed medical practitioner at the end of a weight loss program to help address stubborn areas of fat retention.

These are but a handful of options, there are many more available methods out there to achieve your fitness and health goals. Don't believe any 'gurus' who claim to have the answers or the magic bullet. No one has all the answers, I certainly don't. What I can offer you is a very *solid* starting point, which is to clear out any negative belief systems or old emotional traumas that are preventing you from living your best life/achieving your goals, and then go out and find what works best *for you.*

I also want to take a few paragraphs here and insist that if you want to have any reasonable chance of losing fat/being healthy, it is imperative to remove anything with the word '*diet*' in it, specifically diet sodas. Diet sodas are intentionally engineered and designed in a lab to make you fat. The artificial sweeteners trick your brain into thinking that the body is intaking nutrients and calories that it can use for important metabolic processes, only for it to find itself in a severe deficit later. This triggers a cascade metabolic 'panic' which drives a vicious, never-ending cycle of over-consumption. That is just for starters. The health side effects not just correlated with, but directly associated with, the carcinogenic ingredients in diets sodas are numerous and severe:

- **Aspartame**—artificial sweetener which was twice banned by the FDA (due to concerns over brain tumors in test rats) before the then head of the FDA was fired in 1981 and replaced by an administrative appointee (Dr. Arthur Hayes) who held multiple conflicts of interest, had no previous experience with food additives, and subsequently left his post at the FDA due to being exposed for accepting corporate gifts for political favors. Right before leaving the post, Dr. Hayes managed to override the existing FDA ban under shady circumstances. For the whole story on how Donald Rumsfeld and Dr. Hayes managed to propagate the use of this known carcinogen and excitotoxin, read here:

  https://www.huffingtonpost.com/robbie-gennet/donald-rumsfeld-and-the-s_b_805581.html

  https://www.thankyourbody.com/is-aspartame-dangerous/

https://www.collective-evolution.com/2013/01/19/the-shocking-story-of-how-aspartame-became-legal/

https://grist.files.wordpress.com/2011/02/apm_admini stered_in_feed_am.j.ind.med_2010.pdf

So how dangerous is aspartame? Consider this...aspartame single-handedly accounts for over 75 percent of the adverse reactions to food additives reported to the FDA. Here are just *some* of the different documented symptoms listed in the report as being caused by aspartame:

- Headaches/migraines
- Dizziness/Dehydration
- Seizures
- Nausea
- Numbness
- Muscle spasms
- Weight gain
- Rashes
- Depression
- Fatigue
- Irritability
- Tachycardia
- Insomnia
- Vision Problems
- Heart palpitations
- Breathing difficulties
- Anxiety attacks
- Slurred speech
- Loss of taste
- Vertigo
- Joint pain
- Kidney Stones
- Poor Concentration
- Hypertension

According to researchers and experts who have studied the dangerous effects of aspartame, the following chronic illnesses can be worsened or even triggered by aspartame:

- Brain tumors
- Multiple sclerosis
- Epilepsy
- Chronic fatigue syndrome
- Parkinson's disease
- Alzheimer's
- Lymphoma
- Fibromyalgia
- Birth defects
- Leukemia
- Non-Hodgkin's Lymphoma
- Bone Density Loss
- Metabolic Syndrome

As an anecdotal/personal aside, I cannot begin to tell you just how many people we've had come through the clinic who have been diagnosed with 'Fibromyalgia.' Better than 90% of them are diet Coke addicts. It's gotten to the point where I don't ask Fibromyalgia patients "Do you drink diet soda?". I instead ask them "How many diet Cokes do you drink a day?" They look at me in shock and disbelief... "How did you even know I drink diet Coke?" they ask. I then begin to go through this information you have before you. I tell them that we are happy to treat them for their symptoms, but I pro-offer that perhaps before they waste our time and their money, that they should set the intention to discontinue ingesting one of the most toxic substances known to man. This is often easier said than done (it is, at times, easier to get people off heroin than it is diet Coke because of the withdrawal symptoms). But for the patients who kick the habit, the results are often nothing short of miraculous—and that's before we even begin treatment. Over the years I've had no less than 40 patients who come back 6 weeks after their initial consult, completely overjoyed that they've been 'cured' of Fibromyalgia...which of course is utterly ridiculous. The only thing they were 'cured' of is pouring a poisonous substance into their bodies.

- **Phenylalanine—** Phenylalanine can increase a chemical in the body called tyramine. Large amounts of tyramine can cause high blood pressure. DL-phenylalanine can cause symptoms of anxiety, jitteriness, and hyperactivity in children. Doses higher than 5,000 mg a day may be toxic and can cause nerve damage. High quantities of DL-phenylalanine may cause mild side effects such as nausea, heartburn, and headaches. Phenylalanine can cause mental retardation, brain damage, seizures and other problems in people with PKU.

- **Bisphenol A—**Bisphenol A is found in the hard-plastic bottles and aluminum cans many people use every day. It can imitate the body's hormones as a xenoestrogen, and it can interfere with the production, secretion, transport, action, function, and elimination of natural hormones. BPA can behave in a similar way to estrogen and other hormones in the human body. BPA exhibits toxic, endocrine, mutagenic, and carcinogenic effect in living organisms. BPA elevates risk of obesity, diabetes, and heart disease in humans.

- **Caramel Color IV—**prepared by the controlled heat treatment of carbohydrates with ammonium-containing and sulfite-containing compounds. Other than a dark color, this chemical reaction also yields a carcinogenic chemical called '4-methylimidazole.' Studies on rats/mice fed show significant carcinogenic effects. The evidence is so strong that the state of California added this chemical to the list of "chemicals known to the state to cause cancer." In a can of diet Coke, there are 130mcg of CC4...which is *eight times* *higher* than California's danger threshold. That's for one can. How much worse is it when people are drinking 8 to 10 cans a day of this garbage?

Friends, diet sodas are unequivocally one of the single most toxic things you can conceivably put in your body. Avoid these like the *plague*. According to a study from the University of Miami, regularly drinking diet soda can significantly elevate a risk of a heart attack/coronary event. For pregnant women, just one diet soda a day was associated with a 38 percent risk of preterm delivery. Four diet sodas a day increased the risk by **78 percent**. One study published in the journal General Dentistry showed that the mouth of a habitual diet soda drinker can be just as eroded as a crystal meth user. A study from Boston University showed diet soda drinkers *are up to three times more likely to develop Alzheimer's/dementia or suffer from a stroke* than non-diet soda drinkers. Your liver converts the aspartame from diet soda into methanol, and then into *formaldehyde,* a very well-known carcinogen. I cannot overstate how poisonous, carcinogenic, and deadly these products are. If you value your health, your neurological and cognitive function, and your quality of life whatsoever, don't touch these with a ten-foot pole.

CHAPTER 14A
DIET AND FITNESS ARTICLE
(Art De Vany)

How I Practice Evolutionary Fitness

By Art De Vany
reprinted with permission

Evolutionary Fitness (EF) is the original name that Arthur (Art) De Vany gave to his style of exercise and diet. EF is a way of exercise that uses the body in the manner that our hunter-gatherer ancestors did - which happens to build strength, speed, and a ripped physique.

I practice EF these days since it's...
1. An easy way to stay ripped and get strong, and
2. I understand and respect the science underlying it.

First, What Is Evolutionary Fitness?

EF is a style of exercise designed to work with our genes to bring out peak strength and ability. This will also make us look like the second to last guy in the picture on the next page, and not like chubby at the end.

Our hunter-gatherer ancestors were strong, fast, and didn't have the chronic health problems associated with a 'modern' or 'western' lifestyle and diet. The few tribes that have survived to the present day show these characteristics. EF allows you to emulate the good points of their lifestyle — yet avoid those pesky ice ages.

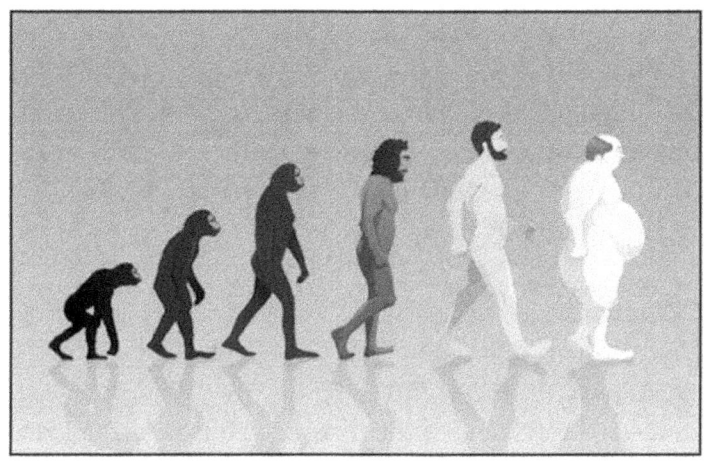

Major Components of Evolutionary Fitness
- Intermittent Fasting (IF)
- Fasted Training
- Intermittent, Brief (But Intense) Weight Training Workouts
- No Post-Workout Drink or Meal
- Eccentrics/Negatives
- Let It Happen

These are the most important components in evolutionary fitness. There are many other finer points, but the six ideas listed above are the essentials.

Another important component is integrating evolutionary fitness with the paleo diet. They were made to be done together and doing one without the other just doesn't give you the same results.

Intermittent Fasting

I've written at lot about intermittent fasting, and the way it's used in EF is very doable. If you're trying to lose weight, skip dinner once a week so you have a mini-fast until breakfast.

Since you're already eating a paleo style diet (mostly vegetables and meat), you will probably be eating fewer calories. And that mini-fast once a week will also accelerate your fat loss.

The key is to avoid going chronically hungry. If you diet down, you're chronically decreasing your calories. This leads to diet relapses, binging, loss of lean body mass, and a host of bad things.

Eating a healthy paleo style diet with occasional periods of starvation is easier on your body. It's a more *sustainable* way of achieving a better body composition.

Fasted Training

Basically, workout when you're hungry. First thing in the morning? A great time to train!

Fasted weight lifting (or other exercise) burns fat, and also trains you not to rely on dietary sugar for your fuel. This will help you break the sugar-crash-sugar-crash cycle of eating that I see in so many people.

Also, there's some preliminary evidence that working out in a fasted state puts more strain on your body and, hence, forces it to work harder to adapt after the workout. Martin Berkhan at LeanGains.com advocates working out in a fasted state too, which helps him stay lean and build muscle.

Intermittent, Brief & Intense Weight Training Workouts

There's more and more evidence to show that brief, intense weight training workouts produce dramatic results for increasing muscle mass and strength. This is used in high intensity interval (HIIT) training, and Doug McGuff advocates this approach in his *Body By Science* book and workout routines (a doctor and exercise expert who I really admire).

Think of exercise like walking. You walk around all day, but that doesn't build strength. It's the hardest things you do (walking up the stairs, squats, jumping, etc.) that actually increase your strength.

Art backs a 15-8-4 sequence for his workouts.[1] 15 Reps with a light weight, 8 with medium weight, and 4 at your max weight. All done with no rests in between, and never going to failure.

So go to the gym, do a few really hard things, and get out.

No Post-Workout Drink or Meal

No post workout recovery meal. Why? Well...

For starters, do you think your ancestors did something really difficult and then had a sugary-protein shake? No.

From a scientific standpoint, brief workouts release lots of growth hormone. And insulin triggered by a sugary workout drink *can* push those levels of growth hormone right down again.

A sugary post-workout drink doesn't always tank your growth hormone - there are studies going both ways. And bodybuilders drink post-workout protein shakes religiously and *do* put on muscle. Just keep in mind that EF works primarily to strengthen your muscles, not to put on lots more muscle mass.

Eccentrics/Negatives

Negatives (also called eccentrics) are when you lower a weight that you don't have the strength to lift (yet). You just do the negative part of the movement.

Using negatives, you can work with a lot more weight than you can with conventional lifting. Like, 40% more!

Also, there is some evidence that doing negatives causes increased expression of your fast twitch type two muscle fiber.[2] That's the stuff that helps you move forcefully at lightning speed.

Negatives are also very safe, since you're just lowering the weight. You don't have the speed and accompanying lack of control, which keeps you from hurting yourself.

Let It Happen

Art brings a wonderful sense of Zen into his ideas about evolutionary fitness. He teaches that you shouldn't be overly focused on reps, sets, or necessarily making progress at every workout.

While that viewpoint might not appeal to you if you are particularly young and crazy, it's a great mentality to bring to your training long-term. It will keep you training for the fun of it.

How I Do Evolutionary Fitness

I do evolutionary fitness because it's relatively simple, and there's lots of evidence for it. On workout days I'll usually skip breakfast and just workout in the morning, and then go lifting in the afternoon or early evening when I get really hungry.

Then I go home and have a good meal! No shakes, but real cooking - which sometimes takes a bit of time. I don't worry about eating within a time window after my workout.

I put negatives at the end of my weight lifting sets and do a brief workout. And if I didn't make progress, I get some rest and come back in a few days or a week. I know I'll get stronger if I just stick with it, and I give it my all when I'm training.

I also do some sprints up a hill near my home. Sprint up, walk down several times, and then switch it up and sprint down to train myself to go faster.

It's a more relaxed mentality to bring to your weight training and exercise. It makes your life more enjoyable. Try it.

References:

1. De Vany, Arthur. 2011. The New Evolution Diet: What Our Paleolithic Ancestors Can Teach Us About Weight Loss, Fitness, And Aging. Emmaus, Pa: Rodale. Pp. 94.

2. Tannerstedt et al. Maximal lengthening contractions induce different signaling responses in the type I and type II fibers of human skeletal muscle. Journal of Applied Physiology (2009) vol. 106 (4) pp. 1412-1418.

CHAPTER 15

GALLBLADDER HEALTH

The gallbladder is located just under the liver on the right side of the abdomen. Its primary function is to concentrate and act as a reservoir for bile, an enzyme that is produced by the liver and used in the breaking down of fats. When dietary fat is ingested, the hormone cholecystokinin is released, which signals the gallbladder to contract, dispensing bile (by way of the bile ducts) into the small intestine to perform its primary task as well as the secondary task of draining waste products from the liver into the duodenum.

An excessive or chronic overage of cholesterol, bile salts or bilirubin can lead to the formation of gallstones, which are hardened/crystalized pieces of bile. Symptoms can range from being completely asymptomatic to acute pain, nausea, dizziness, migraines, and vomiting, especially if a gallstone gets lodged in a bile duct.

Shockingly, the standard protocol to address this very common condition is to *cut out the organ*. Removing the gallbladder (cholecystectomy) is now considered a *routine procedure*. We should take great umbrage with that as healers. Granted, the procedure is significantly less invasive than it was 20 years ago (it's now done laparoscopically and is more or less an out-patient surgery), but that isn't the point, this still falls squarely in the "WTF?" category! We *need* that organ to perform a vital task, that is why it's there in the first place. There are no unnecessary or superfluous organs (not even the appendix, which we've addressed in the pro-biotic chapter). The travesty here is that, in all but the absolute severest of cases, gallstones can be easily and safely expelled via a gallbladder flush. Despite the fact that gallbladder cleanses/flushes have been referenced in mainstream medical journals since the late 1800's, most modern day surgeons are completely oblivious to the concept, and when asked, are dismissive of the cleanse as either being 1) a waste of time and ineffective, 2) of inconsequence because "you don't really need the gallbladder anyways, you might as well have it removed," or 3) that even if you remove the gallstones this time, "you'll just have more of them crop up over time." I have had countless patients come to me asking for a second opinion after hearing one of these 3 inappropriate and uninformed responses. To be fair and to clarify, I'll repeat that there certainly are some severe cases where the gallbladder needs to be removed due to extreme inflammation or outright organ failure, but percentage-wise, I would say it's somewhere in the neighborhood of 10 to 15% of the actual number of cholecys-tectomies performed. There are over *750,000* gallbladder removals performed annually in the United States, making it the most commonly performed elective abdominal procedure, ringing in at a cost of $6.2 billion dollars a year. This is quantitatively and qualitatively absurd and unacceptable. It is time the medical community radically reforms and re-establishes the proper approach for this easily treatable issue. So, that begs the question, what are our options? Glad you asked!

Prevention is the first line of defense. Having a healthier diet is a no brainer, but considering the average western diet and the resistance to change on that front, let's skip ahead:

1. Oral Pro-biotics and Digestive enzymes
These little miracle workers greatly aid in the digestive process, actively breaking down food with high fat content (as well as protein and carbohydrates) and easing the strain on the gallbladder from the start.

2. Bragg's Organic Apple Cider Vinegar w/ Mother
This stuff is worth its weight in gold and has too many benefits to list health-wise, but in this case, it aids at several stages of the digestive process and softens existing gallstones to help them process out. With regular (at least 3x a week) use, ACV goes a very long way towards maintaining optimal gallbladder health. 3) Most importantly, we have the gallbladder cleanse. The oldest and most well-known gallbladder cleanse is the Hulda Clark protocol. It has helped countless patients avoid unnecessary surgery and restore their organ to optimal function. I certainly don't endorse the majority of the often-bizarre teachings of Hulda Clark, but to her credit she was able to help a vast number of patients with gallbladder issues by crafting a very comprehensive gallbladder cleanse/flush. The only issue with her version of the protocol is the slight impracticality of it as it requires multiple days-worth of steps and preparation. We've created a condensed, yet equally safe and effective version of the cleanse that is a little bit more pragmatic and included it at the end of this chapter. Also, certain holistic physicians have modified the cleanse over the years to include the phosphoric acid component, known to help soften gallstones. We've integrated that step as well and feel like our version of the cleanse is the best of both worlds.

We believe that almost everyone can benefit from a periodic gallbladder flush, and that it is an excellent prophylactic measure to employ to prevent the development of serious gallbladder issues from ever occurring. I routinely do one gallbladder flush per season (4 times a year) and it never ceases to amaze us how great I feel afterwards. More specifically, there are certain demographics of people that are genetically pre-disposed to having a weaker functioning gallbladder, and it is all the more essential for those people to address it with diet and preventative maintenance. It's a well-known (albeit crassly and unofficially classified) group that falls into the highest risk category informally known as the 'Four F's': 1) Fat, 2) Female, 3) Fair (Caucasian), and 4) over-Forty. Women who fall into these parameters unfortunately are much more likely to be predisposed to the main symptoms associated with a low functioning gallbladder:

- Inflammation of gallbladder and bile ducts
- Muscular spasms and/or poor contraction of the gallbladder wall
- Stones forming in the liver, gallbladder, and/or bile ducts
- Obstruction to the free flow of bile.

Whether you fall into this category or not, a periodic gallbladder cleanse can be a great tool in your arsenal towards achieving and maintaining optimal health. As always, it is recommended that cleanses of this nature be done under the supervision of a licensed healthcare provider. It is *not* recommended that you attempt this cleanse if you are already in an emergency state of gallbladder blockage or failure. If that's the case, you should seek immediate medical attention at the hospital. Even if you've reached this set of circumstances, it may be possible for the surgeon to remove the obstruction/gallstone and not the whole organ, but that determination will be up to your healthcare provider at that point.

If you have already had your gallbladder removed, all is not lost! But it is imperative to eat a fat-restricted diet, and it is even more critical include supplemental digestive enzymes into your routine.

CHAPTER 15A

GALLBLADDER CLEANSE

Step 1: Drink one big swig/mouthful of organic ACV in the morning about 10am and another big swig about 2pm.

Step 1a: Eat lightly today, avoid fatty foods, and cut off solid foods by 2pm.

Step 2: Around 8pm, drink a generous helping—3 heaping table-spoonfuls of CALM (magnesium citrate) or Epsom Salt (magnesium sulfate) in hot water.

(Optional) Step 2a: Use the Bemer for 8 minutes on Program 1.

(Optional) Step 2b: Do an organic coffee enema for 15 minutes.

Step 3: About 10:00pm, pour 7 ounces of Organic Olive Oil into a glass, and squeeze either a large lemon or a small grapefruit's worth of juice into the glass as well...shake the mixture thoroughly and let it sit for about 5 minutes.

Step 4: Get a Coke or Pepsi or Dr. Pepper **classic/throwback**...the kind with the old school formula with real sugar and not HFCS.

Step 5: Relatively quickly, consume both the olive oil/lemon juice mixture as well as the Pepsi classic. You can alternate them as you drink both if this makes it easier.

Step 6: Immediately lay down in bed on your right side and try to go to sleep for the evening. You want to lay on your right side so that the concoction will pool in your liver/gallbladder and work its magic. You may experience mild waves of nausea, but generally nothing too severe.

Notes:

This is nowhere near as bad as it sounds. I dreaded it going in, but it ended up being only mildly unpleasant. The next morning, when you produce a bowel movement, be sure to check to see what type of stuff came out. If you see the little pea-sized green balls, those are gallstones. Sometimes the older stones that have been lodged in the bile ducts for a long time will be slightly larger and may be brown/black and look like little walnuts.

Over the next couple of days, you should see a marked improvement with respect to how you feel and your overall energy level. It is helpful to continue to drink the Bragg's ACV on a regular basis to continue the cleansing process and to maintain gallbladder support.

Brands I recommend for this cleanse:

- Olive Oil—Newman's Own (USDA organic)
- Apple Cider Vinegar—Bragg's (Organic w/ 'mother')
- Magnesium Citrate (CALM) or Magnesium Sulfate (EPSOM salt)
- Coke/Pepsi/Dr.Pepper **classic only**. This is simply for the phosphoric acid which it contains, you do not want to get the regular version as these contain high fructose corn syrup and other chemicals
- Grapefruit—organic. However, if you take any maintenance medications (i.e. blood pressure, diabetic, anti-histamines blood thinners, etc), then use organic lemon juice. (There is an enzyme in grapefruit—CYP3A4, which can influence blood serum concentrations of certain meds and cause adverse effects.)

CHAPTER 16

GERM THEORY vs TERRAIN THEORY

This is at core of why there still remains antagonism between holistic/integrative and allopathic medicine… Bechamp vs Pasteur, one of the greatest debates of all time.

Holistic/Integrative medicine gives rise to the notion, that if we strengthen the body and give it all it needs, it is nigh invincible, and that germs/pathogens/microbes are nothing but opportunistic clean-up mechanisms that turn harmful once we are already in a compromised state. The mechanism is internal. Allopathic medicine believes that harmful germs are everywhere, and therefore we must sterilize and eradicate all harmful pathogens to truly be safe. It turns the mechanism and responsibility to the external as opposed to the internal. Let's see two quick articles on Pasteur and his contemporaries before we draw a conclusion.

Pasteur vs. Bechamp: An Alternative View of Infectious Disease

(Borrowed with permission from Marone Family Wellness)

> "Le microbe n'est rien, le terrain est tout." (The microbe is nothing; the terrain is everything) –The last words of Louis Pasteur (Father of the "Germ Theory" of disease)

Pasteurization, named after scientist Louis Pasteur who developed it, involves heating raw milk to very high temperatures in order to kill the germs and bacteria inside the milk and prevent infections. The idea is that "germs are bad" and that they are the cause of disease and ill health. Following that assumption, it makes sense that "killing germs" would be the solution to both treating and preventing states of disease. This is the basic concept—that germs (virus, bacteria, etc.) are the cause of illness—upon which Western medicine is based.

But there is a fascinating history behind both the "germ theory" of disease as well as its controversial proponent...Louis Pasteur. I invite you to do your own research by Googling "Pasteur vs. Bechamp" to see the many sources of information on this controversy. Meanwhile I will try to summarize our thoughts on this issue and how it relates to patients who come to us with illness related to chronic infections.

In 19th century France, while Pasteur was advocating the notion of germs as the cause of disease, another French scientist named Antoine Bechamp advocated a conflicting theory known as the "cellular theory" of disease.

Bechamp's cellular theory is almost completely opposite to that of Pasteur's. Bechamp noted that these germs that Pasteur was so terrified of were opportunistic in nature. They were everywhere and even existed inside of us in a symbiotic relationship. Bechamp noticed in his research that it was only when the tissue of the host became damaged or compromised that these germs began to manifest as a prevailing symptom (not cause) of disease.

To prevent illness, Bechamp advocated not the killing of germs but the cultivation of health through diet, hygiene, and healthy lifestyle practices such as fresh air and exercise. The idea is that if the person has a strong immune system and good tissue quality (or "terrain" as Bechamp called it), the germs will not manifest in the person, and they will have good health. It is only when their health starts to decline (due to personal neglect and poor lifestyle choices) that they become victim to infections.

You can see this when a group of people go hiking in the woods. It often seems that the mosquitoes attack only one or two people out of the group. And as it turns out, it's always the same person that always gets attacked by the mosquitoes. This person is usually the one who always catches the latest flu and has the weakest immune system. This is because these germs (including insects) are opportunistic in nature and only attack the weak.

To treat illness, Bechamp's cellular theory also applied. Bechamp was less concerned with killing the infection and focused more on restoring the health of the patient's body through healthy lifestyle choices. Bechamp saw the infection as a **footnote** to the state of illness and not the primary cause. As the person restored health through diet, hygiene, and detoxification the infection went away on its own–without needing measures to kill it.

Pasteur and Bechamp had a long and often bitter rivalry regarding who was right about the true cause of illness. Ultimately Pasteur's ideas were accepted by society and Bechamp was pretty much forgotten. The practice of Western medicine is based on Pasteur's germ phobia which gives rise to the use of vaccinations, antibiotics, and other anti-microbials.

The irony is that towards the end of his life, Pasteur renounced the germ theory and admitted that Bechamp was right all along. In the 1920's medical historians also discovered that most of Pasteur's theories were plagiarized from Bechamp's early research work.

At Marone Family Wellness, we make recommendations to patients analyzed with infectious illness using the guidelines set forth by Antoine Bechamp:

"Treat the patient, not the infection."

We do this through our threefold approach of detoxification, nutritional healing, and restoring internal communication through chiropractic.

We feel that Bechamp was indeed right when he said that as health returns to the patient, the germs and infections leave on their own and do not come back unless health becomes compromised again. We have found this approach to be very satisfying in terms of results for the patient.

We feel that it is a mistake to try to kill the infection directly rather than searching for the cause as to why that person's immune system did not handle the infection on its own. Sadly, Pasteur's approach of killing germs is used by a large number of so-called "natural" healers who use large amounts of anti-microbial herbs in the same philosophical fashion as antibiotics. We feel that if all you do is kill the infection without addressing the dysfunction in the patient's immune system (which allowed the infection to manifest in the first place), the patient will simply become sick again at a later date.

Another problem with this approach is that in chronic infections you almost never see just one type of infection. When a person's immune function becomes compromised, one infection such as a bacterium will open the door to other infections such as viruses, parasites, and fungi. It's like when one burglar enters your home and holds the door open for his friends to come in. When this occurs, as it does in almost all immuno-compromised patients, focusing on treating the infection directly becomes a never-ending nightmare. Once one bug is gone, the next one appears. However, if you focus on treating the body's self-defense mechanism against infections (immune function), the body will handle the infections on its own, as it should have in the first place. We hope you understand how big of a difference in approach it is to treat the patient's immune system and not the infection. Treat the cause of the infectious illness, the underlying dysfunction of the host's immunity, and the infection will leave on its own as the health of the patient's body returns.

> **Disclaimer:** Regarding the controversial topic of vaccinations and antibiotics...we at Marone Family Wellness take a completely neutral stance on the topic. We neither advocate nor discourage their use and leave that

up to the patient to decide. We do this mainly due to legal reasons being that it is against the law for us to advocate one position vs. another. We only ask that you become as educated on this topic as possible and make your own informed decision. We will respect your decision either way.

—Marone Family Wellness

The Causes of Disease: The Great Debate

Ralph Metzner (ralphmetznerblog.com)
Reprinted with permission

Two giants of scientific medicine in the 19th century, both French, propounded radically different paradigms for the understanding and treatment of disease, that are still relevant today.

Louis Pasteur (1822-1895), chemist and microbiologist, put forward the germ theory, according to which diseases are caused by infectious microbes, that impair the functioning and structures of different organ systems. This paradigm is the basis for the use of antibiotics to destroy these invasive microbes and vaccines with low doses of the microbe to challenge the body's immune defenses and thereby prevent systemic infection.

Pasteur's contemporary and friend, the physiologist Claude Bernard (1813-1878), argued instead for the importance of balance in the body's internal environment – what he called le milieu intérieur. "The constancy of the interior environment is the condition for a free and independent life." Bernard thought that the body becomes susceptible to infectious agents only if the internal balance – or homeostasis as we now call it – is disturbed. After all, there are billions of microbes and bacteria inhabiting our guts, our blood, our whole body. Why do we sometimes sicken from them, sometimes not? When a bacterial or viral agent is "going around," as we say, why do some people sicken and others remain healthy?

There is an apocryphal story that Pasteur renounced his germ theory on his death-bed, saying that "Bernard is right. The microbe is nothing. The environment is everything." The renowned 20th century French-American microbiologist René Dubos (1901-1982) agreed with Bernard's principle: "Most microbial diseases are caused by organisms present in the body of a normal individual. They become the cause of disease when a disturbance arises which upsets the equilibrium of the body."

Today, Pasteur's germ theory of disease provides the rationale for the pharmaceutical industry's billions of dollars research and sales programs for ever more potent anti-bacterial and anti-viral drugs, the use of these antibiotics as a feed-additive in the disease-prone, overcrowded environments of industrial farming – with the predictable consequence that bacterial evolution is out-stripping the discovery rate of effective antidotes.

The Bernard/Dubos theory that health and resilience is a function of homeostatic balance in the internal environment is reflected in the growing influence of the ancient medical systems of India and China, as well as the **field of functional and integrative medicine.**

In all these approaches, the maintenance of health and prevention of disease involves conscious attention given to factors of life-style, environment, nutrition, exercise and recreation, as well as psychological well-being and spiritual practice.

Dr. Grisanti's Comments: It is of utmost importance to be grateful for the wonderful discovery of the works of Louis Pasteur. Infectious diseases that were once lethal can now be effectively treated thanks to Louis Pasteur. Unfortunately, his theory of acute disease management has not been fruitful in the treatment of many chronic diseases. Our present medical system still looks for the "one" treatment for many debilitating diseases like diabetes, auto-immune disease, cancer and cardiovascular disease. We constantly see a group of people rallying around the "CURE" for XYZ disease. We are asked for donations to fund a "CURE" for XYZ diseases.

GERM THEORY VS TERRAIN THEORY

Again, this is in line with the faulty theory of Louis Pasteur as it relates to chronic, long-standing health issues. Instead we need to embrace the workings of Claude Bernard. He was absolutely correct in stating we need to spend more of our time in fixing the balance in the body's internal environment. That is the focus of functional medicine. Functional medicine practitioners are passionate in discovering what has gone wrong with the body's internal environment and provide solutions to improve it. The results are amazing with many long-standing health problems resolved.

Remember as stated above, Louis Pasteur recognized the truth behind the workings of Claude Bernard when on his deathbed stated, "Bernard is right. The microbe is nothing. The environment is everything.."

Where do you stand? Are you still looking for the one drug that is going to "CURE" your disease or do you understand that fixing the internal environment of your sick body just may be the solution all along. Investigate functional medicine. It just may be the answer you have been looking for.

The information on this website is not intended to replace a one-on-one relationship with a qualified health care professional and is not intended as medical advice. It is intended as a sharing of knowledge and information from the research and experience of Dr. Grisanti and his functional medicine community. Dr. Grisanti encourages you to make your own health care decisions based upon your research and in partnership with a qualified health care professional. Visit www.FunctionalMedicineUniversity.com for more information on our training in functional medicine. Look for practitioners who have successfully completed the Functional Medicine University's Certification Program (CFMP) www.functionalmedicinedoctors.com. This content may be copied in full, with copyright, contact, creation and information intact, without specific permission, when used only in a not-for-profit format. If any other use is desired, permission in writing from Dr. Grisanti is required.

Conclusion

It is the hope that the reader can see that the answer is fairly obvious; the truth is somewhere in the middle. When one supercharges the immune system, achieves optimal health, and eliminates distractors, the body (i.e. the *terrain*) becomes *almost* invincible, and is certainly capable of holding its own when it comes to duking it out against whatever comes its way. As practitioners, we need to do our best to treat the whole patient, not just the symptoms, and moreover make sure the patient knowns how to treat themselves. But there are times when we must invoke prophylactic or reactive measures to defend against powerful micro-organisms, most notably foreign ones that our immune systems are naïve against and have no pre-developed immunity for.

A key example of this is when the Native Americans had their populations absolutely decimated when European settlers brought epidemics with them like scarlet fever, smallpox, influenza, and bubonic plague.

The most productive method is always to join together our collective strengths, *objectively*, and without conflicts of interests. In doing so weed out our respective weaknesses. We are on the same team with the same goal, and now more than ever, the world needs a new paradigm of *adaptive* healing and true synergy.

The same holds true on the heavily fought battles on controversial topics like vaccines:

The concept of **immunization** is quite scientifically sound. It has been around for over *6,000 years* going back to Druidic medicine, perhaps longer. The current *administration route* of 'vaccination' is absolutely draconian and rife with deleterious side effects. Fifty years from today, we will look back on the year 2017 and think, how quaint and foolish we were back then, putting aluminum and mercury and ethylene glycol (anti-freeze) and nagalase into the vaccines and directly into people's bloodstreams! It is no different than us now looking back at the 18th century and laughing at bloodletting for the flu, or chuckling to ourselves about how doctor's in the 1930's used to recommend specific brands of cigarettes. ("Four out of five doctors recommend this brand of cigarette, it soothes the throat! Not a cough in the car!" proclaimed road-side billboards.) If you really want to see some draconian humor, do a google search on how Dr. Harvey Kellogg invented the well-known cereal Kellogg's Corn Flakes to stop masturbation and prevent teenage boys from committing the 'deadly sin' of touching themselves. (I'm not making that up, that actually happened, it's in the history books and on the Wikipedia page. He also advocated forms of genital mutilation in the name of 'chastity' and 'purity.' That part is not funny, that's quite scary really.) But back then, stuff like that was the 'accepted medical science' of the day. People actually thought like this. How foolish are we to think that we aren't just as susceptible to newer version of the same folly? Just because we have better technology now doesn't mean we don't fall victim to the same human nature, tendencies, and inability to admit our own mistakes. Let's put an end to this vicious cycle, raise our collective consciousness, collectively call for a new era in medicine that truly heals, and stop history from repeating itself once and for all.

CHAPTER 17

HEMOCHROMATOSIS

Staying within the realm of blood/iron for a moment, we will briefly touch on what lies at the complete opposite end of the spectrum from anemia. **Hemochromatosis** is the condition of having too *much* iron accumulating in the blood. This is often a genetic condition, which can present at any point in life. However, it is not very well known that it can also be caused by having a 'backed-up' liver. This typically occurs when the liver becomes over-burdened with toxins and/or pharmaceutical drugs, specifically opioid narcotics. The excess iron causes the already-taxed liver to get inflamed and parts of the phase 2 detoxification pathway (most notably the sulfation pathway) begin to break down and stop working properly. In English that means that the liver is unable to perform its primary function effectively, which is to eliminate toxins from the body. Liver enzymes then become elevated and the patient begins to suffer from the early symptoms of chronic fatigue and joint pain, followed by irregular heart beat/flutters, loss of libido, brain fog, etc. Eventually, this condition can cause cancer and/or other life threatening conditions. Fortunately, there is a relatively easy fix in the short term, but we integrative folks like to use the two-step method to return the patient to optimal health in the long term.

The standard clinical solution is to do **Therapeutic Phlebotomy**, taking a full unit (500cc) of blood from the patient. This helps to immediately bring down the ferritin/iron concentration (about 30ng/ml for every unit taken). A licensed medical practitioner will need to evaluate how often a unit of blood can be taken, based on the urgency of the situation and the health of the patient. The patient's iron/ferritin levels are continually monitored every few weeks via an iron panel/labs, and the TP service is repeated until acceptable levels are reached. The reference range is anywhere from 30 to 400ng/ml for ferritin, however we like to get as close as possible to the optimal range of ~150ng/ml to 200ng/ml.

What we like to do on the integrative side of things is to administer **Intravenous Glutathione** concurrently with the phlebotomy service. We draw the 500cc of blood out, and then, without having to do a separate venipuncture, are able to push 1000mg (200mg/ml) of compounded glutathione into the bloodstream through the same access. Glutathione is the body's master detoxification molecule and it is also the body's master anti-oxidant molecule. (It's normally synthesized from the amino acids N-acetyl-cysteine, glycine, and glutamic acid and made in very small amounts in the liver.) The sulfur component in glutathione is key in helping clean up the liver and giving it the assistance it needs to return to optimal function. It's always amazing and very rewarding to see how quickly the patients typically begin to feel much better, as well as how succinctly their lab values—liver enzymes and iron/ferritin—begin to normalize. The results with glutathione occur much quicker than with the phlebotomy service alone, and with appropriate supporting therapies and modifications to lifestyle/diet/opiate usage, we often see the patient's liver function improve so much that their liver enzymes and iron levels remain stabilized at optimal levels and they no longer require regular phlebotomy services. When patients come in to see their general practitioners for their yearly routine check-up and bloodwork (CMP, CBC, Thyroid Panel, etc), an Iron Panel should also be included. It is extremely cheap to run and includes very important information that often gets overlooked.

For more basic information on this condition, visit the very informative website www.hemochromatosis.org.

CHAPTER 18

HIRUDOTHERAPY

All things ancient under the Sun become 'new' again in the cyclical nature of human history. One of the most powerful treatments known to man for millennia, which is now being rediscovered and re-explored, is hirudotherapy. At first glance, using leeches to treat patients in the context of modern medicine seems perhaps quaint or medieval. And yet the irony should not be lost on the reader that, out of the entire scope of this book, Hirudotherapy is one of the very few FDA approved treatments (for certain applications). Yes, you read that right. The PubMed studies are there (https://www.ncbi.nlm.nih.gov/pmc/articles/PMC5741396/), and there are actually approved allopathic uses for these little creatures. How fascinating! Leeches reached the height of their medicinal use around the 1850s, but in 2004 the FDA granted approval to a French firm seeking to market them as medical devices, and leeches began to return to the limelight. The approved uses include their ability to assist in healing skin grafts via restoring vascular circulation and removal of trapped/pooled blood just under the graft, as well as circumventing the need for amputation in certain instances by facilitating blood flow to wounded limb.

Let's move beyond allopathic recognition and talk about the rest of the powerful benefits that our little friends provide. There are well over 360 bioactive substances in leech saliva, most notably hyaluronidase (which affects the viscosity of interstitial fluid), lipase, antistasin, hirudin, serotonin, Factor Xa inhibitor, calin, acetylcholine, carboxypeptidase A, and many more. When released into the human bloodstream, these substances provide a myriad of benefits, often far outpacing standard pharmaceuticals in their efficacy. There are several sub-species of leeches, the ones most commonly used in medical practice are the standard medical leech (*Hirudo medicinalis*), and the very similar Hungarian leech (*Hirudo Verbana*). They are quite similar in genetic predisposition, appearance, and function, however, anecdotal evidence tends to indicate the Verbana as having slightly more potent qualities to it.

Known uses include (but are not limited to):
- Hypertension, Polycythemia
- Hepatic Disease (including Hepatitis)
- Certain Cancers (Skin, Breast, Lymphatic)
- Vascular and Cardiovascular diseases
- Degenerative Eye and Ear conditions
- Diabetes and Hypertension
- Prostate issues
- Insomnia and Migraines
- Parkinson's Symptoms
- Stroke Recovery
- Arthritis, Osteoarthritis, Tendonitis, R.A.,
- Alopecia
- Skin Grafts and Sport Injury Healing, Upper and Lower Back Pain
- Biliary Dyskinesia and other Gallbladder issues
- G.I. issues (gastritis duodenitis, pancreatitis, ulcers, IBS, colitis, hemorrhoids, motility disturbances, etc.)
- Varicose Veins, Thrombophlebitis

It is recommended that a licensed and trained practitioner performs Hirudotherapy, there are a few but clearly established contraindications (most notably patients with low blood pressure and pregnant women), but in the grand scope of healing, the amalgamation of benefits provided by these wondrous little phlebotomists is too substantial to ignore. When applied to the appropriate zone(s) of the body, leeches intelligently find the nearest reflex/pressure point and get to work. They latch on with a circular row of tiny teeth and (almost painlessly) begin to draw blood while simultaneously releasing their natural anesthetic and healing bio-active substances into the human host. In less than 30 minutes they will have engorged themselves to maximum capacity and will typically detach and fall off. As with most other 'medical devices,' they are to be used one time only on a single patient. A practitioner would not want to use a single leech on multiple patients for the same reason we don't reuse needles on multiple patients, it helps prevent the transmission of any blood-borne illnesses. The proper recommended procedure after they have been used on a patient is to humanely euthanize them with isopropyl alcohol and discard them with bio-medical waste. (As a personal aside, I have hard time from a bio-ethical perspective simply destroying a living creature who has just provided me with such an amazing healing service, so I release them into my 'used' aquarium, where they can live out their retirement in peace. Call me a softy!)

As with many modalities, the benefits of Hirudotherapy are aggregate, and with continued use we've found it to be a powerful tool in our arsenal with respect to the slowing, alleviating, and in certain cases, outright reversal of many common disease states. As we make technological and bio-pharmaceutical breakthroughs at the cutting edge of health care, we can still continue to use and benefit from this centuries' old and proven remedy under the broad scope of *adaptive* medicine.

Blood Viscosity and Hypertension

A specifically noteworthy group of patients that Hirudotherapy can benefit remarkably are those who suffer from chronic hypertension (high blood pressure) and/or high blood viscosity from polycythemia.

One of the primary substances released by the medical leeches during therapy is *hirudin*—clinically shown to be nearly *ten times* more effective than heparin at thinning blood, as well as providing multiple benefits that pharmaceutical blood thinners (Heparin, Coumadin) cannot. There are several co-factors and enzymes in leech saliva that can both permanently lower blood pressure (over the course of multiple treatments) as well as completely dissolve any thrombus (blood clot) in a patient's system, thus drastically reducing the risk of stroke. This is a much healthier alternative than the traditional daily regimen of aspirin, which we now know can damage kidneys, increase the risk of pancreatic cancer (Schernhammer 2004), and increase the risk of gastrointestinal bleeding or of a hemorrhagic (bleeding) stroke. By permanently lowering blood pressure, Hirudotherapy also has the potential to wholly remove the need for the traditional ace inhibitor, beta blocker, and calcium channel blocker classes of blood pressure medications, and by proxy their respective side effects.

As a side note for those who do not have access to, or do not wish to go the route of hirudotherapy to address high blood viscosity, thrombi (clots), or platelet aggregation, there is yet another readily available and viable preventative option that is superior to taking warfarin/coumadin or aspirin. That is to take between at least 400iu of *natural* vitamin E as part of your daily regimen. There are several conflicting studies and opinions on this topic, and the arguments concerning the use of Vitamin E for heart health have been ongoing for well over half a century. But most of those arguments and conflicting studies seem to always miss that the devil is once again *in the details*. The studies that seem to disprove the effectiveness of Vitamin E (and also tout its dangers) without fail only test the **synthetic** form of Vitamin E, which is *dl-alpha-tocopherol*. The studies that seem to prove the effectiveness and therapeutic value of Vitamin E (at high enough doses) exclusively use the **natural** form of Vitamin E, which is *d-alpha-tocopherol*. This little 'one-letter' detail on paper may seem trivial, but in a living organism, it makes all the difference in the world.

Anecdotally, I've had several patients who only come to our integrative clinic for 'adjunct therapy' (i.e. the occasional B12 shot or something minor), yet they are holistically minded in general. Meanwhile their hematologist has them on the toxic drug Coumadin for blood thinning purposes. Many of those patients have, of their own accord, simply switched to high-dose, practitioner-grade *natural* vitamin E, yet continue to have their hematologist monitor their partial thromboplastin time (PTT) and prothrombin time (PT). Based on the consistent results, the doctor simply thinks they are still on the pharmaceutical blood thinner and is none-the-wiser that they discontinued the drug months and sometimes years prior. (For the record, I do not advocate patients withholding information like this from any of their other healthcare providers, but this still serves as powerful demonstration of what can be achieved from taking a simple vitamin at the appropriate dose and in the appropriate (natural) form.)

CHAPTER 19

HOMEOPATHY

Ok here's one we can readily admit that most of us don't fully understand. At first glance it smells, looks, and tastes like snake oil, and I'm sure, as with all forms of medicine, that *some* of it is. It does not appear to be anywhere close to the 'functional' medicine that most of us practice as Integrative practitioners. But we also cannot fully discount the sheer number of people who swear by it and claim to get results and benefits from this type of therapy. It has absolutely no place in emergency or urgent medicine, and it is utterly challenging to quantify what is actually happening, if anything, when this type of treatment regimen is undertaken.

But we do know a few variables that we can plug in as part of our thought experiment so that over time we can make an intelligent decision on whether we need to integrate this sort of modality or not:

- Certain publications like www.homeopathyjournal.net seem to make a very solid case for scientific validation by carrying out and publishing their own version of "PubMed-style" studies to prove what they are doing has a measurable effect. That certainly carries more weight than listening to anecdotes from the hippy at the front desk of Mother Mary's Herbal Cauldron down the street.

- The placebo effect is an actual effect. In controlled, doubled blind studies, when you give a patient with arrhythmia a placebo/sugar pill, it can regulate the heart beat nearly 30%

of the time. That's just a glimpse of how powerful the mind is and how drastically it can affect biochemistry and other physiological processes.

- Homeopathy could potentially work very subtly on a quantum level. The famous "double slit" experiment taught in every Physics 101 class could explain how that works. (You can look up videos on Youtube on this experiment). Basically, the act of observing or expecting can influence an outcome or result. This is known as quantum entanglement, and also lends itself to extrapolating the probability that people who don't believe in homeopathy will most likely not receive benefit from it, whereas people who are open to it may potentially receive *some* benefit from it. Even if this was the case, it makes for a somewhat unstable model considering the fickle nature of the human mind, as well as the fact the homeopathy practitioner's *intent* could also influence the outcome, instead of just the substance he/she is prescribing.

- Another potentially influencing factor is how toxic someone is. If they are 'dense' with toxic residue, if they are severely injured, are suffering life threatening illness, or are overall in a significantly compromised state (mental, physical, or emotional), then they may not have the ability to be overtly influenced by such a subtle form of treatment, which has no more than a trace amount of any sort of active ingredient. Sometimes less is more, but sometimes more is more.

We cannot fully pass judgment on Homeopathy, and we can once again admit that most of us don't fully understand the precepts behind it. To me personally, even if it works, it feels kind of like 'playing in the kiddie pool' when we've got access to much more powerful, more effective options. But we've got to be wise enough to be ok with the fact that there is no reason to deny people their right to receive a benefit from it if they believe it's helping them.

CHAPTER 20

HORMONE REPLACEMENT THERAPY

To continue on in the same vein of endocrine therapy and support, we next address the sex hormones, how they affect our health and what we can do to address the decline of the optimal balance of sex hormones as we age.

Sex hormones are what potentiate the libido and reproductive process—we all know this, but they are vital for so much more. They play a large role in composing and sustaining our constitution, our drive, our energy levels, mood, immune system, cognitive function, homeostatic conditions like core body temperature, the ability to get restful sleep, as well as staving off the aging process and degenerative conditions like type II diabetes. Moreover, hormones in general are a key component in the generation of what we know as *life force*. They are a fundamental element of sustaining life from beginning to end. To give example, we now know (through recent discovery) that when a newborn is nursing from a mother, the chemoreceptors on the mother's nipples actively sample the baby's saliva in real time for illness. The mother's body then modulates the composition of the anti-bodies in the milk/colostrum to give the child the immunological support they need to withstand the illness since they haven't developed an immune system yet. The mother's body even makes different blends of breast milk depending upon whether the child is male or female! This is all done hormonally.

On the other end of the spectrum, thanks to hormone replacement therapy, age-related decline of the sex hormones—

testosterone, estrogen(s), progesterone, DHEA, pregnenolone, and androstenedione—is no longer the hindrance to quality of life it once was. We've got the ability to augment and replace what's lost and restore optimal levels. It now becomes a matter of 'good, better, best' with regard to how exactly we go about it. The intent of this chapter is to diagram how to reach the desired patient outcome while eliminating the oversights, pitfalls, and side effects of inadequate understanding or gross oversimplification of this process.

First item of business—diagnosing properly. Blood/Serum draws have been the gold standard for testing hormones for a very long time. But lately, there has been a raging debate as to whether saliva collection is now superior to blood collection when it comes to getting the most accurate hormonal measurements. The technology of saliva collection has advanced tremendously since it was first introduced in the 1980's, and it is now a valuable tool in our arsenal. Roughly 97% of steroid/sex hormones circulating in the bloodstream are bound to carrier proteins. Saliva contains the bioavailable 'unbound' portion of those hormones. Hence the theory is that reading the concentrations found in saliva better represents the levels of circulating free hormones.

The truth of the matter is that there are inherent strengths and weaknesses in both blood and saliva assays (and in some cases, urine assays). They are all highly valuable objective measurements. The best philosophy is the one that uses all available options. If we have a 50-year-old male as a new patient and he is interested in Testosterone replacement therapy, we are going draw a blood serum lab for Free/Total Testosterone, *and* we are going to have him to do a saliva collection for a Male Hormone Panel. Both are very affordable and we are able to take the amalgamated data from two types of assays and see how they inter-relate to each other. More importantly we are able to give the patient the exact solution that they need. Synergy is always the best method.

Second order of business—the absolute worst thing a practitioner can do when it comes to HRT is to *overcorrect*. Giving someone too much testosterone, estrogen, or progesterone is a good way to give them cancer. Overcorrecting with HRT is unequivocally worse than doing nothing at all and should be avoided at all costs. I cannot begin to describe how frequently we run hormone panels on patients (both male and female) who have been referred to us from primary care, and their hormone levels are through the roof! Family doctors often mean well but are often overburdened with patient load, are under-educated on HRT, and are quick to write a prescription based on symptomology alone. Not enough labs and monitoring are conducted, hormone levels get pushed to completely unnatural levels, and patients begin to suffer adverse reactions in a big way. Compounding the problem is that the prescriptions often prescribed are synthetic, i.e. a chemical clone of naturally occurring hormones like estrogen and testosterone. These pharmaceutical doppelgangers, such as Premarin and Androgel, produce nearly the same immediate hormonal expression as naturally occurring hormones do, but over time they are not very well tolerated by the body and produce many known negative side effects.

To quote a descriptive excerpt from *Myer's Medical Pharmacy*:

> Hormone treatments such as Premarin, Prempro and Cenestin are synthetic, i.e. they are **not** true hormones. Molecular differences between synthetic progestins and progesterone result in differences in their pharma-cological effects on breast tissue. Some of the pro-carcinogenic effects of synthetic progestins contrast with the anti-carcinogenic properties of progesterone, which result in disparate clinical effects on the risk of breast cancer. In other words, bio-identical hormones are associated with lower risks of breast cancer and cardiovascular disease, and are more efficacious than their synthetic and animal derived counterparts.

What this means is that a much better (here is the 'better' in 'good-better-best') option is the use of **Compounded** Bio-Identical

Hormone Replacement Therapy. The reason compounded bio-identicals are better than manufactured drugs are three-fold. Reason one is that the dosages are individually titrated and specifically dosed based on the need of the patient. Second is the ability to blend multiple ingredients into same topical cream, including precursors. A common example would be a custom Estrogen/Progesterone/DHEA/Test blend (assuming that the particular patient needed all four ingredients). Third is that they are much better tolerated long term, have better efficacy, and are *more* naturally sourced, even though they do have some processed and refined ingredients.

This brings us to our 'best' option, which is all but outright overlooked in modern medicine…and that is to stimulate the body to produce more of its own hormones, naturally. This is the 'best' option because it is the most natural, and it most notably does not shut off what remains of the body's production of its own hormones, which is what often occurs when exogenous hormones are introduced. The reader is encouraged to go to either Youtube or to MarsVenus.com and watch/listen to what Dr. John Gray (PhD), author of *Men are from Mars, Women are from Venus,* has to say in his videos on this topic. The videos are free to watch, and contain an absolute wealth of information on this topic, almost enough to fill a book in its own right. Adaptogenic herbs, the star of another chapter, are also included in some of his talks.

However, there is one specific issue Dr. Gray touches on that is important to mention here. Within the scope of endocrine function, I believe this is the single biggest disruption and threat to healthy endocrine function for everyone, but especially to males. This is the overtly toxic exposure we now experience with something called **XenoEstrogens**. Doctors, physicians, healers, ARNPs, D.O.M.s, biologists, medicine men, shamans, gurus, whoever you are, hear me now: Laser etch this word into your brains. This is **the** cause of the endocrine disease state of the future, and it's here now. We need to address it with due haste, and with a vengeance.

An average 40-year-old male today, in the year 2017, has the testosterone level of an average 70-year-old male in the 1980's.........not the 1890's mind you, the 1980's. That is an asymptotically steep curve in the wrong direction. What the *hell* happened? The emergence of and exposure to xeno-estrogens have begun a war path with a clear destination of destroying the adolescent male body's ability to properly develop during puberty and is crippling the ability of the adult male to sustain proper testosterone production. It's one of the reasons we are seeing a dramatic spike in gender confusion at a young age and little boys growing breast tissue. It's part of why both males and females, children and adults (even physically active ones) are storing fat at an exponentially higher rate than we ever have before. Excess estrogen(s), whether they are synthetic or not, signal fat storage and they also signal the brain to lower testosterone.

What exactly are xeno-estrogens and how do we stop them? (This time, I'm *really* glad you asked!)

Xeno-estrogens are synthetic chemicals that mimic estrogens when absorbed by the human body. They are now everywhere and in everything. They are in the pesticides we spray. They are the parabens in sunscreens and lotions we slather on. They are the phthalates and BPA/PCBs in the plastics we use that leach into our bottled water. They are in the flame-retardants on the couch you are probably sitting on at the moment. They are in the artificial ingredients and preservatives (that didn't exist 30 years ago) in the processed foods we feed our children. They are in the brand name detergents and chlorine-based cleaning agents we use. (Attached to the end of this chapter is a handy guide borrowed from the blog *womeninbalance.org* that has helpful tips on how to avoid or at least minimize further exposure to xeno-estrogens.)

But once we understand how to minimize exposure, how do we *undo* the damage/exposure we already have? Currently and thankfully, we are blessed with a couple of powerful tools at our disposal in the form of supplemental therapies that are able to help purge excess and xeno-estrogens from our systems. The TCM supplement **Myomin** (by Chi's Enterprise) is composed of three herbs (Astragalus membranaceus, Curcuma zeodaria, Cyperus rotundus), and they work in concert to cleanse and eliminate excess estrogens from the liver, as well as help balance the hormonal metabolic pathways for both men and women. Another supplement we have that can be used in tandem with Myomin is known as **DIM**. This is short for *Diindolylmethane*, a powerful compound derived from the digestion of indole-3-carbinol, which is found in cruciferous vegetables such as broccoli, kale, cabbage, and Brussel sprouts. (The product we carry at our clinic is "Dimmension3" by Xymogen, which is broccoli sourced.) DIM blocks estrogen metabolism a little higher up in the metabolic pathway than Myomin does, and together they are a one-two punch to address this issue over the course of a few months of daily usage. A third option, popular with both body-builders and with patients employing certain holistic cancer therapies, is **Calcium D Glucarate**, which specifically lowers estrogens and helps to facilitate certain components of body detoxification. As I mentioned in the first line of this book, I believe in what works, I don't believe in quackery or rogue pseudoscience. These supplements all have a longstanding record of being safe and effective. As a physician you have the ability to run labs before, during, and after supplementation on patients who have elevated estrogen levels. When you see those levels come down and normalize and the overall improvement in your patients' health, you'll be able to clearly surmise the safety and efficacy thereof. (Also, intravenous Glutathione and intravenous Alpha Lipoic Acid can assist in this liver clean-up process, but we will touch more on that in a later chapter.) To learn more about Myomin, I will again refer you to Dr. John Gray and his free 10-minute video available on Youtube and MarsVenus.com. (Full disclosure I have no vested interest in Myomin, Chi's Enterprise or Dr. John Gray or MarsVenus.com.)

To take this one step further—after we've brought the estrogen(s) down in males to an acceptable reference level and removed estrogenic side effects as a *distractor*, we can also assist the male body in naturally restoring the production more of their own testosterone. We do this with *practitioner grade* nutraceutical supplements like **Maca** and **Tongkat Ali**, which are adaptogenic herbs in their own right but also help stimulate the pituitary gland to signal the upregulation of testosterone production. We put an emphasis on the terms *practitioner grade* and *nutraceutical* because there is big difference on potency, safety, quality, and efficacy when it comes supplements of this nature. Practitioner grade means that you typically have to be an MD, a DO, a DC, or a DOM to carry these lines of supplements. The quality control is generally much more stringent, and the supplements are usually made in accordance with CGMP, which stands for "Current Good Manufacturing Practices," i.e. they are produced in an FDA approved facility under the strict guidelines laid forth by the FDA with regard to strength, quality, purity, proper processing of raw materials, etc. These nutraceutical supplements are often from an entirely different realm than the unregulated (and often junk quality) garden-variety supplements that you find at a local vitamin store which may bear the same name.

As a side note, I believe this is why many allopathic physicians often throw their hands up in dismissal at the concept of integrating supplements into their practice. With there being no baseline of information on the subject being taught in med school (which is a travesty), the knowledge hasn't been made ubiquitous, agreed upon, or readily available, nor has been the safety record, studies, or quality assurances that come with a practitioner grade product. But those times are over, all of those appropriations are at long last in place, and it is time for us to join the forces as health care providers in order to step out of the dark and practice true medicine.

DHEA

As one final note on testosterone and general hormonal support, we sometimes integrate the precursor or 'parent' hormone DHEA (when the labs indicate that it's necessary). Think of it as building block or a blank slate. It's at the very beginning of the hormonal pathway and the body can convert it into any sex hormone that it needs. Sometimes, if DHEA is insufficient, the body struggles to produce enough testosterone, estrogen, progesterone, etc. We've found that when we add in this precursor, the process of regenerating optimal endocrine function often goes a lot easier and smoother. It's easier to build a building when you have bricks, and it's easier to build a fire when you have wood to burn. The logic here is the same.

IGF-1 Boosters

Transitioning into more of the anti-aging side of endocrine function, we move on to maintaining optimal levels of Human Growth Hormone. We know that age-related HGH decline and age-related testosterone decline go hand in hand, and that both lead to sub-optimal energy levels, vitality, and quality of life. When laboratory levels and symptomology indicate the need, we try to support HGH levels in the best way possible, which is to 1) make sure we *don't overcorrect*, and 2) that we stimulate the body to make more of its own. IGF-1 (insulin-like growth factor) is a precursor to HGH, and introducing an IGF-1 boosting supplement is an excellent way to return HGH to youthful levels. We typically either use practitioner grade VAE (velvet antler extract) as an oral supplement, or we prescribe injectable Sermorelin. Sermorelin comes in (double analog peptide GHRP-2/GHRP-6) injectable form and is made at an FDA approved compounding pharmacy. It functions as a growth hormone secretagogue, promotes healthy function of the pituitary gland, and helps the body make more of its own HGH. It's noteworthy that this is a *completely and fundamentally different approach* than injecting straight HGH into a patient, which is rife with potential side effects and reduces the body's own production of HGH via a negative feedback loop mechanism. We do *not* inject or prescribe HGH (with perhaps the exception of the rare conditions that it's actually indicated for, like dwarfism).

Thyroid

Shifting gears once again, we move on to the thyroid, the body's thermostat. Many books have been written both holistically and allopathically on thyroid function, and its general utility is well understood. What we can add to that abundance of knowledge is simply to point out that often times, the usual assessment and treatment of thyroid problems is a little bit obtuse, outdated and grossly over-simplified. So we will quickly and succinctly expound on what's missing.

The thyroid needs iodine to function properly. There are times when poor thyroid function is incorrectly attributed to glandular insufficiency, when it really just needs a little bit of proper dual-form iodine/iodide (and possibly some adaptogenic therapy). Add in the missing ingredient when appropriate (when the labs or old-school topical iodine test indicate) and lo and behold about 3 to 4 weeks later things begin upregulating and returning to optimal function, sans the use of prescription drugs.

Next, the lab work. The basic (T3 Uptake, T4, TSH) thyroid panel sucks and it's equivalent to looking through a soda straw. Looking at TSH and outdated reference ranges as a primary indicator of thyroid function is no longer acceptable, it is a failure. When we run labs, we run an 'expanded' (or what I consider 'normal') thyroid panel. We look at:
- Free T3, Free T4
- Total T3, Total T4
- Reverse T3

- T3 Uptake
- TSH
- TPO and TGA anti-bodies (which help us determine auto-immune response)
- Thyroglobulin (dysregulation of normal Tg function has recently been associated with multiple thyroid diseases including autoimmune and thyroid cancer)

With these multiple layers of information, we can better ascertain whether a patient is dealing with hypothyroidism, and whether they need T4 by itself or if they need a compounded time-release T3 in tandem with T4. Also, for the patients that need thyroid correction, we avoid (like the plague) prescribing the synthetics—Synthroid, Levothyroxine, and Cytomel, and Tirosint, which can lead to death of whatever remaining thyroid function a hypothyroid patient has remaining. We only prescribe natural desiccated thyroid, compounded when appropriate, or one of the Amour Throid, NatureThroid, or WestThroid brands. These are naturally (either bovine or porcine) sourced and are much better tolerated by the human body long term. Through this more comprehensive and *patient specific* methodology, we are able to achieve far more optimal outcomes for our patients with thyroid insufficiency.

CHAPTER 20A

XENOESTROGENS ARTICLE
(Amy LaRue, ND)

Xenoestrogens –
What are they? How to avoid them.

Amy LaRue, ND
reprinted with permission

Xenoestrogens are found in a variety of everyday items. Many of us don't think twice about the makeup we wear each day or the plastic container we use to pack our lunch. We know organic food is supposed to be better for us, but sometimes we just don't want to pay the extra money. Unfortunately, all of the above may be altering the way our body naturally functions because they all contain endocrine disruptors called, xenoestrogens.

Endocrine disruptors are a category of chemicals that alter the normal function of hormones. Normally, our endocrine system releases hormones that signal different tissues telling them what to do. When chemicals from the outside get into our bodies, they have the ability to mimic our natural hormones; blocking or binding hormone receptors. This is particularly detrimental to hormone sensitive organs like the uterus and the breast, the immune and neurological systems, as well as human development.

Xenoestrogens are a sub-category of the endocrine disruptor group that specifically have estrogen-like effects. Estrogen is a natural hormone in humans that is important for bone growth, blood clotting and reproduction in men and women. The body regulates the amount needed through intricate biochemical pathways. When xenoestrogens enter the body they increase the total amount of estrogen resulting in a phenomenon called, estrogen dominance. Xenoestrogens are not biodegradable so, they are stored in our fat cells. Build up of xenoestrogens have been indicated in many conditions including: breast, prostate and testicular cancer, obesity, infertility, endometriosis, early onset puberty, miscarriages and diabetes.

Below is a list of some of the sources of xenoestrogens, but it is by no means exhaustive. We are constantly exposed to these substances in the world we live in. Examples of everyday items that may include xenoestrogens are: fruits and vegetables sprayed with pesticides, plastic water bottles and Tupperware, nail polish, makeup, birth control and on and on.

Here are some of the chemicals that are xenoestrogens:

- Skincare:
    - **4-Methylbenzylidene camphor** (4-MBC) (sunscreen lotions)
    - **Parabens** (methylparaben, ethylparaben, propylparaben and butylparaben commonly used as a preservative)
    - **Benzophenone** (sunscreen lotions)

- Industrial products and Plastics:
    - **Bisphenol A** (monomer for polycarbonate plastic and epoxy resin; antioxidant in plasticizers)
    - **Phthalates** (plasticizers)
    - **DEHP** (plasticizer for PVC)
    - **Polybrominated biphenyl ethers** (PBDEs) (flame retardants used in plastics, foams, building materials, electronics, furnishings, motor vehicles).
    - **Polychlorinated biphenyls** (PCBs)

- Food:
    - Erythrosine / FD&C Red No. 3
    - Phenosulfothiazine (a red dye)
    - Butylated hydroxyanisole / BHA (food preservative)

- Building supplies:
    - Pentachlorophenol (general biocide and wood preservative)
    - Polychlorinated biphenyls / PCBs (in electrical oils, lubricants, adhesives, paints)

- Insecticides:
    - Atrazine (weed killer)
    - DDT (insecticide, banned)
    - Dichlorodiphenyldichloroethylene (one of the breakdown products of DDT)
    - Dieldrin (insecticide)
    - Endosulfan (insecticide)
    - Heptachlor (insecticide)
    - Lindane / hexachlorocyclohexane (insecticide, used to treat lice and scabies)
    - Methoxychlor (insecticide)
    - Fenthion
    - Nonylphenol and derivatives (industrial surfactants; emulsifiers for emulsion polymerization; laboratory detergents; pesticides)

- Other:
    - Chlorine and chlorine by-products, Propyl gallate
    - **Ethinylestradiol** (combined oral contraceptive pill)
    - Metalloestrogens (a class of inorganic xenoestrogens)
    - **Alkylphenol** (surfactant used in cleaning detergents)

So what can you do to avoid these common chemicals? The following list was adapted from the organic excellence website.

Guidelines to minimize your personal exposure to xeno-estrogens:

- Food:
    - Avoid all pesticides, herbicides, and fungicides.
    - Choose organic, locally-grown and in-season foods.
    - Peel non-organic fruits and vegetables.
    - Buy hormone-free meats and dairy products to avoid hormones and pesticides.

- Plastics:
    - Reduce the use of plastics whenever possible.
    - Do not microwave food in plastic containers.
    - Avoid the use of plastic wrap to cover food for storing or microwaving.
    - Use glass or ceramics whenever possible to store food.
    - Do not leave plastic containers, especially your drinking water, in the sun.
    - If a plastic water container has heated up significantly, throw it away.
    - Don't refill plastic water bottles.
    - Avoid freezing water in plastic bottles to drink later.

- Household Products:
    - Use chemical free, biodegradable laundry and household cleaning products.
    - Choose chlorine-free products and unbleached paper products (i.e. tampons, menstrual pads, toilet paper, paper towel, coffee filters).
    - Use a chlorine filter on shower heads and filter drinking water

- Health and Beauty Products:
    - Avoid creams and cosmetics that have toxic chemicals and estrogenic ingredients such as parabens and stearalkonium chloride.

- ▫ Minimize your exposure to nail polish and nail polish removers.
- ▫ Use naturally based fragrances, such as essential oils.
- ▫ Use chemical free soaps and toothpastes.
- ▫ Read the labels on condoms and diaphragm gels.

- At the Office:
  - ▫ Be aware of noxious gas such as from copiers and printers, carpets, fiberboards, and at the gas pump.

To learn more about ingredients and xenoestrogens check out the following website: Better Nutrition

1. Cheryl S. Watson, Yow-Jiun Jeng, Jutatip Guptarak. Endocrine disruption via estrogen receptors that participate in nongenomic signaling pathways. *The Journal of Steroid Biochemistry and Molecular Biology*, Volume 127, Issues 1–2, October 2011, Pages 44-50, ISSN 0960-0760, 10.1016/j.jsbmb.2011.01.015. (http://www.sciencedirect.com/science/article/pii/S0960076011000 288)

2. Sam De Coster, Nicolas van Larebeke. Endocrine-Disrupting Chemicals: Associated Disorders and Mechanisms of Action. *Journal of Environmental and Public Health.*

Published online 2012 September 6. Doi: 10.1155/2012/713696.

1. Xenoestrogens and How to Minimize Your Exposure. Accessed October 15, 2012.

—

[1] http://www.breastcancer.org/symptoms/unde rstand_bc/statistics.jsp.

–By Amy LaRue ND

https://womeninbalance.org/2012/10/26/xenoestrogens-what-are-they-how-to-avoid-them/

CHAPTER 21

INFLAMMATION

We spend billions of dollars (both allopathically and holistically) every year managing it. Inflammation is at the core of just about every major degenerative condition. The inflammation pathways are very well defined, it's how we address it that needs to be re-evaluated and restructured. As mentioned in the previous (allergy) chapter, inflammation is not the true enemy, it's a symptom and part of an incredibly well-engineered system designed to protect us and keep us alive. In urgently acute cases, it may be necessary to use pharmaceuticals to bring excessive inflammation under control, but we've got to get away from the model that prescribes taking 8 ibuprofen tablets a day. While that may continue to keep pain/inflammation at bay, it is palliative at best, doesn't address the underlying root cause, and there is always a trade-off. NSAIDS like ibuprofen and Celebrex may do a great job of knocking down Cox-I and/or Cox-II inflammation, but we now know that we also need those Cox enzymes to protect the heart from cardiac arrest. (The prolonged use of NSAIDS also greatly increases the risk of bleeding ulcers within the gastro-intestinal lining.)

So how about we define a better approach, let's integrate a more thorough and rational set of methods and tactics to help the body naturally lower its own inflammation, instead of chemically forcing it to do so with the added expense of adverse side effects. Let's remember the notion that the very definition of insanity is doing the same thing over and over and expecting it to yield a different or improved result...yet that's exactly what doctors are doing by prescribing daily NSAID regimens in perpetuity with no true resolution in sight.

One of the biggest obstacles when it comes to addressing inflammation is that doctors aren't trained adequately on all the different *origins* of the inflammatory process. We all know that physical injuries cause inflammation. But less than a fourth of our conventionally trained physicians will even think to mention an inflammatory diet as a potential source, and exceedingly fewer of them will mention *emotional* injuries as a basis for inflammation, even though negative emotional states (specifically emotional stress) have been clearly and clinically established as a causative factor within the context of inducing a biochemical inflammatory response.

So let's begin undoing these bad habits and readdress each of the primary origins.

- **Physical injury**—for any of us that have ever played sports long term, the acronym R.I.C.E. is well known when we experience a minor injury. This stands for Rest, Ice, Compression, Elevation and it can be a great help. I would be lying/hypocritical if I said I didn't throw Aleve (naproxen) in there *for the first day or two* immediately following an injury. But as the initial swelling is controlled, it's time to bring in the truly *healing* methods that don't just address the symptoms. It's time to slather on the Arnica Gel (which is plant based and actively aids/accelerates the healing process). It's time to go see the Acupuncturist, who can aid/accelerate the healing process by amplifying the bio-electrical signal and voltage to the injured area. It's time to do an ice bath (or if you have access, a cryo-chamber treatment) to bring down *full body* inflammation. (Just because a single body part is inflamed/injured doesn't mean the inflammatory biochemicals are isolated to that area.) It's time to use the pulsed electromagnetic field device (the Bemer) to increase microcirculation and get extra blood-flow, oxygen, and nutrients to the affected area. It's time to bring in some practitioner-grade turmeric/curcumin to naturally bring down the swelling/inflammation/swelling/soreness. If there is excess pain, it's time to (sparingly) use pure grade Kratom, which is a healthier natural alternative to synthetic opioid narcotics like Hydrocodone. (Kratora.com is an excellent source for pure grade.) If the injury is to a joint, it might be time to go have a Platelet Rich Plasma (PRP) injection done (once the swelling is under control) to help regenerate the soft tissue and complete the healing. (PRP is a form of de facto stem cell therapy that utilizes stem cells and healing co-factors via harvesting them from a few vials of the patient's own blood. They are then concentrated via a centrifuge, and that concentrated serum is re-injected into the affected area on the patient.) Lastly, it's time remove inflammatory foods from our diet, at least temporarily, to aid in the recovery/healing process. The body has a much slower, harder task repairing an injury if it's also having to actively manage a completely different set of inflammatory components from our poor diets.

- **Dietary Inflammation**—As mentioned in the allergy chapter, it's time to eliminate the 'big 4' in order to help our body lower inflammation naturally. Sugar, Dairy, Gluten, and Alcohol need to be eliminated, at least temporarily, if we want to heal and repair our bodies to optimal health. Switching to a plant-based diet or at least a 'pescatarian' diet, which is mostly plant-based but adds in cold-water sourced fish, goes a long way towards this end after just a few weeks. I love a good steak, a cold beer, and desert as much as the next person, but it's amazing how good you feel when you give up the big 4, give up meat, and stick with foods like organic avocado and hummus for a little while. I'll reiterate the importance of considering the "Master Cleanse" and a good probiotic. An imbalance of bacteria and fungi in your gastrointestinal tract, known as **dysbiosis**, can cause the immune system to overreact with an inflammatory response as well.

- **Emotional Inflammation**—This is the one that needs vastly more acknowledgement within the medical community at large. Emotional Inflammation is a different way of saying *psychological stress*. Stress kills. (Just ask any of my fellow saltwater reef aquarium enthusiasts, stress the fish out, and they die!) We now have multiple studies that back this up. We know that stress can raise the stress hormone cortisol, but there is so much more to it than that, including the link between stress, inflammation, and depression. Let's borrow an excerpt from a 2014 PubMed study by George Slavich and Michael Irwin titled "From Stress to Inflammation and Major Depressive Disorder: A Social Signal Transduction Theory of Depression."

> ...In this review, we propose a biologically plausible, multilevel theory that describes neural, physiologic, molecular, and genomic mechanisms that link experiences of social-environmental stress with internal biological processes that drive depression pathogenesis. Central to this social signal transduction theory of depression is the hypothesis that experiences of social threat and adversity up-regulate components of the immune system involved in inflammation. The key mediators of this response, called pro-inflammatory cytokines, can in turn elicit profound changes in behavior, which include the initiation of depressive symptoms such as sad mood, anhedonia, fatigue, psychomotor retardation, and

social-behavioral withdrawal. This highly conserved biological response to adversity is critical for survival during times of actual physical threat or injury. However, this response can also be activated by modern-day social, symbolic, or imagined threats, leading to an increasingly pro-inflammatory phenotype that may be a key phenomenon driving depression pathogenesis and recurrence, as well as the overlap of depression with several somatic conditions including asthma, rheumatoid arthritis, chronic pain, metabolic syndrome, cardiovascular disease, obesity, and neurodegeneration. Insights from this theory may thus shed light on several important questions including how depression develops, why it frequently recurs, why it is strongly predicted by early life stress, and why it often co-occurs with symptoms of anxiety and with certain physical disease conditions. This work may also suggest new opportunities for preventing and treating depression by targeting inflammation.

As a society we desperately need to be more proactive regarding making better choices and taking measures to mitigate stress, specifically chronic stress. As practitioners, it is vital that we offer patients effective options and resources to help them understand the very real physiological dangers of stress and how to manage, reduce, and eliminate it as much as possible. We need to point them in the direction of healing, anti-inflammatory diets, anti-stress outlets like yoga, meditation, full body massage, acupuncture, and spiritual retreats. More specifically, the human body is designed to handle acute/short term stress. It is *not* designed to handle chronic stress. There is a very clear dichotomy there. Here is another excerpt from a study published in 2012 by Sheldon Cohen and his research team at Carnagie Mellon University:

Stress wreaks havoc on the mind and body. For example, psychological stress is associated with greater risk for depression, heart disease and infectious diseases. But, until now, it has not been clear exactly how stress influences disease and health.

A research team led by Carnegie Mellon University's Sheldon Cohen has found that chronic psychological stress is associated with the body losing its ability to regulate the inflammatory response. Published in the Proceedings of the National Academy of Sciences, the research shows for the first time that the effects of psychological stress on the body's ability to regulate inflammation can promote the development and progression of disease.

"Inflammation is partly regulated by the hormone cortisol and when cortisol is not allowed to serve this function, inflammation can get out of control," said Cohen, the Robert E. Doherty Professor of Psychology within CMU's Dietrich College of Humanities and Social Sciences.

Cohen argued that prolonged stress alters the effectiveness of cortisol to regulate the inflammatory response because it decreases tissue sensitivity to the hormone. Specifically, immune cells become insensitive to cortisol's regulatory effect. In turn, runaway inflammation is thought to promote the development and progression of many diseases.

Cohen, whose groundbreaking early work showed that people suffering from psychological stress are more susceptible to developing common colds, used the common cold as the model for testing his theory. With the common cold, symptoms are not caused by the virus -- they are instead a "side effect" of the inflammatory response that is triggered as part of the body's effort to fight infection. The greater the body's inflammatory response to the virus, the greater is the likelihood of experiencing the symptoms of a cold.

In Cohen's first study, after completing an intensive stress interview, 276 healthy adults were exposed to a virus that causes the common cold and monitored in quarantine for five days for signs of infection and illness. Here, Cohen found that experiencing a prolonged stressful event was associated with the inability of immune cells to respond to hormonal signals that normally regulate inflammation. In turn, those with the inability to regulate the inflammatory response were more likely to develop colds when exposed to the virus.

In the second study, 79 healthy participants were assessed for their ability to regulate the inflammatory response and then exposed to a cold virus and monitored for the production of pro-inflammatory cytokines, the chemical messengers that trigger inflammation. He found that those who were less able to regulate the inflammatory response as assessed before being exposed to the virus produced more of these inflammation-inducing chemical messengers when they were infected.

"The immune system's ability to regulate inflammation predicts who will develop a cold, but more importantly it provides an explanation of how stress can promote disease," Cohen said. "When under stress, cells of the immune system are unable to respond to hormonal control, and consequently, produce levels of inflammation that promote disease. Because inflammation plays a role in many diseases such as cardiovascular, asthma and autoimmune disorders, this model suggests why stress impacts them as well."

He added, "Knowing this is important for identifying which diseases may be influenced by stress and for preventing disease in chronically stressed people."

In addition to Cohen, the research team included CMU's Denise Janicki-Deverts, research psychologist; Children's Hospital of Pittsburgh's William J. Doyle; University of British Columbia's Gregory E. Miller; University of Pittsburgh School of Medicine's Bruce S. Rabin and Ellen Frank; and the University of Virginia Health Sciences Center's Ronald B. Turner.

The National Center for Complementary and Alternative Medicine, National Institute of Mental Health, National Heart, Lung and Blood Institute and the MacArthur Foundation Research Network on Socioeconomic Status and Health funded this research.

CHAPTER 22

LYME DISEASE

This one has been a real can of worms (literally and figuratively speaking) over the past 25 years or so. It has been an absolute travesty that so many patients have suffered and languished for so long from a (very treatable) disease that modern medicine refused to admit even existed for quite some time. To this day, insurance companies often refuse to pay the treatment costs of patients that have been clinically diagnosed with Lyme disease. You almost can't blame them due to all the conflicting information out there, compounded by the fact that most labs designed to detect the primary Lyme infection and its 10 or more possible co-infections are expensive, and some are unreliable and don't have a high enough confidence interval for diagnosis even with a positive result. The available labs today include the CD-57, Western Blot, Advanced Labs Poly-Borrelia culture, ELISA test, and the IGeneX, which all test via different methods and for different strains and co-infections (Borrelia, Babesia, Spirochetes, etc) and have varying degrees of accuracy. As of this writing in 2017, there are more hi-tech (and hopefully more reliable) labs on the horizon being developed for the near future. We are of the opinion that none of these tests has the slightest chance of any sort of accuracy without doing what we call a 'provocation' first. A provoked test in this case would be administering an IV anti-biotic (most likely doxycycline or minocycline), which would then theoretically agitate sometimes dormant or hidden pathogenic components of the disease so that they would actually show up on the testing. An even better alternative would be to stop suppressing the use of **Dark Field Microscopy**, which is a much more capable method of determining whether someone has Lyme disease, because it gives you the ability to see the moving spirochetes in real time.

Furthermore, there is some controversial but very prevailing evidence that certain degenerative neurological conditions like ALS (Lou Gehrig's disease) and MS are actually a form of neurospirochetosis (specific Lyme infection) at its core, and that all the subsequent symptoms are just that, downstream symptoms. Both older and recent autopsy findings have found that all deceased MS patients' brains tested to date harbored live Lyme spirochetes. This is another way of saying Lyme Disease and MS might be the same thing. (This is by no means 'hard evidence,' but it should also not be lost on the reader that Lou Gehrig had a holiday home in Lyme, Connecticut, and spent a lot of time in the outdoors there...'there' being the biggest Lyme hotspot on the Earth at the time.)

Ok so let's imagine that at some point in the near future we get this Lyme diagnosis conundrum figured out, and Lyme disease is much better understood. How do we address it? We in the integrative world do not claim to have a cure for Lyme disease, but we've gotten pretty damn good at knocking it down hard and possibly opening the window for some patients to experience a radical reversal of the condition and symptoms, even if some component of the Borrelia goes dormant in the tissues. How do we do that? Glad you asked!

We can use a synergy of IV therapies and oral supplements to attack it on all sides:

- **Umbilical Cord Sourced** Stem Cell Therapy (anti-pathogenic and regenerative therapy)
- **Silver Hydrasol (Argentyn23) IV's** (anti-pathogenic, anti-bacterial, anti-viral therapy)
- **UVLrx Ultraviolet Blood Irradiation** (UV light anti-pathogenic, anti-inflammatory therapy)

- **Glutathione IV's** (master liver cleanser, master anti-oxidant, neurological and cognitive function potentiator
- **Kambo** (South American Peptide anti-viral, anti-pathogen, anti-inflammatory therapy)
- **Serretia** (serrapeptase oral supplement to break down biofilms)
- **LDN** (naltrexone in small doses has shown promise with reversing the chronic fatigue/energy production issues seen with Lyme patients)
- **Doxycycline IV's** (anti-biotic IV therapy, only known class of anti-biotics to have any sort of real effectiveness against Lyme disease. Some doctors do incorporate cefuroxime in tandem. Doxycycline therapy works best if administered within the first few months of exposure/infection)
- **Herbal Parasite Cleanse** (G.I. Synergy by Apex Energetics combined with Lauracidin/Monolaurin)
- **GcMaf** (macrophage activation and vitamin D carrier molecule that restores maximum immune function)

To date, the Umbilical Stem Cell therapy seems to be the most powerfully effective standalone option, and we often see a big reversal of symptomology in certain patients following the administration of multiple stem cell treatments over the course of a few months, especially if it's used in tandem with some of the other mentioned therapies. In time, and with synergy, we will develop, discover, or rediscover the cure for Lyme disease and be able to outright eradicate it. It's a reversible, killable scourge. But it's going to take the best that all of us as practitioners have to give, and we are going to have to collectively get rid of the roadblocks, red tape, bean counters, political lobbyists, and any other obstructionists who actively impede the road to getting patients the effective diagnosis and treatments that they deserve.

CHAPTER 23

MOLD TOXICITY and MYCOTOXINS

One of the greatest 'distractors' from optimal health that often gets 'lost in the shuffle' or goes undiagnosed/unrecognized is mold toxicity. It is an especially prevalent issue in humid regions (like here in Florida). The symptoms are myriad, ranging from undetectable to extreme, including flu-like symptoms severe respiratory and/or psychiatric distress. For a brief, but thorough overview on household molds, check here:

https://aerindustries.com/blog/2017/03/28/common-types-mold-in-home/

In more recent on-going scientific studies, it is starting to become more well-known that upwards of 20% of the population genetically lack the ability to fully detox from mold toxicity/illness, even when they are removed from a mold saturated environment.

In a clinical setting, we have excellent results helping patients afflicted with mold toxicity/illness via various methods at our disposal, including:

- Silver Hydrasol
- UltraViolet Blood Irradiation
- Intravenous Myer's Cocktail
- Bio-Film destroyers (Serrapeptase and Monolaurin)
- Hydrogen Peroxide Therapy
- Far Infrared Sauna
- Ozone Therapy
- Intravenous Glutathione
- Stem Cell Therapy

If you believe you suffer from mold toxicity, it is wise to have both your home and yourself tested. There are effective blood and culture labs that can be performed by mold specialists to determine not only if you have been exposed to mold, but specifically what strain(s) you may be dealing with, which then makes treatment/therapy more specific and direct.

For more information on mold toxicity, testing, and remedies, the reader is invited to access the comprehensive information within these extensively researched and well-written resources on the subject:

- *Toxic: Heal Your Body from Mold Toxicity, Lyme Disease, Multiple Chemical Sensitivities, and Chronic Environmental Illness* by Neil Nathan

- *Break the Mold: 5 Tools to Conquer Mold and Take Back Your Health* by Dr. Jill Crista

- *Mold & Mycotoxins: Current Evaluation and Treatment 2016* by Neil Nathan

- *Nature's Mold Rx, the Non-Toxic Solution to Toxic Mold* by Edward R. Close, PhD

- www.naturesmoldrx.com (Edward R. Close, PhD)

There is enough information on mold to fill volumes, but we are just now at a point medically where we are beginning to realize just how many people are affected by mold toxicity/illness. Once you've had your home tested (and professional mold removal performed if necessary) and you've had yourself tested (and the appropriate remedies have been administered if necessary), I recommend investing $150 or so and having a UV-light filter installed in your airducts. Typically, the people who perform professional mold-removal service also offer this as an additional service. I also recommend investing in high quality air filtering devices for your home. My current favorite is the Ionic Breeze Quadra by Sharper Image, but there are many excellent ones available.

CHAPTER 24

MEDICINAL MARIJUANA

Unless you've been living under a rock for the past several years, you are probably well aware of the now known health benefits of marijuana. Patients with PTSD, cancer, glaucoma, anxiety, inflammation and countless other conditions are getting relief through medical cannabis when everything else has failed them. We are finally moving past the ignorant crusades of the 80's and 90's that linked the 'dangers' of marijuana to being a 'gateway drug' to stuff like heroin and crack. There is no LD-50 (lethal dose) of marijuana, the effects are self-limiting. The benefits of it are numerous, and it has been used for thousands of years for its medicinal properties. Because of the commonality of this knowledge, it isn't necessary to take up much space in this book on the subject, other than to say it is an amazing plant. For just a moment though let's expound upon the lesser known aspects of marijuana:

There is an entire metabolic pathway within human beings seemingly dedicated to the uptake and use of the active ingredient(s) and alkaloids in marijuana...the human **Endocannabinoid System.** (Another 90's reference here—I don't think McGruff the Crime Dog had this information when he was so fervently trying to prevent us from smoking a dooby back in the day!) As an aside though, I will mention that to receive the full benefit of the wondrous molecules of this plant species, it needs to be ingested orally, and not smoked. Some of the benefits can still be attained through smoking the herb, but some of them are lost. Furthermore, many studies have shown that smoking marijuana can lead to harmful side effects in the lungs and in the brain.

For those of you that want to know more on the Endocannabinoid system, let's take the easy way out and borrow the Wikipedia page on this:

Endocannabinoid system
From Wikipedia, the free encyclopedia

The endocannabinoid system (ECS) is a group of endogenous cannabinoid receptors located in the mammalian brain and throughout the central and peripheral nervous systems, consisting of neuro-modulatory lipids and their receptors. Known as "the body's own cannabinoid system",[1] the ECS is involved in a variety of physiological processes including appetite, pain-sensation, mood, and memory, and in mediating the psychoactive effects of cannabis.[2] The ECS is also involved in voluntary exercise[3] and may be related to the evolution of the runner's high in human beings and related aspects of motivation or reward for locomotor activity in other animals.[4]

Two primary endocannabinoid receptors have been identified: CB1, first cloned in 1990; and CB2, cloned in 1993. CB1 receptors are found predominantly in the brain and nervous system, as well as in peripheral organs and tissues, and are the main molecular target of the endocannabinoid ligand (binding molecule), Anandamide, as well as its mimetic phytocannabinoid, THC. One other main endocannabinoid is 2-Arachidonoylglycerol (2-AG) which is active at both cannabinoid receptors, along with its own mimetic phytocannabinoid, CBD. 2-AG and CBD are involved in the regulation of appetite, immune system functions and pain management.[1][5][6]

Contents
[show]

Basic overview[edit]

The endocannabinoid system, broadly speaking, includes:

- The endogenous arachidonate-based lipids, anandamide (N-arachidonoylethanolamide, AEA) and 2-arachidonoylglycerol (2-AG); these are known as "endocannabinoids" and are physiological ligands for the cannabinoid receptors. Endocannabinoids are all eicosanoids.[7]

- The enzymes that synthesize and degrade the endocannabinoids, such as fatty acid amide hydrolase or monoacylglycerol lipase.

- The cannabinoid receptors CB1 and CB2, two G protein-coupled receptors that are located in the central and peripheral nervous systems.

The neurons, neural pathways, and other cells where these molecules, enzymes, and one or both cannabinoid receptor types are all colocalized from the endocannabinoid system.

The endocannabinoid system has been studied using genetic and pharmacological methods. These studies have revealed that cannabinoids act as neuromodulators[8][9][10] for a variety of processes, including motor learning,[11] appetite,[12] and pain sensation,[13] among other cognitive and physical processes. The localization of the CB1 receptor in the endocannabinoid system has a very large degree of overlap with the orexinergic projection system, which mediates many of the same functions, both physical and cognitive.[14] Moreover, CB1 is colocalized on orexin projection neurons in the lateral hypothalamus and many output structures of the orexin system,[14][15] where the CB1 and orexin receptor 1 (OX1) receptors physically and functionally join together to form the CB1–OX1 receptor hetero-dimer.[14][16][17]

Expression of receptors[edit]

For more details on receptor localization, see Cannabinoid receptor type 1 (CB1) and Cannabinoid receptor type 2 (CB2).

Cannabinoid binding sites exist throughout the central and peripheral nervous systems. The two most relevant receptors for cannabinoids are the CB1 and CB2receptors, which are expressed predominantly in the brain and immune system respectively.[18] Density of expression varies based on species and correlates with the efficacy that cannabinoids will have in modulating specific aspects of behavior related to the site of expression. For example, in rodents, the highest concentration of cannabinoid binding sites are in the basal ganglia and cerebellum, regions of the brain involved in the initiation and coordination of movement.[19]In humans, cannabinoid receptors exist in much lower concentration in these regions, which helps explain why cannabinoids possess a greater efficacy in altering rodent motor movements than they do in humans.

A recent analysis of cannabinoid binding in CB1 and CB2 receptor knockout mice found cannabinoid responsiveness even when these receptors were not being expressed, indicating that an additional binding receptor may be present in the brain.[19] Binding has been demonstrated by 2-arachidonoylglycerol (2-AG) on the TRPV1 receptor suggesting that this receptor may be a candidate for the established response.[20]

In addition to CB1 and CB2, certain orphan receptors are known to bind endocannabinoids as well, including GPR18, GPR55 (a regulator of neuroimmune function), and GPR119. CB1 has also been noted to form a functional human receptor heterodimer in orexin neurons with OX1, the CB1–OX1 receptor, which mediates feeding behavior and certain physical processes such as cannabinoid-induced pressor responses which are known to occur through signaling in the rostral ventrolateral medulla.[21][22]

Endocannabinoid synthesis, release, and degradation[edit]
During neurotransmission, the pre-synaptic neuron releases neurotransmitters into the synaptic cleft which bind to cognate receptors expressed on the post-synaptic neuron. Based upon the interaction between the transmitter and receptor, neurotransmitters may trigger a variety of effects in the post-synaptic cell, such as excitation, inhibition, or the initiation of second messenger cascades. Based on the cell, these effects may result in the on-site synthesis of endogenous cannabinoids anandamide or 2-AG by a process that is not entirely clear, but results from an elevation in intracellular calcium.[18] Expression appears to be exclusive, so that both types of endocannabinoids are not co-synthesized. This exclusion is based on synthesis-specific channel activation: a recent study found that in the bed nucleus of the stria terminalis, calcium entry through voltage-sensitive calcium channels produced an L-type current resulting in 2-AG production, while activation of mGluR1/5 receptors triggered the synthesis of anandamide.[20]

Evidence suggests that the depolarization-induced influx of calcium into the post-synaptic neuron causes the activation of an enzyme called transacylase. This enzyme is suggested to catalyze the first step of endocannabinoid biosynthesis by converting phosphatidylethanolamine, a membrane-resident phospholipid, into N-acyl-phosphatidylethanolamine (NAPE). Experiments have shown that phospholipase D cleaves NAPE to yield anandamide.[23][24] This process is mediated by bile acids.[25] In NAPE-phospholipase D (NAPEPLD)-knockout mice, cleavage of NAPE is reduced in low calcium concentrations, but not abolished, suggesting multiple, distinct pathways are involved in anandamide synthesis.[26] The synthesis of 2-AG is less established and warrants further research.

Once released into the extracellular space by a putative endocannabinoid transporter, messengers are vulnerable to glial cell inactivation. Endocannabinoids are taken up by a transporter on the glial cell and degraded by fatty acid amide hydrolase (FAAH), which cleaves anandamide into arachidonic acid and ethanolamineor monoacylglycerol lipase (MAGL), and 2-AG into arachidonic acid and glycerol.[27] While arachidonic acid is a substrate for leukotriene and prostaglandinsynthesis, it is unclear whether this degradative byproduct has unique functions in the central nervous system.[28][29] Emerging data in the field also points to FAAH being expressed in postsynaptic neurons complementary to presynaptic neurons expressing cannabinoid receptors, supporting the conclusion that it is major contributor to the clearance and inactivation of anandamide and 2-AG after endocannabinoid reuptake.[19] A neuropharmacological study demonstrated that an inhibitor of FAAH (URB597) selectively increases anandamide levels in the brain of rodents and primates. Such approaches could lead to the development of new drugs with analgesic, anxiolytic-like and antidepressant-like effects, which are not accompanied by overt signs of abuse liability.[30]

Binding and intracellular effects[edit]

Cannabinoid receptors are G-protein coupled receptors located on the pre-synaptic membrane. While there have been some papers that have linked concurrent stimulation of dopamine and CB1 receptors to an acute rise in cyclic adenosine monophosphate (cAMP) production, it is generally accepted that CB1 activation via cannabinoids causes a decrease in cAMP concentration by inhibition of adenylyl cyclase and a rise in the concentration of mitogen-activated protein kinase(MAP kinase).[7][19] The relative potency of different cannabinoids in inhibition of adenylyl cyclase correlates with their varying efficacy in behavioral assays. This inhibition of cAMP is followed by phosphorylation and subsequent activation of not only a suite of MAP kinases (p38/p42/p44), but also the PI3/PKB and MEK/ERK pathway (Galve-Roperh et al., 2002; Davis et al., 2005; Jones et al., 2005; Graham et al., 2006). Results from rat hippocampal gene chip data after acute administration of tetrahydrocannabinol (THC) showed an increase in the expression of transcripts encoding myelin basic protein, endoplasmic proteins, cytochrome oxidase, and two cell adhesion molecules: NCAM, and SC1; decreases in expression were seen in both calmodulin and ribosomal RNAs (Kittler et al., 2000). In addition, CB1 activation has been demonstrated to increase the activity of transcription factors like c-Fos and Krox-24 (Graham et al., 2006).

Binding and neuronal excitability[edit]

 This section **provides insufficient context for those unfamiliar with the subject**. Please help *improve the article* with a *good introductory style*. (January 2014) (*Learn how and when to remove this template message*)

The molecular mechanisms of CB1-mediated changes to the membrane voltage have also been studied in detail.

Cannabinoids reduce calcium influx by blocking the activity of voltage-dependent N-, P/Q- and L-type calcium channels.[31][32] In addition to acting on calcium channels, activation of Gi/o and Gs, the two most commonly coupled G-proteins to cannabinoid receptors, has been shown to modulate potassium channel activity. Recent studies have found that CB1 activation specifically facilitates potassium ion flux through GIRKs, a family of potassium channels.[32] Immunohistochemistry experiments demonstrated that CB1 is co-localized with GIRK and Kv1.4 potassium channels, suggesting that these two may interact in physiological contexts.[33]

In the central nervous system, CB1 receptors influence neuronal excitability, reducing the incoming synaptic input.[34] This mechanism, known as presynaptic inhibition, occurs when a postsynaptic neuron releases endocannabinoids in retrograde transmission, which then bind to cannabinoid receptors on the presynaptic terminal. CB1 receptors then reduce the amount of neurotransmitter released, so that subsequent excitation in the presynaptic neuron results in diminished effects on the postsynaptic neuron. It is likely that presynaptic inhibition uses many of the same ion channel mechanisms listed above, although recent evidence has shown that CB1 receptors can also regulate neurotransmitter release by a non-ion channel mechanism, i.e. through Gi/o-mediated inhibition of adenylyl cyclase and protein kinase A.[35] Direct effects of CB1 receptors on membrane excitability have been reported, and strongly impact the firing of cortical neurons.[36] A series of behavioral experiments demonstrated that NMDAR, an ionotropic glutamate receptor, and the metabotropic glutamate receptors(mGluRs) work in concert with CB1 to induce analgesia in mice, although the mechanism underlying this effect is unclear.[citation needed]

Functions of the endocannabinoid system[edit]

Memory[edit]

Mice treated with tetrahydrocannabinol (THC) show suppression of long-term potentiation in the hippocampus, a process that is essential for the formation and storage of long-term memory.[37] These results concur with anecdotal evidence suggesting that smoking Cannabis impairs short-term memory.[38] Consistent with this finding, mice without the CB1 receptor show enhanced memory and long-term potentiation indicating that the endocannabinoid system may play a pivotal role in the extinction of old memories. One study found that the high-dose treatment of rats with the synthetic cannabinoid HU-210 over several weeks resulted in stimulation of neural growth in the rats' hippocampus region, a part of the limbic system playing a part in the formation of declarative and spatial memories, but did not investigate the effects on short-term or long-term memory.[39] Taken together, these findings suggest that the effects of endocannabinoids on the various brain networks involved in learning and memory may vary.

Role in hippocampal neurogenesis[edit]

In the adult brain, the endocannabinoid system facilitates the neurogenesis of hippocampal granule cells.[39][40] In the subgranular zone of the dentate gyrus, multipotent neural progenitors (NP) give rise to daughter cells that, over the course of several weeks, mature into granule cells whose axons project to and synapse onto dendrites on the CA3 region.[41] NPs in the hippocampus have been shown to possess fatty acid amide hydrolase (FAAH) and express CB1 and utilize 2-AG.[40] Intriguingly, CB1 activation by endogenous or exogenous cannabinoids promote NP proliferation and differentiation; this activation is absent in CB1 knockouts and abolished in the presence of antagonist.[39][40]

Induction of synaptic depression[edit]

The inhibitory effects of cannabinoid receptor stimulation on neurotransmitter release have caused this system to be connected to various forms of depressant plasticity. A recent study conducted with the bed nucleus of the stria terminalis found that the endurance of the depressant effects was mediated by two different signaling pathways based on the type of receptor activated. 2-AG was found to act on presynaptic CB1 receptors to mediate retrograde short-term depression(STD) following activation of L-type calcium currents, while anandamide was synthesized after mGluR5 activation and triggered autocrine signalling onto postsynapic TRPV1 receptors that induced long-term depression (LTD). Similar post-synaptic receptor dependencies were found in the striatum, but here both effects relied on presynaptic CB1 receptors.[20] These findings provide the brain a direct mechanism to selectively inhibit neuronal excitability over variable time scales. By selectively internalizing different receptors, the brain may limit the production of specific endocan-nabinoids to favor a time scale in accordance with its needs.

Appetite[edit]

Evidence for the role of the endocannabinoid system in food-seeking behavior comes from a variety of cannabinoid studies. Emerging data suggests that THC acts via CB1 receptors in the hypothalamic nuclei to directly increase appetite.[42] It is thought that hypothalamic neurons tonically produce endocannabinoids that work to tightly regulate hunger. The amount of endocannabinoids produced is inversely correlated with the amount of leptin in the blood.[43] For example, mice without leptin not only become massively obese but express abnormally high levels of hypothalamic endocannabinoids as a compensatory mechanism.[12] Similarly, when these mice were treated with an endocannabinoid inverse agonists, such as rimonabant, food intake was reduced.[12] When the CB1 receptor is knocked out in mice, these animals tend to be leaner and less hungry than wild-type mice. A related study examined the effect of THC on the hedonic (pleasure) value of food and found enhanced dopamine release in the nucleus accumbens and increased pleasure-related behavior after administration of a sucrose solution.[44] A related study found that endocannabinoids affect taste perception in taste cells[45] In taste cells, endocannabinoids were shown to selectively enhance the strength of neural signaling for sweet tastes, whereas leptin decreased the strength of this same response. While there is need for more research, these results suggest that cannabinoid activity in the hypothalamus and nucleus accumbens is related to appetitive, food-seeking behavior.[42]

Energy balance and metabolism[edit]
The endocannabinoid system has been shown to have a homeostatic role by controlling several metabolic functions, such as energy storage and nutrient transport. It acts on peripheral tissues such as adipocytes, hepatocytes, the gastrointestinal tract, the skeletal muscles and the endocrine pancreas. It has also been implied in modulating insulin sensitivity. Through all of this, the endocannabinoid system may play a role in clinical conditions, such as obesity, diabetes, and atherosclerosis, which may also give it a cardiovascular role.[46]

Stress response[edit]

While the secretion of glucocorticoids in response to stressful stimuli is an adaptive response necessary for an organism to respond appropriately to a stressor, persistent secretion may be harmful. The endocannabinoid system has been implicated in the habituation of the hypothalamic-pituitary-adrenal axis (HPA axis) to repeated exposure to restraint stress. Studies have demonstrated differential synthesis of anandamide and 2-AG during tonic stress. A decrease of anandamide was found along the axis that contributed to basal hypersecretion of corticosterone; in contrast, an increase of 2-AG was found in the amygdala after repeated stress, which was negatively correlated to magnitude of the corticosterone response. All effects were abolished by the CB1 antagonist AM251, supporting the conclusion that these effects were cannabinoid-receptor dependent.[47] These findings show that anandamide and 2-AG divergently regulate the HPA axis response to stress: while habituation of the stress-induced HPA axis via 2-AG prevents excessive secretion of glucocorticoids to non-threatening stimuli, the increase of basal corticosterone secretion resulting from decreased anandamide allows for a facilitated response of the HPA axis to novel stimuli.

Exploration, social behavior, and anxiety[edit]

Prolonged, systemic exposure to cannabinoids has often been associated with anti-social effects.[citation needed] To investigate this theory, a cannabinoid receptor-knockout mouse study examined the effect that these receptors play on exploratory behavior. Researchers selectively targeted glutamatergic and GABAergiccortical interneurons and studied results in open field, novel object, and sociability tests. Eliminating glutamatergic cannabinoid receptors led to decreased object exploration, social interactions, and increased aggressive behavior. In contrast, GABAergic cannabinoid receptor-knockout mice showed increased exploration of objects, socialization, and open field movement.[48] These contrasting effects reveal the importance of the endocannabinoid system in regulating anxiety-dependent behavior. Results suggest that glutamatergic cannabinoid receptors are not only responsible for mediating aggression, but produce an anxiolytic-like function by inhibiting excessive arousal: excessive excitation produces anxiety that limited the mice from exploring both animate and inanimate objects. In contrast, GABAergic neurons appear to control an anxiogenic-like function by limiting inhibitory transmitter release. Taken together, these two sets of neurons appear to help regulate the organism's overall sense of arousal during novel situations.

Immune function[edit]
Evidence suggests that endocannabinoids may function as both neuromodulators and immunomodulators in the immune system. Here, they seem to serve an autoprotective role to ameliorate muscle spasms, inflammation, and other symptoms of multiple sclerosis and skeletal muscle spasms.[7] Functionally, the activation of cannabinoid receptors has been demonstrated to play a role in the activation of GTPases in macrophages, neutrophils, and BM cells. These receptors have also been implicated in the proper migration of B cells into the marginal zone (MZ) and the regulation of healthy IgM levels.[49] Interestingly, some disorders seem to trigger an upregulation of cannabinoid receptors selectively in cells or tissues related to symptom relief and inhibition of disease progression, such as in that rodent neuropathic

pain model, where receptors are increased in the spinal cord microglia, dorsal root ganglion, and thalamic neurons.[18]

Multiple sclerosis[edit]

Historical records from ancient China and Greece suggest that preparations of Cannabis indica were commonly prescribed to ameliorate multiple sclerosis-like symptoms such as tremors and muscle pain. Modern research has confirmed these effects in a study on diseased mice, wherein both endogenous and exogenous agonists showed ameliorating effects on tremor and spasticity. It remains to be seen whether pharmaceutical preparations such as dronabinol have the same effects in humans.[50][51] Due to increasing use of medical Cannabis and rising incidence of multiple sclerosis patients who self-medicate with the drug, there has been much interest in exploiting the endocannabinoid system in the cerebellum to provide a legal and effective relief.[38] In mouse models of multiple sclerosis, there is a profound reduction and reorganization of CB1 receptors in the cerebellum.[52] Serial sections of cerebellar tissue subjected to immunohistochemistry revealed that this aberrant expression occurred during the relapse phase but returned to normal during the remitting phase of the disease.[52] Other studies suggest that CB1 agonists promote the survival of oligodendrocytes in vitro in the absence of growth and trophic factors; in addition, these agonist have been shown to promote mRNA expression of myelin lipid protein. (Kittler et al., 2000; Mollna-Holgado et al., 2002). Taken together, these studies point to the exciting possibility that cannabinoid treatment may not only be able to attenuate the symptoms of multiple sclerosis but also improve oligodendrocyte function (reviewed in Pertwee, 2001; Mollna-Holgado et al., 2002). 2-AG stimulates proliferation of a microglial cell line by a CB2 receptor dependent mechanism, and the number of microglial cells is increased in multiple sclerosis.[53]

Female reproduction[edit]
See also: Cannabis in pregnancy
The developing embryo expresses cannabinoid receptors early in development that are responsive to anandamide secreted in the uterus. This signaling is important in regulating the timing of embryonic implantation and uterine receptivity. In mice, it has been shown that anandamide modulates the probability of implantation to the uterine wall. For example, in humans, the likelihood of miscarriage increases if uterine anandamide levels are too high or low.[54] These results suggest that intake of exogenous cannabinoids (e.g. marijuana) can decrease the likelihood for pregnancy for women with high anandamide levels, and alternatively, it can increase the likelihood for pregnancy in women whose anandamide levels were too low.[55][56]

Autonomic nervous system[edit]
Peripheral expression of cannabinoid receptors led researchers to investigate the role of cannabinoids in the autonomic nervous system. Research found that the CB1 receptor is expressed presynaptically by motor neurons that innervate visceral organs. Cannabinoid-mediated inhibition of electric potentials results in a reduction in noradrenaline release from sympathetic nervous system nerves. Other studies have found similar effects in endocannabinoid regulation of intestinal motility, including the innervation of smooth muscles associated with the digestive, urinary, and reproductive systems.[19]

Analgesia[edit]

At the spinal cord, cannabinoids suppress noxious-stimulus-evoked responses of neurons in the dorsal horn, possibly by modulating descending noradrenalineinput from the brainstem.[19] As many of these fibers are primarily GABAergic, cannabinoid stimulation in the spinal column results in disinhibition that should increase noradrenaline release and attenuation of noxious-stimuli-processing in the periphery and dorsal root ganglion.

The endocannabinoid most researched in pain is palmitoylethanolamide. Palmitoylethanolamide is a fatty amine related to anandamide, but saturated and although initially it was thought that palmitoylethanolamide would bind to the CB1 and the CB2 receptor, later it was found that the most important receptors are the PPAR-alpha receptor, the TRPV receptor and the GPR55 receptor. Palmitoylethanolamide has been evaluated for its analgesic actions in a great variety of pain indications[57] and found to be safe and effective. Basically these data are proof of concept for endocannabinoids and related fatty amines to be therapeutically useful analgesics; palmitoylethanolamide is available under the brand names Normast and PeaPure as nutraceuticals.

Endocannabinoids are involved in placebo induced analgesia responses.[58]

Thermoregulation[edit]

Anandamide and N-arachidonoyl dopamine (NADA) have been shown to act on temperature-sensing TRPV1 channels, which are involved in thermoregulation.[59] TRPV1 is activated by the exogenous ligand capsaicin, the active component of chili peppers, which is structurally similar to endocannabinoids. NADA activates the TRPV1 channel with an EC50 of approximately of 50 nM.[clarify]

The high potency makes it the putative endogenous TRPV1 agonist.[60] Anandamide has also been found to activate TRPV1 on sensory neuron terminals, and subsequently cause vasodilation.[19] TRPV1 may also be activated by methanandamide and arachidonyl-2'-chloroethylamide (ACEA).[7]

Sleep[edit]

Increased endocannabinoid signaling within the central nervous system promotes sleep-inducing effects. Intercerebroventricular administration of anandamide in rats has been shown to decrease wakefulness and increase slow-wave sleep and REM sleep.[61] Administration of anandamide into the basal forebrain of rats has also been shown to increase levels of adenosine, which plays a role in promoting sleep and suppressing arousal.[62] REM sleep deprivation in rats has been demonstrated to increase CB1 receptor expression in the central nervous system.[63] Furthermore, anandamide levels possess a circadian rhythm in the rat, with levels being higher in the light phase of the day, which is when rats are usually asleep or less active, since they are nocturnal.[64]

Experimental use of CB1 -/- phenotype[edit]

Neuroscientists often utilize transgenic CB1 knockout mice to discern novel roles for the endocannabinoid system. While CB1 knockout mice are healthy and live into adulthood, there are significant differences between CB1 knockout and wild-type mice. When subjected to a high-fat diet, CB1 knockout mice tend to be about sixty percent leaner and slightly less hungry than wildtype.[65] Compared to wildtype, CB1 knockout mice exhibit severe deficits in motor learning, memory retrieval, and increased difficulty in completing the Morris water maze.[11][66][67] There is also evidence indicating that these knockout animals have an increased incidence and severity of stroke and seizure.[68][69]

See also[edit]

- Endocannabinoid enhancer
- Endocannabinoid reuptake inhibitor
- Cannabinoid receptor antagonist

References[edit]

1. Grotenhermen, Franjo (23 Jul 2012). "The Therapeutic Potential of Cannabis and Cannabinoids". Dtsch Arztebl Int. 109 (PMC3442177): 495–501. PMC 3442177 . PMID 23008748. doi:10.3238/arztebl.2012.0495.

2. Aizpurua-Olaizola, Oier; Elezgarai, Izaskun; Rico-Barrio, Irantzu; Zarandona, Iratxe; Etxebarria, Nestor; Usobiaga, Aresatz (2016). "Targeting the endocannabinoid system: future therapeutic strategies". Drug Discovery Today. PMID 27554802. doi:10.1016/j.drudis.2016.08.005.

3. Thompson, Z., D. Argueta, T. Garland, Jr., and N. DiPatrizio. 2017. Circulating levels of endocannabinoids respond acutely to voluntary exercise, are altered in mice selectively bred for high voluntary wheel running, and differ between the sexes. Physiology & Behavior 170:141–150.

4. Kuhn, S. L., D. A. Raichlen, and A. E. Clark. 2016. What moves us? How mobility and movement are at the center of human evolution. Evolutionary Anthropology: Issues, News, and Reviews 25:86–97.

5. Blázquez, C; Chiarlone, A; Bellocchio, L; Resel, E; Pruunsild, P; García-Rincón, D; Sendtner, M; Timmusk, T; Lutz, B; Galve-Roperh, I; Guzmán, M (20 February 2015). "The CB1 cannabinoid receptor signals striatal neuroprotection via a PI3K/Akt/mTORC1/BDNF pathway". Cell Death and Differentiation. 22(10): 1618–1629. doi:10.1038/cdd.2015.11.

6. Russo, Ethan B (August 2011). "Taming THC: potential cannabis synergy and phytocannabinoid-terpenoid entourage effects". British Journal of Pharmacology. 163 (7): 1344–1364. PMC 3165946 . PMID 21749363. doi:10.1111/j.1476-5381.2011.01238.x.

7. Pertwee RG (April 2006). "The pharmacology of cannabinoid receptors and their ligands: an overview". Int J

Obes (Lond). 30 (Suppl 1): S13–8. PMID 16570099. doi:10.1038/sj.ijo.0803272.

8. Fortin DA, Levine ES (2007). "Differential effects of endocannabinoids on glutamatergic and GABAergic inputs to layer 5 pyramidal neurons". Cereb. Cortex. 17 (1): 163–74. PMID 16467564. doi:10.1093/cercor/bhj133.

9. Good CH (2007). "Endocannabinoid-dependent regulation of feedforward inhibition in cerebellar Purkinje cells". J. Neurosci. 27 (1): 1–3. PMID 17205618. doi:10.1523/JNEUROSCI.4842-06.2007.

10. Hashimotodani Y, Ohno-Shosaku T, Kano M (2007). "Presynaptic monoacylglycerol lipase activity determines basal endocannabinoid tone and terminates retrograde endocannabinoid signaling in the hippocampus". J. Neurosci. 27 (5): 1211–9. PMID 17267577. doi:10.1523/JNEUROSCI.4159-06.2007.

11. Kishimoto Y, Kano M (2006). "Endogenous cannabinoid signaling through the CB1 receptor is essential for cerebellum-dependent discrete motor learning". J. Neurosci. 26 (34): 8829–37. PMID 16928872. doi:10.1523/JNEUROSCI.1236-06.2006.

12. Di Marzo V, Goparaju SK, Wang L, Liu J, Bátkai S, Járai Z, Fezza F, Miura GI, Palmiter RD, Sugiura T, Kunos G (April 2001). "Leptin-regulated endocannabinoids are involved in maintaining food intake". Nature. 410 (6830): 822–5. PMID 11298451. doi:10.1038/35071088.

13. Cravatt BF, et al. (July 2001). "Supersensitivity to anandamide and enhanced endogenous cannabinoid signaling in mice lacking fatty acid amide hydrolase". Proc. Natl. Acad. Sci. U.S.A. 98 (16): 9371–6. Bibcode:2001PNAS...98.9371C. JSTOR 3056353. PMC 55427 . PMID 11470906. doi:10.1073/pnas.161191698.

14. Flores A, Maldonado R, Berrendero F (2013). "Cannabinoid-hypocretin cross-talk in the central nervous system: what we know so far". Front Neurosci. 7: 256. PMC 3868890 . PMID 24391536. doi:10.3389/fnins.2013.00256. Direct CB1-HcrtR1 interaction was first proposed in 2003 (Hilairet et al., 2003). Indeed, a 100-fold increase in the potency of hypocretin-1 to activate the ERK signaling was observed when CB1 and HcrtR1 were co-expressed ... In this study, a higher potency of hypocretin-1 to regulate CB1-HcrtR1 heteromer compared with the HcrtR1-HcrtR1 homomer was reported (Ward et al., 2011b). These data provide unambiguous identification of CB1-HcrtR1 heteromerization, which has a substantial functional impact. ...

The existence of a cross-talk between the hypocretinergic and endocannabinoid systems is strongly supported by their partially overlapping anatomical distribution and common role in several physiological and pathological processes. However, little is known about the mechanisms underlying this interaction.

• Figure 1: Schematic of brain CB1 expression and orexinergic neurons expressing OX1 or OX2

• Figure 2: Synaptic signaling mechanisms in cannabinoid and orexin systems

• Figure 3: Schematic of brain pathways involved in food intake

15. Watkins BA, Kim J (2014). "The endocannabinoid system: helps to direct eating behavior and macronutrient metabolism". Front Psychol. 5: 1506. PMC 4285050 . PMID 25610411. doi:10.3389/fpsyg.2014.01506. CB1 is present in neurons of the enteric nervous system and in sensory terminals of vagal and spinal neurons in the gastrointestinal tract (Massa et al., 2005). Activation of CB1 is shown to modulate nutrient processing, such as gastric secretion, gastric emptying, and intestinal motility. ... CB1 is shown to co-localize with the food intake inhibiting neuropeptide, corticotrophin-releasing hormone, in the paraventricular nucleus of the hypothalamus, and with the two orexigenic peptides, melanin-concentrating hormone in the lateral hypothalamus and with pre-pro-orexin in the ventromedial hypothalamus (Inui, 1999; Horvath, 2003). CB1 knockout mice showed higher levels of CRH mRNA, suggesting that hypothalamic EC receptors are involved in energy balance and may be able to mediate food intake (Cota et al., 2003). ... The ECS works through many anorexigenic and orexigenic pathways where ghrelin, leptin, adiponectin, endogenous opioids, and corticotropin-releasing hormones are involved (Viveros et al., 2008).

16. Thompson MD, Xhaard H, Sakurai T, Rainero I, Kukkonen JP (2014). "OX1 and OX2 orexin/hypocretin receptor pharmacogenetics". Front Neurosci. 8: 57. PMC 4018553 . PMID 24834023. doi:10.3389/fnins.2014.00057. OX1–CB1 dimerization was suggested to strongly potentiate orexin receptor signaling, but a likely explanation for the signal potentiation is, instead, offered by the ability of OX1 receptor signaling to produce 2-arachidonoyl glycerol, a CB1 receptor ligand, and a subsequent co-signaling of the receptors (Haj-Dahmane and Shen, 2005; Turunen et al., 2012; Jäntti et al., 2013). However, this does not preclude dimerization.

17. Jäntti MH, Mandrika I, Kukkonen JP (2014). "Human orexin/hypocretin receptors form constitutive homo- and heteromeric complexes with each other and with human CB1 cannabinoid receptors". Biochem. Biophys. Res. Commun. 445 (2): 486–90. PMID 24530395. doi:10.1016/j.bbrc.2014.02.026. Orexin receptor subtypes readily formed homo- and hetero(di)mers, as suggested by significant BRET signals. CB1 receptors formed homodimers, and they also heterodimerized with both orexin receptors. ... In conclusion, orexin receptors have a significant propensity to make homo- and heterodi-/oligomeric complexes. However, it is unclear whether this affects their signaling. As orexin receptors efficiently signal via endocannabinoid production to CB1 receptors, dimerization could be an effective way of forming signal complexes with optimal cannabinoid concentrations available for cannabinoid receptors.

18.Pertwee RG (January 2008). "The diverse CB1 and CB2 receptor pharmacology of three plant cannabinoids: delta9-tetrahydrocannabinol, cannabidiol and delta9-tetrahydrocannabivarin". Br. J. Pharmacol. 153 (2): 199–215. PMC 2219532 . PMID 17828291. doi:10.1038/sj.bjp.0707442.

19. Elphick MR, Egertová M (March 2001). "The neurobiology and evolution of cannabinoid signalling". Philos. Trans. R. Soc. Lond., B, Biol. Sci. 356 (1407): 381–408. PMC 1088434 . PMID 11316486. doi:10.1098/rstb.2000.0787.

20. Puente N, Cui Y, Lassalle O, Lafourcade M, Georges F, Venance L, Grandes P, Manzoni OJ (December 2011). "Polymodal activation of the endocannabinoid system in the extended amygdala". Nat. Neurosci. 14 (12): 1542–7. PMID 22057189. doi:10.1038/nn.2974.

21. Ibrahim BM, Abdel-Rahman AA (2014). "Cannabinoid receptor 1 signaling in cardiovascular regulating nuclei in the brainstem: A review". J Adv Res. 5 (2): 137–45. PMC 4294710 . PMID 25685481. doi:10.1016/j.jare.2013.03.008.

22. Ibrahim BM, Abdel-Rahman AA (2015). "A pivotal role for enhanced brainstem Orexin receptor 1 signaling in the central cannabinoid receptor 1-mediated pressor response in conscious rats". Brain Res. 1622: 51–63. PMC 4562882 . PMID 26096126. doi:10.1016/j.brainres.2015.06.011. Orexin receptor 1 (OX1R) signaling is implicated in cannabinoid receptor 1 (CB1R) modulation of feeding. Further, our studies established the dependence of the central CB1R-mediated pressor response on neuronal nitric oxide synthase (nNOS) and extracellular signal-regulated kinase1/2 (ERK1/2)

phosphorylation in the RVLM. We tested the novel hypothesis that brainstem orexin-A/OX1R signaling plays a pivotal role in the central CB1R-mediated pressor response. Our multiple labeling immunofluorescence findings revealed co-localization of CB1R, OX1R and the peptide orexin-A within the C1 area of the rostral ventrolateral medulla (RVLM). Activation of central CB1R following intracisternal (i.c.) WIN55,212-2 (15μg/rat) in conscious rats caused significant increases in BP and orexin-A level in RVLM neuronal tissue. Additional studies established a causal role for orexin-A in the central CB1R-mediated pressor response

23. Okamoto Y, Morishita J, Tsuboi K, Tonai T, Ueda N (February 2004). "Molecular characterization of a phospholipase D generating anandamide and its congeners". J. Biol. Chem. 279 (7): 5298–305. PMID 14634025. doi:10.1074/jbc.M306642200.

24. Liu J, Wang L, Harvey-White J, Osei-Hyiaman D, Razdan R, Gong Q, Chan AC, Zhou Z, Huang BX, Kim HY, Kunos G (September 2006). "A biosynthetic pathway for anandamide". Proc. Natl. Acad. Sci. U.S.A. 103 (36): 13345–50. Bibcode:2006PNAS..10313345L. PMC 1557387 . PMID 16938887. doi:10.1073/pnas.0601832103.

25. Magotti P, Bauer I, Igarashi M, Babagoli M, Marotta R, Piomelli D, Garau G (2014). "Structure of Human N-Acylphosphatidylethanolamine-Hydrolyzing Phospholipase D: Regulation of Fatty Acid Ethanolamine Biosynthesis by Bile Acids". Structure. 23 (3): 598–604. PMC 4351732 . PMID 25684574. doi:10.1016/j.str.2014.12.018.

26. Leung D, Saghatelian A, Simon GM, Cravatt BF (April 2006). "Inactivation of N-acyl phosphatidylethanolamine phospholipase D reveals multiple mechanisms for the biosynthesis of endocannabinoids". Biochemistry. 45 (15): 4720–6. PMC 1538545 . PMID 16605240. doi:10.1021/bi0601631.

27. Pazos MR, Núñez E, Benito C, Tolón RM, Romero J (June 2005). "Functional neuroanatomy of the endocannabinoid system". Pharmacol. Biochem. Behav. 81(2): 239–47. PMID 15936805. doi:10.1016/j.pbb.2005.01.030.

28. Yamaguchi T, Shoyama Y, Watanabe S, Yamamoto T (January 2001). "Behavioral suppression induced by cannabinoids is due to activation of the arachidonic acid cascade in rats". Brain Res. 889 (1–2): 149–54. PMID 11166698. doi:10.1016/S0006-8993(00)03127-9.

29. Brock TG (December 2005). "Regulating leukotriene synthesis: the role of nuclear 5-lipoxygenase". J. Cell. Biochem. 96 (6): 1203–11. PMID 16215982. doi:10.1002/jcb.20662.

30. Clapper JR, Mangieri RA, Piomelli D (2009). "The endocannabinoid system as a target for the treatment of cannabis dependence". Neuropharmacology. 56(Suppl 1): 235–43. PMC 2647947 . PMID 18691603. doi:10.1016/j.neuropharm.2008.07.018.

31. Twitchell W, Brown S, Mackie K (1997). "Cannabinoids inhibit N- and P/Q-type calcium channels in cultured rat hippocampal neurons". J. Neurophysiol. 78 (1): 43–50. PMID 9242259.

32. Guo J, Ikeda SR (2004). "Endocannabinoids modulate N-type calcium channels and G-protein-coupled inwardly rectifying potassium channels via CB1 cannabinoid receptors heterologously expressed in mammalian neurons". Mol. Pharmacol. 65 (3): 665–74. PMID 14978245. doi:10.1124/mol.65.3.665.

33. Binzen U, Greffrath W, Hennessy S, Bausen M, Saaler-Reinhardt S, Treede RD (2006). "Co-expression of the voltage-gated potassium channel Kv1.4 with transient receptor potential channels (TRPV1 and TRPV2) and the cannabinoid receptor CB1 in rat dorsal root ganglion neurons". Neuroscience. 142 (2): 527–39. PMID 16889902. doi:10.1016/j.neuroscience.2006.06.020.

34. Freund TF, Katona I, Piomelli D (2003). "Role of endogenous cannabinoids in synaptic signaling". Physiol. Rev. 83 (3): 1017–66. PMID 12843414. doi:10.1152/physrev.00004.2003.

35. Chevaleyre V, Heifets BD, Kaeser PS, Südhof TC, Purpura DP, Castillo PE (2007). "ENDOCANNABINOID-MEDIATED LONG-TERM PLASTICITY REQUIRES cAMP/PKA SIGNALING AND RIM1α". Neuron. 54 (5): 801–12. PMC 2001295 . PMID 17553427. doi:10.1016/j.neuron.2007.05.020.

36. Bacci A, Huguenard JR, Prince DA (2004). "Long-lasting self-inhibition of neocortical interneurons mediated by endocannabinoids". Nature. 431 (7006): 312–6. Bibcode:2004Natur.431..312B. PMID 15372034. doi:10.1038/nature02913.

37. Hampson RE, Deadwyler SA (1999). "Cannabinoids, hippocampal function and memory". Life Sci. 65 (6–7): 715–23. PMID 10462072. doi:10.1016/S0024-3205(99)00294-5.

38. Pertwee RG (2001). "Cannabinoid receptors and pain". Prog. Neurobiol. 63(5): 569–611. PMID 11164622. doi:10.1016/S0301-0082(00)00031-9.

39. Jiang W, Zhang Y, Xiao L, Van Cleemput J, Ji SP, Bai G, Zhang X (2005). "Cannabinoids promote embryonic and adult hippocampus neurogenesis and produce anxiolytic- and antidepressant-like effects". J. Clin. Invest. 115 (11): 3104–16. PMC 1253627 . PMID 16224541. doi:10.1172/JCI25509.

40. Aguado T, Monory K, Palazuelos J, Stella N, Cravatt B, Lutz B, Marsicano G, Kokaia Z, Guzmán M, Galve-Roperh I (2005). "The endocannabinoid system drives neural progenitor proliferation". FASEB J. 19 (12): 1704–6. PMID 16037095. doi:10.1096/fj.05-3995fje.

41. Christie BR, Cameron HA (2006). "Neurogenesis in the adult hippocampus". Hippocampus. 16 (3): 199–207. PMID 16411231. doi:10.1002/hipo.20151.

42. Kirkham TC, Tucci SA (2006). "Endocannabinoids in appetite control and the treatment of obesity". CNS Neurol Disord Drug Targets. 5 (3): 272–92. PMID 16787229. doi:10.2174/187152706777452272.

43. Di Marzo V, Sepe N, De Petrocellis L, Berger A, Crozier G, Fride E, Mechoulam R (December 1998). "Trick or treat from food endocannabinoids?". Nature. 396(6712): 636–7. Bibcode:1998Natur.396..636D. PMID 9872309. doi:10.1038/25267.

44. De Luca MA, Solinas M, Bimpisidis Z, Goldberg SR, Di Chiara G (July 2012). "Cannabinoid facilitation of behavioral and biochemical hedonic taste responses". Neuropharmacology. 63 (1): 161–8. PMC 3705914 . PMID 22063718. doi:10.1016/j.neuropharm.2011.10.018.

45. Yoshida R, et al. (January 2010). "Endocannabinoids selectively enhance sweet taste". Proc. Natl. Acad. Sci. U.S.A. 107 (2): 935–9. Bibcode:2010PNAS..107..935Y. JSTOR 40535875. PMC 2818929 . PMID 20080779. doi:10.1073/pnas.0912048107.

46. Bellocchio L, Cervino C, Pasquali R, Pagotto U (June 2008). "The endocannabinoid system and energy metabolism". J. Neuroendocrinol. 20 (6): 850–7. PMID 18601709. doi:10.1111/j.1365-2826.2008.01728.x.

47. Hill MN, McLaughlin RJ, Bingham B, Shrestha L, Lee TT, Gray JM, Hillard CJ, Gorzalka BB, Viau V (May 2010). "Endogenous cannabinoid signaling is essential for stress adaptation". Proc. Natl. Acad. Sci. U.S.A. 107 (20): 9406–11.

Bibcode:2010PNAS..107.9406H. PMC 2889099 . PMID 20439721. doi:10.1073/pnas.0914661107.

48. Häring M, Kaiser N, Monory K, Lutz B (2011). Burgess HA, ed. "Circuit specific functions of cannabinoid CB1 receptor in the balance of investigatory drive and exploration". PLoS ONE. 6 (11): e26617. Bibcode:2011PLoSO...626617H. PMC 3206034 . PMID 22069458. doi:10.1371/journal.pone.0026617.

49. Basu S, Ray A, Dittel BN (December 2011). "Cannabinoid receptor 2 is critical for the homing and retention of marginal zone B lineage cells and for efficient T-independent immune responses". J. Immunol. 187 (11): 5720–32. PMC 3226756 . PMID 22048769. doi:10.4049/jimmunol.1102195.

50. Baker D, Pryce G, Croxford JL, Brown P, Pertwee RG, Huffman JW, Layward L (2000). "Cannabinoids control spasticity and tremor in a multiple sclerosis model". Nature. 404 (6773): 84–7. PMID 10716447. doi:10.1038/35003583.

51. Baker D, Pryce G, Croxford JL, Brown P, Pertwee RG, Makriyannis A, Khanolkar A, Layward L, Fezza F, Bisogno T, Di Marzo V (2001). "Endocannabinoids control spasticity in a multiple sclerosis model". FASEB J. 15(2): 300–2. PMID 11156943. doi:10.1096/fj.00-0399fje.

52. Cabranes A, Pryce G, Baker D, Fernández-Ruiz J (August 2006). "Changes in CB1 receptors in motor-related brain structures of chronic relapsing experimental allergic encephalomyelitis mice". Brain Res. 1107 (1): 199–205. PMID 16822488. doi:10.1016/j.brainres.2006.06.001.

53. Carrier EJ, Kearn CS, Barkmeier AJ, Breese NM, Yang W, Nithipatikom K, Pfister SL, Campbell WB, Hillard CJ (April 2004). "Cultured rat microglial cells synthesize the endocannabinoid 2-arachidonylglycerol, which increases proliferation via a CB2 receptor-dependent mechanism". Mol. Pharmacol. 65 (4): 999–1007. PMID 15044630. doi:10.1124/mol.65.4.999.

54. Maccarrone M, Valensise H, Bari M, Lazzarin N, Romanini C, Finazzi-Agrò A (2000). "Relation between decreased anandamide hydrolase concentrations in human lymphocytes and miscarriage". Lancet. 355 (9212): 1326–9. PMID 10776746. doi:10.1016/S0140-6736(00)02115-2.

55. Das SK, Paria BC, Chakraborty I, Dey SK (1995). "Cannabinoid ligand-receptor signaling in the mouse uterus". Proc. Natl. Acad. Sci. U.S.A. 92 (10): 4332–6. Bibcode:1995PNAS...92.4332D. PMC 41938 . PMID 7753807. doi:10.1073/pnas.92.10.4332.

56. Paria BC, Das SK, Dey SK (1995). "The preimplantation mouse embryo is a target for cannabinoid ligand-receptor signaling". Proc. Natl. Acad. Sci. U.S.A. 92 (21): 9460–4. Bibcode:1995PNAS...92.9460P. PMC 40821 . PMID 7568154. doi:10.1073/pnas.92.21.9460.

57. Hesselink JM (2012). "New Targets in Pain, Non-Neuronal Cells, and the Role of Palmitoylethanolamide". The Open Pain Journal. 5 (1): 12–23. doi:10.2174/1876386301205010012.

58. Colloca, Luana (2013-08-28). Placebo and Pain: From Bench to Bedside (1st ed.). Elsevier Science. pp. 11–12. ISBN 9780123979315.

59. Ross RA (November 2003). "Anandamide and vanilloid TRPV1 receptors". Br. J. Pharmacol. 140 (5): 790–801. PMC 1574087 . PMID 14517174. doi:10.1038/sj.bjp.0705467.

60. Huang SM, Bisogno T, Trevisani M, Al-Hayani A, De Petrocellis L, Fezza F, Tognetto M, Petros TJ, Krey JF, Chu CJ, Miller JD, Davies SN, Geppetti P, Walker JM, Di Marzo V (June 2002). "An endogenous capsaicin-like substance with high potency at recombinant and native vanilloid VR1 receptors". Proc. Natl. Acad. Sci. U.S.A. 99 (12): 8400–5. Bibcode:2002PNAS...99.8400H. PMC 123079 . PMID 12060783. doi:10.1073/pnas.122196999.

61. Murillo-Rodríguez E, Sánchez-Alavez M, Navarro L, Martínez-González D, Drucker-Colín R, Prospéro-García O (November 1998). "Anandamide modulates sleep and memory in rats". Brain Res. 812 (1–2): 270–4. PMID 9813364. doi:10.1016/S0006-8993(98)00969-X.

62. Santucci V, Storme JJ, Soubrié P, Le Fur G (1996). "Arousal-enhancing properties of the CB1 cannabinoid receptor antagonist SR 141716A in rats as assessed by electroencephalographic spectral and sleep-waking cycle analysis". Life Sci. 58 (6): PL103–10. PMID 8569415. doi:10.1016/0024-3205(95)02319-4.

63. Wang L, Yang T, Qian W, Hou X (January 2011). "The role of endocannabinoids in visceral hyposensitivity induced by rapid eye movement sleep deprivation in rats: regional differences". Int. J. Mol. Med. 27 (1): 119–26. PMID 21057766. doi:10.3892/ijmm.2010.547.

64. Murillo-Rodriguez E, Désarnaud F, Prospéro-García O (May 2006). "Diurnal variation of arachidonoylethanolamine, palmitoylethanolamide and oleoylethanolamide in the brain of the rat". Life Sci. 79 (1): 30–7. PMID 16434061. doi:10.1016/j.lfs.2005.12.028.

65. Ravinet Trillou C, Delgorge C, Menet C, Arnone M, Soubrié P (2004). "CB1 cannabinoid receptor knockout in mice leads to leanness, resistance to diet-induced obesity and enhanced leptin sensitivity". Int. J. Obes. Relat. Metab. Disord. 28 (4): 640–8. PMID 14770190. doi:10.1038/sj.ijo.0802583.

66. Varvel SA, Lichtman AH (2002). "Evaluation of CB1 receptor knockout mice in the Morris water maze". J. Pharmacol. Exp. Ther. 301 (3): 915–24. PMID 12023519. doi:10.1124/jpet.301.3.915.

67. Niyuhire F, Varvel SA, Martin BR, Lichtman AH (2007). "Exposure to marijuana smoke impairs memory retrieval in mice". J. Pharmacol. Exp. Ther. 322 (3): 1067–75. PMID 17586723. doi:10.1124/jpet.107.119594.

68. Parmentier R, Ohtsu H, Djebbara-Hannas Z, Valatx JL, Watanabe T, Lin JS (September 2002). "Anatomical, physiological, and pharmacological characteristics of histidine decarboxylase knockout mice: evidence for the role of brain histamine in behavioral and sleep-wake control". J. Neurosci. 22 (17): 7695–711. PMID 12196593.

69. Marsicano G, Goodenough S, Monory K, Hermann H, Eder M, Cannich A, Azad SC, Cascio MG, Gutiérrez SO, van der Stelt M, López-Rodriguez ML, Casanova E, Schütz G, Zieglgänsberger W, Di Marzo V, Behl C, Lutz B (October 2003). "CB1 cannabinoid receptors and on-demand defense against excitotoxicity". Science. 302 (5642): 84–8. Bibcode:2003Sci...302...84M. PMID 14526074. doi:10.1126/science.1088208.

Further reading[edit]

• Neumeister A, Normandin MD, Pietrzak RH, Piomelli D, Zheng MQ, Gujarro-Anton A, Potenza MN, Bailey CR, Lin SF, Najafzadeh S, Ropchan J, Henry S, Corsi-Travali S, Carson RE, Huang Y (2013). "Elevated brain cannabinoid CB1 receptor availability in post-traumatic stress disorder: A positron emission tomography study". Molecular Psychiatry. 18 (9): 1034–40. PMC 3752332 . PMID 23670490. doi:10.1038/mp.2013.61. Lay summary – ScienceDaily(May 14, 2013).

• Földy C, Malenka RC, Südhof TC (May 2013). "Autism-associated neuroligin-3 mutations commonly disrupt tonic endocannabinoid signaling". Neuron. 78(3): 498–509. PMC 3663050 . PMID 23583622. doi:10.1016/j.neuron.2013.02.036. Lay summary – ScienceDaily (April 11, 2013).

• Puighermanal E, Marsicano G, Busquets-Garcia A, Lutz B, Maldonado R, Ozaita A (September 2009). "Cannabinoid modulation of hippocampal long-term memory is mediated by mTOR signaling". Nat. Neurosci. 12 (9): 1152–8. PMID 19648913. doi:10.1038/nn.2369. Lay summary – ScienceDaily (August 4, 2009).

• Niehaus JL, Liu Y, Wallis KT, Egertová M, Bhartur SG, Mukhopadhyay S, Shi S, He H, Selley DE, Howlett AC, Elphick MR, Lewis DL (December 2007). "CB1 cannabinoid receptor activity is modulated by the cannabinoid receptor interacting protein CRIP 1a". Mol. Pharmacol. 72 (6): 1557–66. PMID 17895407. doi:10.1124/mol.107.039263. Lay summary – ScienceDaily (November 30, 2007).

CHAPTER 25
MTHFR—
THE METHYLATION EQUATION

The Human Genome Project was started in 1990 and completed in 2003. It produced an overwhelmingly expansive treasure trove of new information on the role genetics play, and it ventured into a neoteric frontier of understanding with regard to the make-up and function of our DNA sequencing. This project constitutes one of the greatest scientific accomplishments and human achievements of all time, the implications of which are vast and boundless. To date we have only begun to scratch the surface when it comes to understanding all of the data yielded. This research is the progenitor of the now emerging field of science (and medicine) known as '**Epigenetics**,' which seeks to understand and control gene expression in order to improve our life-span and reverse chronic illnesses. (I'm sure the next book will have a chapter on this as new therapies become available! In the meantime, the reader is invited to read the very well-written book: **The Epigenetics Revolution** by Nessa Carey in order to grasp the basic science behind how it all works.)

One of the key discoveries that surfaced as result of the HGP is a genetic defect known as the MTHFR Mutation. There is a lot of complicated biochemistry (which we we'll skip for now) involved, but one of the main manifestations of having this mutated sequence is the inability for the body to make the proper form of folate, i.e. 5-

methyltetrahydrofolate (*not* folic acid**), which leads to a folate deficiency. The mutation also either partially hinders or outright subverts the methylation process that converts vitamins like B6 and B12 into usable form. The effects of deficient levels of folate (vitamin B9), B6, and B12 are well known, including everything from impaired cognitive function/neurotransmitter production to sluggish digestion, poor sleep, low sex drive and eventually lead to chronic health conditions like coronary heart disease, migraines, IBS and many others. But the one we wish to most specifically address in this chapter is **Pernicious Anemia**, which occurs when the body cannot make enough healthy red blood cells by way of not having enough B12.

Often times patients will be initially diagnosed with 'true' anemia after a basic iron panel (serum iron, ferritin, transferrin, total iron binding capacity) is run and their levels are found to be insufficient. Anemia is technically the accurate diagnosis here, but it isn't true anemia, it is an 'indirect' anemia—the patient actually has enough iron in their system, however they are *unable to use* that iron to produce things like ferritin and hemoglobin (oxygen-transport protein in red blood cells) because of a B12/Folate deficiency as a result of the genetic methylation issue. Unfortunately, this still often goes misdiagnosed and the patient is simply given a prescription for more iron (in the form of ferrous sulfate or ferrous gluconate). This is a band-aid at best and eventually over-burdens the liver and gastro-intestinal tract with the damaging effects of too much dietary iron. Conversely, if patients are properly diagnosed, they can be given adequate folate/ B12 and their iron/ferritin/transferrin/TIBC levels can be returned to normal over time, thus effectively absolving them of anemia altogether in many cases.

Fortunately, more and more practitioners (both holistic and allopathic) are being made aware of the simple blood tests available to determine whether a patient is B12/Folate deficient, and more importantly of the simple (genetic) blood test available to determine if a patient has the MTHFR mutation(s).

Testing, proper diagnosing, and plenty of B12/B6/Folate— got it! So tell us, what else do we need to know if we are practitioners treating patients for this condition? (Glad you asked!)

Details. The devil is *always* in the details and this issue is a prime example:

1. The MTHFR mutation presents at two different genes: **C677T** and **A1298C**. The lab test you run should include *both*.

2. Some patients will have neither, some patients will have one, some patients will have both. For each of these two gene mutations, a patient can present as either *heterozygous* or *homozygous*, meaning a patient can have either a single copy of a gene (from one parent), or they could be unfortunate enough to have inherited two copies (from both parents), respectively. If a patient is homozygous, they typically suffer more pronounced symptoms than heterozygous patients. If a patient ends up being homozygous for both the C677T *and* A1298C, well then they've been dealt an unlucky hand and will likely require the most effort supplementally to alleviate their condition.

3. The **proper form** of vitamin therapy is of the utmost importance to address this issue. Most doctors are only familiar with the prescribable/over-the-counter form of B12 known as *cyanocobalamin*, whether it's injectable or an oral supplement. This is the synthetic form, and for patients with the genetic mutation, it's utterly useless. Let's examine why that is:

    The liver has to convert *cyanocobalamin* up two steps in the pathway in order for it to be a usable form of vitamin B12. It converts it first from cyano-cobalamin to *hydroxy-cobalamin*. (Hydroxycobalamin is the form we naturally encounter from eating fruits and vegetables.) From *hydroxycobalamin,* the liver then has to 'methylate' it into the final usable form known as **methylcobalamin**. Therein lies the core of the issue. These patients do not have the ability to 'methylate' properly, therefore they cannot use the (synthetic) cyano- or the (food-sourced) hydroxy- very effectively. We as holistic practitioners order (through compounding pharmacies all around the nation) the injectable form of *methylcobalamin,* and it is typically the only form we administer. (Why not use the best even for regular patients?)

The methyl B12 is then administered to the patient via an intramuscular injection or in an intravenous solution known as a "Myer's Cocktail" (which also contains other water-soluble vitamins and minerals). Since the methyl B12 is pre-methylated and is also by-passing digestive absorption en route directly into the bloodstream, nothing is lost/wasted in either digestion or conversion, ensuring that the patient receives and uptakes nearly 100% of the dose.

4. The proper dosage/frequency of Methyl-B12 for MTHFR mutation patients, especially those with pernicious anemia, constitutes a significant increase over the exogenous/sup-plemental requirement of regular patients. P.A. patients are constantly depleting their reserves and are unable to replenish them dietarily. Furthermore, all water soluble vitamins (vitamin C and B vitamins) more or less fully metabolize in the human body in approximately 3 to 4 days, and it is virtually impossible to overdose on them (the kidneys pass whatever the body doesn't use). So to ensure a patient with pernicious anemia is adequately covered, the *optimal solution is to give them a Methyl B12 (2mg/ml)*

injection every 3 days at the minimum. (Regular doctor's offices typically only prescribe B12 injections—it being synthetic cyanocobalamin at that—at a maximum of once a month, which is woefully inadequate.) We've seen dramatic improvements in literally every single pernicious anemia patient we've treated at the twice a week Methyl B12 dosage. (We've also had a few severe cases where the patients showed an even greater improvement at a 3x a week dosage.)

The other important new piece of information is that Methylcobalamin is interconverted back and forth at a cellular level into **Adenosylcobalamin**. Both forms are converted from hydroxycobalamin and are co-enzymes of each other, used to facilitate different functions. (Methylcobalamin is found in the cytosol of cells and predominates in blood/other fluids, whereas Adenosylcobalamin is the major form of B12 stored in the mitochondria of cellular tissues.) Adenosyl B12 is not yet available in injectable form, however it is available in oral supplementation. *We've been able to achieve the best results/ optimal patient outcomes by combining both forms (methyl and adenosyl) into our therapies along with the 5-MTHF form of folate.*

The best oral formula we've found so far for our pernicious anemia patients is "**Methyl Protect**" by Xymogen. It contains 25mg of Riboflavin (as riboflavin 5'-phosphate sodium), 10mg of B6 (as pyroxidal 5'-phosphate), Folate (1mg as calcium folinate and 1mg as 5-MTHF), 1mg of B12 (methylcobalamin), and 500mg of trimethylglycine. We also have the patient separately take one capsule (2mg) of the **Adenosyl B12/Hydroxy B12** product by Pure Encapsulations.

Lastly, if a patient truly is iron deficient—whether they have pernicious anemia or regular anemia—we recommend a product called **Hema-Plex**, which has a pre-chelated iron complex. This form is much gentler on the stomach lining, doesn't cause constipation, and has enhanced absorption as compared to the standard ferrous sulfate or ferrous gluconate forms.

** (As a side note, it is necessary to mention that 'folic acid' is synthetic and should not be taken. It's very poorly converted into a usable form by humans and recent studies have linked it to the proliferation of certain types of cancer. It can also cause the symptom(s) suffered by patients with the MTHFR mutation to be compounded. The proper form of folate supplementation is the 5-MTHF, i.e. 'methyl folate' form.)

Once again the details mean *everything*.

CHAPTER 26

PARASITES, CANDIDA, MIGRAINES, DIABETES, AND ASTHMA

You probably looked at the title of this chapter and thought something to the effect of 'what strange bedfellows', is this the leftover or miscellaneous section? And who could blame you? Rest assured that it's not, and that there can be, and often is, an interrelation, correlation, and sometimes, causation amongst these disease states. Let's address each one individually, and see what type of helpful information we can come up with, shall we?

Parasites. For some reason, when this word is uttered, it often conjures stereotypical images of third-world countries with terrible living conditions, or it reminds us of that crazy aunt we all have who has 12 cats and is convinced that she has millions of bugs crawling under her skin (when really it's just the *toxoplasmosis* burrowing into her brain).

That is not what is being referenced here. I personally was blessed with the good fortune of having an amazing Anatomy/Physiology teacher when I was in college. For some reason (that I don't remember), she had an extensive background and interest in the field of parasitology. Much to my benefit (but chagrin at the time), she somehow managed to shoehorn a ton of information about parasitology *on top* of the already existing curriculum that we were required to learn for A&P. I'm not really sure what the deal was with that or how it reconciled with learning the basic structure(s) of anatomy/physiology, but dammit it was important to her so we had to learn it anyways. May I just pause for a moment and laugh at how the Universe has a funny way of helping us out *if* we are simply willing to *listen* and *receive* what it has for us. Nothing happens by coincidence. Not too many years later this information *saved my life* as well as many of my patients and a few family/friends. (I'll describe how at the end of the chapter.) I won't mention her last name for privacy reasons, but Theresa, wherever you are out there, thank you from my entire being for teaching us about parasitology *in an A&P class*. You have no idea the impact you ended up having on me, and untold countless others. I hope I can somehow repay that benefit in some small way by passing on that valuable wisdom and teaching to others via this book and whatever other opportunities present themselves.

Let's begin the lesson.

Parasites/Parasitology

We all have them. It's perfectly normal, they co-exist in harmony with us like so many millions of harmless viruses and bacteria, and they have done so for all of human history. Some of them are beneficial and some of them aren't. It's nothing to be squeamish about, and it can't be avoided (sorry to any germ-a-phobes out there, hopefully this type of stuff doesn't keep you up at night.) If you've every walked barefoot in the grass, you have them. If you've ever played with a dog, swam in a lake, or eaten sushi or pork you have them. If you haven't lived your life in a sterile containment field, you have them.

But something in the last 50 to 60 years has changed, and it's drastically altered our relationship with common parasites. Before we talk about what's changed, let's understand their life cycle first. For the sake of getting to the point and instead of boring you with the overly-complicated intricacies of the developmental stages of all the different types of common parasites, let's simplify it here:

Think of the life cycle of a butterfly. Everyone is familiar with that…Caterpillar→Cocoon→Adult Butterfly. A lot of parasite life cycles are the same way, but some of them can have either 4, 5, or 6 life stages within the cycle instead of just 3. For all of human history, our immune systems have managed them pretty well, and certain species typically only live *very specific stages of their* life cycles within the human body, before they are passed by the liver/kidneys out of the body via excrement, and make their way into the next host, be it a snail or frog or whatever. Easy enough right? So what's changed?

In the past 50 or 60 years, humans have introduced a whole new world of endocrine and micro-biome disrupting compounds, most of which we've already touched on in both the cancer chapter and the endocrine chapter. So, whether it's by way of hairspray, parabens, triclosan, iso-propyl alcohol, food additives, or thousands of other potentially disruptive synthetic chemicals, those endocrine, metabolic, and cellular disruptions don't just affect us, i.e. the *host*. It also affects the life cycle and hormonal signaling of the common (and sometimes not so common) parasites within us. We've entered into a heretofore unknown realm of (normally) harmless parasites suddenly becoming harmful because they behave differently or prematurely go into the next life stage; whereas in centuries past, they would have left our bodies long before they matured, laid eggs, or performed whatever other stage-specific action(s) they normally only carry out *after* they've left us as human hosts.

On the other side of the coin we have the parasites who were already somewhat harmful to begin with, now becoming more harmful and migrating to organs they don't normally migrate to, excessively proliferating/over-infesting due to the 'steroid' effect, or creating more cystic formations/bio-films, or even dying prematurely and exposing us unnecessary toxin release. Combine this with the candida yeast/fungal epidemic we now deal with in western culture from (gluten-induced) leaky gut, over-prescribing of anti-biotics, and the massive over-consumption of sugar, and suddenly we have a lot of minor 'bugs' turning into major problems...so much so that many people are being treated with medications for diseases they don't actually have. This occurs when someone presents with symptoms commonly associated with a particular disease, when in reality they just have an overblown parasite infection (examples include certain forms of asthma, migraines, and diabetes) that can be easily remedied, *permanently*. We'll talk more about that shortly.

We just mentioned **Candida**. A lot of people have heard of it but don't know what it is. It is a particular type of fungus/yeast, and it goes hand-in-hand with parasites. A small amount of it in our gut is perfectly normal, we all have it. What happens is another case of a relatively minor thing over-proliferating, going systemic, and becoming harmful. It's a well-known side effect that, after completing a course of anti-biotics, patients often come down with a yeast infection, (oral) thrush, or full-blown systemic **candidiasis**. This can also open the door to other opportunistic fungal co-infections like the tinea (ring worm, jock itch, athlete's foot) fungus. Anti-biotics compromise our immune systems by killing off the good bacteria in our guts, which normally keep fungal forms like candida at bay. Candida thrives on sugar, and in order to sustain itself when it goes systemic, it begins to manipulate biochemical reactions that make you the *host* crave sugar much more than you normally would. Additionally, candida, once it has left the gut and gone systemic in the bloodstream, has the ability to form a chitinous-like shell/biofilm around itself so that it can further resist the immune response trying to kill it, and it becomes more resilient against anti-fungal medications. So how do we get rid of this two-headed spectre of parasite/candida systemic overload? Glad you asked! It's time for a parasite/candida cleanse. I personally do one of these once a year preventatively, and it has served me and countless patients quite well. Again, I'm not a germ-a-phobe...I'll pick up a piece of food I dropped off the floor and eat it (5-second rule!) and I'm not paranoid about things crawling under my skin (hell, I play with leeches!). But despite the stereotypes of this being considered a 'fringe' element of medicine, it would actually greatly serve us, reduce health-care costs dramatically, and ease a lot of various symptomology if they simply made a parasitology class required curriculum at every med school. I would venture to say that any western/allopathic doctor who happens to be a parasitologist would agree with me. Onward to the cleanse shall we?

Years ago, it would have been necessary to source a bunch of individual anthelmintic (anti-parasite) herbs/ingredients from a local herb shop or get them online to do this cleanse. But now we have an excellent practitioner-grade formula from Apex Energetics called **G.I. Synergy**:

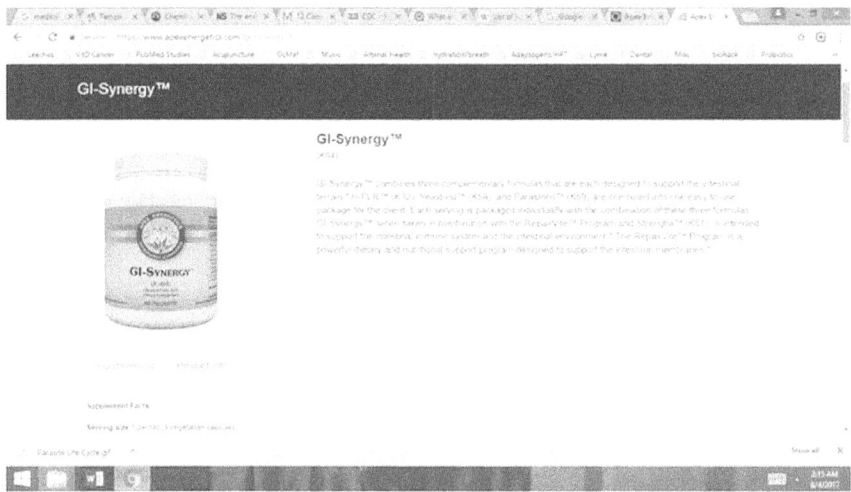

GI-Synergy (k64) Facts: 1 packet (3 vegetarian capsules) contain: **Proprietary Blend:** 2200 mg
- Wormwood Extract (leaf)
- Black Walnut Extract (hull)
- Undecylenic Acid (as calcium undecylenate)
- Caprylic Acid (as magnesium caprylate)
- Barberry Extract (root) (Berberis vulgaris
- Berberis aristata)

- Olive Extract (leaf) (standardized to 18% oleuropein)
- Garlic Extract (bulb) (standardized to 1% allicin)
- Uva Ursi Extract (leaf) (standardized to 20% arbutin)
- Cat's Claw Extract (bark) (standardized to 3% oxindole alkaloids)
- Pau D'Arco Extract (bark)
- Goldenseal Extract (root)
- Oregano Extract (leaf)
- Oregon Grape extract (root)
- Chinese Goldthread Extract (root)
- Yerba Mansa Extract (leaf).

Also contains: Vegetarian capsule (HPMC). Contains Walnut (black walnut hull extract).

This is the main parasite cleanse formula, and we combine it with one other ingredient (*from Lauricidin.com*):

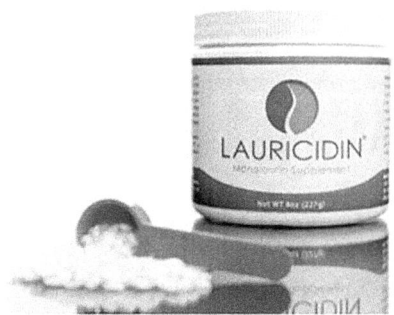

Lauricidin (monolaurin) is a concentrated coconut oil extract. It has very powerful anti-fungal properties to it and is the only thing we have found that can effectively break down the chitinous shell/biofilm that systemic candida encapsulates itself with. It also is beneficial towards the parasite cleanse and towards improving general immune function.

Our tried and true cleanse is as follows:

- GI Synergy—1 packet 3x a day for **30 days**

- Lauricidin (monolaurin)—1 teaspoonful 3x a day for **30 days**

- If patients are experiencing a *severe* overgrowth of candida, we will give them a series of 3 Fluconazole IV's (anti-fungal medication) over the course of 6 days, beginning concurrently with the start of the cleanse (If Fluconazole IV's are not available then you can substitute a 10-day prescription of Fluconazole 200mg tablets (one daily):

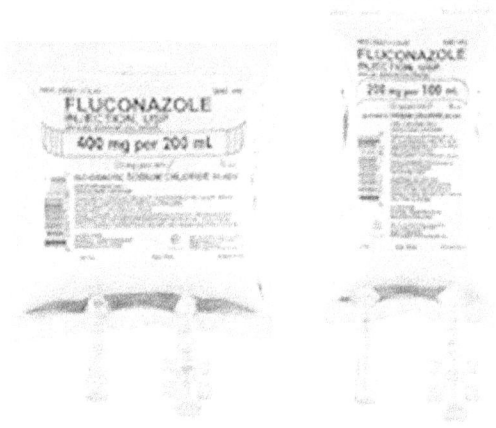

- If the patient is suffering from *severe* overgrowth of tinea fungus (ringworm, athletes foot, jock itch), you can prescribe a 30-day course of Terbinafine 250mg tablets (one daily) to be begun concurrently with the parasite cleanse. This anti-fungal med is a tad harsh on the liver, so be sure to monitor the patient for elevated liver enzymes and/or any minor side effects. (At the completion of the course of Terbinafine, we typically have the patient do a series of 2 to 3 IV Glutathione infusions to detox the liver from any drug residue/stress.) Lamisil (terbinafine) cream can concurrently be applied topically to the infected area(s) during the cleanse.

- The patient is to eliminate simple sugars (junk food, starchy carbs, high-glycemic fruits), gluten (all bread products), and preferably dairy and alcohol from the diet for the entire 30 days, and stay extra hydrated.

- It may be necessary to ease into the cleanse at a slower rate if the patient begins to experience what is known as a **Herxheimer** reaction, also known as a 'die-off' reaction. As heavy loads of parasites/candida are killed off, it is not uncommon for a 1 or 2-degree fever, and to experience mild flu-like symptoms like body aches, sore throat, joint/muscle pain, low-energy, etc. If these symptoms become too much for the patient, you may initially have to drop back to 2 or even 1 dose a day of the parasite herbs for the first few days of the cleanse.

- It is also beneficial to add in a powerful probiotic to restore the balance of the gut flora once the candida/parasites have been eliminated. Our favorite one to date is **Primal Defense Ultra** by Garden of Life, which not only re-populates the microbiome, but actively shields (via saccharomyces) against reinfection of candida. The entirety of all this is what we call a *permanent* solution. So many patients struggle mightily with reoccurring/chronic candida infections and can't seem to get any help from their primary care physicians, who *may* write them an Rx for a single fluconazole tablet. As practitioners, we must do better than that, and address the entire issue—i.e. grasp the scope of the actual problem, educate the patient to the fullest extent possible, correct the dietary component and any other underlying root causes, and then successfully help the body *heal itself* and *rid itself* of the chronic infection, *permanently*.

Diabetes (Type II)

To be entirely honest, we happened upon the improvement (and sometimes outright reversal) in this condition by sheer accident, and then did some more research (into eastern remedies) and found out what was actually happening. We had several patients over the years come into the clinic for help with candida/parasites who also happened to be Type II (adult onset) Diabetic. Upon completion of the 30-day parasite cleanse, they were highly shocked (as were we) at how drastically their diabetic symptoms had improved. (Many of these patients were on high doses of rapid acting insulin (Humalog/Novolog), short-acting insulin (Humulin/Novolin), or long-acting insulin (Lantus, Levemir) to help control their diabetes in tandem with oral drugs like Metformin which are used to help control blood sugar levels. They would often have to check their blood sugar 5 to 6 times a day in severe cases.) After the 30 days, several of them were dumbfounded...they would keep checking their blood sugar throughout the day and it was *self-regulating* again. Patients that were on large amounts of short and long acting insulin were able to completely drop out their short acting insulin, and cut back significantly on their long-acting insulin, to roughly *one-fourth* the amount they were prescribed. Many other patients who used only moderate amounts of insulin were able to ***completely discontinue the insulin altogether*** and either stick with just the Metformin or discontinue diabetic medicine outright.

So what the heck happened here? Well, it is a little-known morsel of information that virtually 100% (as in, every single one of them that has ever been tested) of Type-II diabetics have a common fluke parasite, Eurytrema pancreaticum. This is more widely known as a pancreatic fluke (commonly found in cattle). Conventional medicine considers this a rare type of infection for humans to have, but then again they don't often test for it either. (If they did, they wouldn't consider it rare anymore.) With the increase in exposure to environmental toxins like methanol (methyl alcohol) and certain other ingredients (mostly discussed in the cancer chapter) that have disruptive metabolic properties, pancreatic fluke infections are now much more prevalent in humans. During an infection, the pancreatic duct can become inflamed/enlarged. In cases of heavy organ saturation/infestation, the duct can get completely blocked (full occlusion) and the pancreatic tissues can suffer damage. The pancreas has tiny clusters of cells called the **islets of Langerhans**. These specialized groups of cells produce and **secrete insulin** (as well as the opposing hormone, glucagon) when needed. If the pancreas itself is damaged/infested/occluded/inflamed and stressed to its limits, that generally means that it is going to have a reduced/diminished capacity (via the islets of Langerhans) to produce insulin, and possibly lose that ability outright.

But an astonishing thing happens when you do a hardcore parasite cleanse and purge the pancreas of the flukes...you see, the human body is a remarkably resilient and incredibly well-engineered machine. Remove the *distractor*, remove the parasites, and in many patients the islets of Langerhans start to come back online and regain their ability to produce insulin. The pancreas begins to heal and regain function and throttles back up to optimal capacity. **We didn't 'cure' diabetes** (the word 'cure' is rather stale and inaccurate anyways), what we did was *remove the distractor*, give the patient the support they needed, and ***the body began to heal itself***. Cool stuff. Really, really cool.

(As an additional side note, we've found that using the *Bemer* for pulsed emf/ micro-circulatory therapy has also significantly improved diabetic symptoms like poor circulation and diabetic neuropathy.)

Ok so what's next on the list? **Asthma**—this paragraph doesn't need to be nearly as long because it would be pretty similar to the last one. Transient (usually helminth worm) parasites that end up in the lungs can cause an immune response that tries to contain these foreign invaders being somewhere they shouldn't be. Do a parasite cleanse and often times asthma (as well as allergy) symptoms are drastically reduced, if not outright eliminated. We've been blessed to see this occur in many of our (previously) asthmatic patients. To once again clarify, we *didn't cure asthma, we helped the body heal itself by removing a distractor.* Here is a 2010 study published by the University of Pennsylvania that clearly articulates the science behind this phenomenon.

Immune cells that fight parasites may promote allergies and asthma

Date: March 12, 2010
Source: University of Pennsylvania
reprinted with permission

Summary:
Millions of people in both the developing and developed world may benefit from new immune-system research findings that identify a cell population that fights off parasitic infections but also causes allergies and asthma.

Millions of people in both the developing and developed world may benefit from new immune-system research findings from the University of Pennsylvania School of Veterinary Medicine.

The Penn Vet researchers, studying how the immune system operates, have discovered a previously unidentified cell population that may be the body's double-edged sword, fighting off parasitic infections but also causing the harmful immune responses that can lead to allergies and asthma.

This cell population, termed multipotent progenitor cells, or MPP, appears to be activated in the context of allergies or infection with parasitic worms and may be one of the earliest cellular events in the developing immune response. The research published by David Artis, assistant professor in the Department of Pathobiology at Penn Vet, and colleagues may identify an important process in the immune response to helminth parasites and allergies.

A better understanding of what regulates the development of this cell population and what promotes its activation and function may aid in the development of drugs.

The research could benefit two patient populations: Those in developing countries still wrestling with parasitic worm infections and those in more industrialized environments where parasites are less prevalent but where immune responses can run amok, leading to a higher prevalence of allergies and asthma.

Millions worldwide struggle with health problems due to parasitic worms. These helminth worm parasites thrive in unsanitary conditions, in uncooked meat and in contaminated water. In more sanitary regions with fewer helminth parasites, the immune response that evolved to fight these infections may be redundant. It has been proposed that, due to reduced exposure to helminth parasites, the inactive immune response may inappropriately respond to substances like pollen, pollutants and some contents of food, resulting in exaggerated rates of asthma and allergy.

The National Institutes of Health estimates that as many as 40 to 50 million Americans suffer from allergic diseases. Consistent with this theory of redundancy, there are reports that show equatorial regions with an abundance of helminth parasites have populations that encounter lower rates of asthma and allergies.

"From an evolutionary perspective, it is likely that we evolved a complex immune response to fight parasitic worms, but our more sanitized environment no longer has this same population of parasites," Artis said. "This newly identified cell population could represent one of the earliest events in this type of immune response, which offers potential new targets for treatment of infection and allergic inflammation."

The research team demonstrated that a molecule called IL25, a member of the IL17 cytokine family, promotes the accumulation of a lineage-negative multipotent progenitor cell population in the intestine that promotes T cell responses associated with asthma and helminth infection. The resulting cell population gives rise to cells of macrophage and granulocyte lineages. The ability of IL25 to induce the emergence of an MPP cell population identifies a link between the IL17 cytokine family and extramedullary haematopoiesis and suggests a previously unrecognized innate immune pathway that promotes TH2 cytokine responses at mucosal sites.

The study, published in the current issue of *Nature*, was conducted by Artis, Steven A. Saenz, Mark C. Siracusa, Jacqueline G. Perrigoue and Sean P. Spencer of the Department of Pathobiology at Penn; Taku Kambayashi and Avinash Bhandoola of the Department of Pathology and Laboratory Medicine at Penn; Joseph F. Urban Jr. of the U.S. Department of Agriculture; Joel E. Tocker and Alison L. Budelsky of the Department of Inflammation Research at Amgen; and Melanie A. Kleinschek and Robert A. Kastelein of Discovery Research at Schering-Plough Biopharma.

The research was funded by the National Institutes of Health, the Burroughs Wellcome Fund, a National Institute of Diabetes and Digestive Kidney Disease Center Grant and the University of Pennsylvania.

Tocker and Budelsky are stockholding employees of Amgen. Kleinschek and Kastelein are employees of Schering-Plough Biopharma, a subsidiary of Merck & Co. Inc.

Story Source:
Materials provided by University of Pennsylvania. Note: Content may be edited for style and length.

Journal Reference:
1. Steven A. Saenz, Mark C. Siracusa, Jacqueline G. Perrigoue, Sean P. Spencer, Joseph F. Urban Jr, Joel E. Tocker, Alison L. Budelsky, Melanie A. Kleinschek, Robert A. Kastelein, Taku Kambayashi, Avinash Bhandoola & David Artis. IL25 elicits a multipotent progenitor cell population that promotes TH2 cytokine responses. Nature, 2010; DOI: 10.1038/nature08901

Cite This Page:
University of Pennsylvania. "Immune cells that fight parasites may promote allergies and asthma." ScienceDaily. ScienceDaily, 12 March 2010. <www.sciencedaily.com/releases/2010/03/10031113175 8.htm>.

Migraines

I personally have had the very good fortune to be healthy in the truest sense of the word for most of my life. I've almost always felt good, no matter what life threw my way. That's why this issue is so near and dear to my heart...it's the only serious health issue I've ever suffered...the scourge known as **migraine**. I cannot imagine a worse pain or a greater degree of suffering. To those of you fortunate enough to have never suffered one, be thankful. This is not a 'bad headache'. This is a lightning bolt attached to a chainsaw blade boring into the side of your skull with the intensity of a jackhammer. I was 22 when they began. The first time it happened, I thought I was having a brain hemorrhage and deliriously stumbled into the Emergency Room barely able to form coherent words and unable to see. It was 3:45am and they admitted me right away and ordered a CT scan...but nothing appeared to be wrong. WTF? How could there be nothing wrong? I felt like I was *dying*, and the pounding/throbbing/stabbing pain was not abating. They hooked me up to an IV bag of fluids, and once the CT scan came back the doctor realized what it was, a really intense migraine. I owe that doctor a cold beer if I ever see him again, because he took pity on me and pushed a dose of Nubain (nalbuphine) through my IV; I went from the most intense pain imaginable to feeling really good in about 30 seconds (a little *too* good in fact. Nubain is an emergency room (mild/non-scheduled) pain med that they use when they don't need the heavy stuff like Morphine or Dilaudid). To this day, it's the only thing I know of (short of Morphine) that can stop a migraine dead in its tracks.

I drove home feeling good physically, but really scared. What the hell just happened? Why did my body attack itself so randomly in the middle of the night? Am I at risk of an aneurism or stroke? What could have caused this? I was hoping it was just a freak thing or a fluke. Before that night I had no idea what a migraine was. And I hoped to never know it again. Two nights later I had another one...went back to the E.R., same thing happened only this time they didn't have to run a CT scan. The doctor on duty wrote me a prescription for Augmentin (anti-biotic) because he thought all this might have been caused by a sinus infection. It didn't help, and I continued to suffer in agony, miss work, and writhe in pain in a dark room for hours on end. I never knew when a migraine would strike, but approximately once every 2 days one would come in and run me over like a freight train. I grew up with (relatively) holistically minded parents, so I knew I had to do some research, and I felt like I was running out of time because this thing was actually going to kill me if I let it. My heart rate and blood pressure and adrenaline would get so elevated from the hours of intense pain that I would sometimes verge on a hypertensive crisis, and then crash for about 16 hours afterwards from the adrenal fatigue. (Fortunately, I was healthy otherwise and I was able to manage.) I tried the conventional stuff (Imitrex, Maxalt) for migraines, nothing worked. I tried holistic remedies like taking massive doses of CoQ10. I tried the essential oil lavender. I took apple cider vinegar, Butterbur, Migranol, Magnesium, deep breathing, ice packs and a few other things. That stuff actually did help some and give me a measure of relief (i.e. less intensity, less frequency), but it did not address the root cause. I was told I would just have to learn to live with the condition and manage it by a neurologist. I told him (as politely as I could) that that was a bullshit answer. Even then, with virtually no medical knowledge at the time, I knew that the body didn't just randomly attack itself. That concept was utterly unacceptable to me then, and it still is now. It was insulting, and I resolved myself to finding a real solution. But then, miraculously, after a couple months, the migraines completely disappeared, almost as though they were never there...I was ecstatic to be out of the woods, maybe it was just some late stage growing pain or a freak rare infection or temporary chemical imbalance or something. It wasn't...it was just my body finding a way to *manage* the condition. Everything was going well again until almost exactly 3 years later at age 25 when they returned. I was so disheartened and upset. I had gotten *past* this, why had it come back to haunt me? What did I do to deserve this? I missed work, self-medicated, had a completely irregular sleep cycle, and generally felt miserable for 6 weeks...but then I had a breakthrough...I had more of an understanding of the human body at this point and had access to research. I discovered the link between several causative factors and migraines.

One of them was the mercury amalgam link. I had 4 mercury amalgams in my mouth, and they were all on the left side of my mouth (two upper molars, two lower molars). I only ever experienced migraines on the left side of my head. I went to see a biological dentist, spent all the money I had to my name, and had the mercury fillings extracted and replaced with either composite material or porcelain crowns. The migraines ceased immediately. I felt strange the next couple of days, like someone had taken a 50lb weight off my back. I had really strong mood swings and hormonal swings (which was highly atypical for me). But I felt tremendously healthier and *better* within 48 hours. I was so relieved to have gotten some answers.

But then 3 years later, at age 28, the migraines showed up again like clockwork. They weren't as bad this time around, they were more manageable, but why were they back? What caused migraines to *go dormant* for 3 whole years and then show up out of the blue? I was missing something. By this time, I was working at the clinic and in the midst of holistic medicine. I wanted answers, the *final* answers, and I wanted to remove all possible causes. I did a round of heavy duty intravenous chelations (both EDTA and DMPS) to remove all heavy metals from my system. I did well over two hundred hours of research, scouring studies, looking for commonalities, talking to doctors, ruling certain things out, examining causes and treatments, talking with patients who also suffered from migraines, reviewing biochemistry books from college, studying the effects of vasodilators and vasoconstrictors on trigeminal nerve spasming (which is a component of the action of migraines), etc.

I did it all. You probably could have filmed an 80's movie-style montage (think Rocky Balboa) showing someone furiously typing at a computer, reading books, doing sit-ups in the snow, and flipping their desk upside down in frustration, but refusing to take no for an answer. That was me, just without *Eye-of-the-Tiger* playing in the background.

Then I found it, right in front of my nose, the final answer that had alluded me all these years. It was the specific genus (which has

53 members) of parasite *strongyloides*, that my A&P teacher had first taught me about in college. I had been doing some research on studies done overseas (as well as anecdotal stories) and actually found my way back to some American PubMed studies that helped support my theory. But it was the stuff that Professor Theresa had felt it so important for us to learn about parasites in A&P class that tied it all together for me and kept me from completely missing the solution. Again, thank you, and thank you to all the good teachers out there who make a difference. They don't pay you enough.

Strongyloides is a very common class of parasite, we pretty much all get exposed to them. Walk barefoot outside in the grass, and the infectious larvae penetrate your skin when it makes contact with the soil. They are highly attracted to the Urocanic acid on the bottom of your feet. Again, I'll reiterate that this isn't a cause to freak out, we pretty much all have them, but we do need to be aware that they can *cross the blood brain barrier*. The research shows (see PubMed study below) that when there is an active infection (and I'm guessing the resulting bacteria and detritus when they die as well) cause neurological symptoms, *most often a persistent headache*. It is my heavily researched theory and life experience that there is a sizeable percentage of the population that 1) has this infection and 2) suffers more than just a 'persistent headache', but *major neurological symptoms including, but not limited to, extreme migraine and/or trigeminal nerve spasming.*

The happy ending to this story is that parasite cleanse seems to have been the *final solution* to my migraines because it removed one of the major underlying root causes, i.e. the primary distractor. This ties together with the mercury amalgams, because many species of parasites use heavy metals (i.e. the secondary distractor) to create *bio-films* and protect themselves from the human body's immune system that normally manages them. Remove the source of the parasites' refuge, then remove the parasites themselves.

So in summary, what are the major points we can take away from this?

- Based on my personal experience, PubMed research, and the experiences of numerous patients and doctors I've worked with, the overwhelming majority of migraines are precipitated by 3 major root causes: **1) chiropractic issues** (i.e. subluxations or herniated cervical disks) **2) mercury amalgams/fillings** that have become galvanized and **3) unchecked parasitic infection**—specifically strongyloides. I cannot definitively state that these cause 100% of the migraines in people, but I can confidently state that if a patient eliminates all 3 of these potential *distractors*, their condition will most likely dramatically improve, and has a high likelihood of being completely reversed.

- It is very important to understand and differentiate for patients the clear dichotomy between *causes* and *triggers*. The items mentioned above are causative. Hormonal swings, chocolate, caffeine, stress, food additives, bright strobe lights, loud noises, etc., are *triggers*. Triggers can be minimized or eliminated, but that doesn't solve the issue long term because it doesn't address the underlying root cause.

- Migraines, and any malady for that matter, are not necessarily always attributable to one singular cause. We have got to start internalizing and applying this in the medical field, and treating the whole person, not the singular symptom. It is a disease of the analytical human mind to feel the need to grossly oversimplify any one problem, whether it be medical or otherwise, and put it in one specific box. Issues like migraines can come from a perfect storm of multiple, seemingly unrelated distractors (mercury fillings and parasites in my case).

- As an addendum to the parasite cleanse information, I feel it is necessary to mention that I believe this particular parasite cleanse works so well, not just because of the ingredients, but because of the *duration* of the cleanse. The herbs slowly elevate in blood serum concentration for a full 30 days, and the 'saturation' effect seems to provide optimal efficacy with regard to reducing the parasite/fungal load. In extreme cases of migraine sufferers who may be dealing with a heavy *systemic strogyloidiasis*, it is also warranted to consider integrating the anti-parasitic drugs Stromectol (Ivermectin) and Albenza (albendazole) in with the parasite cleanse (and using IV glutathione to clean up any drug residue/liver stress following the course of therapy). These are broad spectrum, typically used for roundworms, hookworms, pinworms, etc, and do have some cross-sensitivity with strongyloides. It is possible to address the blood/brain barrier issue with this parasite by incorporating intravenous DMSO and/or intravenous Mannitol. In rare cases, we've had to bring these in for patients, but met with good success.

- Parallel to removing distractors and parasitic infections, it is highly recommended that patients who are recovering from systemic parasitic infections never, not even once or on birthdays, eat pork. It is a diseased meat. Yes, I know bacon is awesome, I love it too, but I force myself to find good turkey bacon and eat that instead. You cannot cook all the parasites out of pork because of the cystic nature of the parasite eggs which makes them heat resistant. The three main parasites that pork 'brings to the table' are Trichinella spiralis, Taenia solium (pork tapeworm), and Toxoplasma gondii. There are also multiple low-level viruses transmitted by pork (Hepatitis E, Nipah virus, and Menangle virus). Our immune systems are temporarily over-taxed for about 2 to 4 months every single time we consume it. There is no healthy way to prepare pork. Pigs used for pork are also given a drug called Racopamine, which speeds up growth rates. This has been shown to cause restlessness, anxiety, and elevated heart rate in humans.

To those who are interested, here are the strongyloides PubMed studies, the strongyloides Wikipedia page and the Wikipedia page detailing all of the common human parasites. I don't expect you to actually read through all of this, but it serves as a powerful reference point when needed:

Semin Neurol. Author manuscript; available in PMC 2009 May 6.

Published in final edited form as:
Semin Neurol. 2005 Sep; 25(3): 252–261.
doi: 10.1055/s-2005-917662

PMCID: PMC2678030
NIHMSID: NIHMS109772

Neuroparasitic Infections: Nematodes
M.D. Walker, M.D.[1] and J.R. Zunt, M.D., M.P.H.[1,2]
Author information • Copyright and License information

The publisher's final edited version of this article is available at Semin Neurol

See other articles in PMC that cite the published article.

Go to:

Abstract
Nematodes, commonly known as "roundworms" because of their round cross section, comprise the second largest phylum in the animal kingdom. Nematodes can live freely but many parasitize humans, most often as accidental hosts. With increasing globalization and exotic travel, parasitic infection of the central nervous system (CNS), once considered a "tropical" infection, is becoming increasingly more prevalent in all parts of the world. In

addition, immunosuppression increases susceptibility to opportunistic parasitic infection. Although infected individuals may remain asymptomatic for many years, a higher parasite burden is correlated with greater morbidity and mortality. The epidemiology, pathophysiology, clinical presentation, and recommended diagnostic evaluation and treatment for selected nematode infections are reviewed in this article (Table 1).

Parasite	Type of Lesion	Location	Other Features
Angiostrongylus	Faint T1 signal in focal ganglia and in cerebral peduncles	White matter, deep gray matter of cortex	Meningeal enhancement, edema; CT may show magnetizing lesions
Baylisascaris	Diffuse atrophy, patchy lesions of T1 hyperintensity	White matter of cerebral cortex and cerebellum	Ventriculomegaly, acute chiasma, acidulous than white
Gnathostoma	Small clusters of rounded hyperintensities on FLAIR and T1	Deep gray-white junction of cerebral cortex	Usually bilateral; CT may show subarachnoid hemorrhage
Strongyloides	Diffuse atrophy, patchy molecular white matter hyperintensities on T1 and FLAIR	White matter, spinal cord	Abnormal gray matter, usually unilateral; meningeal enhancement may be seen especially in spinal lesions; can represent tumors and other lesions
Toxocara	Single or multiple lesions, which are low-signal on T1, hyperintense on T2-weighted MR images, and homogeneously enhancing	Gray and white matter, cortical and subcortical, may occur in the spinal cord	Hypodense foci on CT with variable enhancement patterns; can be mistaken for glioma

Table 1 Imaging Findings of Selected Nematode Infections of the CNS

ANGIOSTRONGYLUS (ALICATA'S DISEASE)
Epidemiology
The earliest reported infection with Angiostrongylus cantonensis occurred in the rat population of Canton, China in 1933 and went virtually unnoticed until the first human case was reported in Taiwan in 1945.1Human infection is caused by ingestion of infected aquatic or terrestrial snails (usually Lymnaea catascopium), of slime produced by an infected snail or slug, or of certain shrimp and freshwater fish.2Infection with Angiostrongylus spp. is often asymptomatic and remains undetected for years, so recall of dietary history is often problematic. Abdominal disease due to A. costaricensis infection was recently reported in the Caribbean and Central America, but concomitant involvement of the CNS was not noted.[3,4]

Pathophysiology
Mature Angiostrongylus worms reside in the pulmonary arteries of rodents and are thus commonly called "rat lung worms."[5] After entry into a host rat, adult female parasites lay eggs in the pulmonary vasculature. The eggs

then hatch into young larvae that migrate to the pharynx, where they are swallowed and eventually excreted in the feces. Freshwater scavengers, such as shrimp, snails, crabs, and some fish, are invaded by the larvae and harbor the developing larvae. Mucus produced by infected snails also can be infective. Once ingested by a human host, the larvae migrate to the lungs or brain and die. A. costaricensis, unlike A. cantonensis, usually remains in the intestines. Tissue damage is common during migration, in part due to the host's inflammatory response to proteins secreted by the worm. Host immune status does not appear to affect disease severity.[6]

Clinical Findings

Symptoms typically develop after an incubation period of up to 2 weeks. Although systemic infection is rare, acute abdominal discomfort similar to appendicitis has been reported.[7] Most infections produce neurological symptoms, most often a persistent headache. Additional symptoms are common and depend upon the extent of invasion and host inflammatory response.2 There may be involvement of the cranial nerves, spinal cord, or the eye.[8] Ocular involvement can occur with or without invasion of the CNS.[9] Intraocular invasion can affect vision through destruction of tissue during migration or by causing retinal detachment. Although most infections present acutely, a chronic pain syndrome due to Angiostrongylusinfection has also been reported.[10] In addition, one-third of patients will develop hyperesthesia involving a limb or the trunk.[11]

Diagnosis

Angiostrongylus spp. is one of several parasites that causes eosinophilic meningitis.[12] Cerebrospinal fluid (CSF) pleocytosis is common, with pronounced eosinophilia, increased protein concentration, and elevated opening pressure.[13] Spinal fluid eosinophilia is usually present 2 to 4 weeks after symptoms develop, then wanes, returns again between weeks 6 and 8, then declines toward the end of the third month.11 Definitive diagnosis is achieved by detecting larvae in biopsy tissue, or, more rarely, in the CSF. The diagnosis is more often based on clinical findings and exposure history. Detection of anti–A. cantonensis antibodies is both sensitive and specific, with sensitivity higher in CSF than in serum.[14,15]

Neuroimaging

Computed tomography (CT) imaging may reveal hyper-intensities in the basal ganglia or contrast enhancement of the meninges.[16] T1-weighted magnetic resonance imaging (MRI) postcontrast administration often demonstrates leptomeningeal enhancement and thickening, increased signal in the basal ganglia, as well as small hemorrhages seen with gradient imaging (Fig. 1).[16] Chronic infection often produces a granulomatous lesion that can be mistaken for tuberculosis.

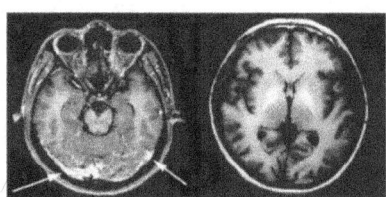

Figure 1 Patient with Angiostrongylus infection. Axial T1 contrast-enhanced images demonstrate meningeal enhancement (left, arrows) and markedly increased signal intensity within the globus pallidus (right). (Reprinted with permission from Tsai HC, Liu YC, Kunin)

Treatment

Treatment is supportive, with most infections being self-limited. Steroids and antiparasitic medications are ineffective. Older studies recommended periodic drainage of CSF to remove the nematode and any eggs that might be present; however, this therapy is no longer widely practiced.[17] Recovery is usually complete, with children faring slightly better than adults.

Go to:

BAYLISASCARIS
Epidemiology

The raccoon roundworm, Baylisacaris procyonis, is endemic in raccoon populations of North America and present in up to 80% of raccoons in the bicoastal and Midwestern United States.[18] In a recent study of California communities reporting high densities of raccoons, 28 to 49% of surveyed properties had raccoon scat containing B. procyonis eggs.[19] Only mild intestinal infection occurs in the raccoon, but parasites can reside within the small bowel of the raccoon for many years. Female adult procyonids produce millions of eggs per day, which are shed with the feces. These eggs are very resilient and can remain viable in the environment for years.[20] Ingestion of eggs by species other than the raccoon results in extraintestinal migration of the larvae, with 5 to 7% of migration leading to the brain, causing "neural larval migrans."[21] Children with pica, developmental delay, or exposure to raccoons are at highest risk for contracting Baylisascaris infection and resultant CNS infection.[22] Severity of human disease is directly proportional to the number of larvae migrating to the brain, thus to the number of eggs ingested.[23]

Pathophysiology

B. procyonis eggs are ingested by humans in the adult form. Larvae are infrequent in human infection, and unlike other parasites (such as Toxocara), the parasite

273

grows as it migrates from the gastrointestinal tract to the CNS, with the adult size reaching up to 2 mm in length.[24] During migration to the CNS, neurotoxins are secreted by the developing procyonid and contribute to the formation of eosinophilic granulomas.

Clinical Findings

B. procyonis infection has been associated with eosinophilic meningoencephalitis, cardiac pseudotumor, and retinitis.[25] Children may develop retinitis, with or without concomitant encephalopathy.[26] Although adults rarely develop clinical signs of infection, mild cases of ocular larva migrans have been reported.[27] Children occasionally have a slowly progressive disease course, and the presence of a profound developmental delay without explanation should raise concern for this infection. Most infections are fatal or neurologically devastating.

Diagnosis

Definitive diagnosis is obtained through identification of B. procyonis larvae in a tissue sample.[28] CSF and peripheral eosinophilia are sometimes present but nonspecific. Stool examination is not helpful because eggs and larvae are not shed in stool. Anti–B. procyonis antibodies in CSF and serum can be detected via enzyme-linked immunosorbent assay or indirect fluorescent antibody, but neither test is available commercially.18 Both tests are specific for procyonids and do not cross-react with other ascarids (e.g., Toxocara).

Neuroimaging

Although often initially normal, with progression of infection the MRI eventually reveals deep white matter abnormalities and global atrophy (Fig. 2).[29] Head CT is usually normal.

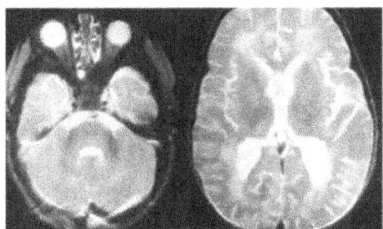

Figure 2 Thirteen month-old patient with Baylisascaris infection. Bilateral, patchy T2 hyperintensity is seen predominantly in the white matter, including the periventricular regions and corpus medullaris of the cerebellum. (Images courtesy of Dr. Howard Rowley.)

Treatment

Unfortunately, Baylisascaris infection does not respond to treatment with antihelminthics. Early diagnosis is uncommon and when infection does become clinically evident, the extent of neurological damage is usually severe and, for the most part, irreversible. Ivermectin can reduce CNS eosinophilia but does not alter disease course.30 Anti-inflammatory medications may be useful early in the course of disease but have not improved outcome. As treatment is largely ineffective, prevention is the best approach to reducing Baylisascaris infection.[30] Raccoons should be discouraged from nesting or eating pet food around children's play areas or residential backyards. Toys exposed to animal excrement should be destroyed because Baylisascaris is resistant to formalin and other typical decontamination efforts.[31]

Go to:

GNATHOSTOMIASIS

Epidemiology

The definitive hosts for Gnathostoma spp. infection include dogs, cats, lions, leopards, minks, and raccoons.[32] Travel through or residence in areas of endemic G. spinigerum infection, such as Southeast Asia and South America, increases the risk of contracting infection. Certain regional specialties are more likely to contain the parasite, including dishes containing raw fish (ceviche) in Latin America, sashimi in Japan, or fresh water eel (sumfak) in Thailand.[33,34] Food handlers in endemic regions are at especially high risk of contracting infection through skin penetration. The parasite is not killed by soaking in lime, even after 5 days. Effective methods for eradication of larva include boiling in water for 5 minutes and soaking in vinegar for at least 6 hours or in soy sauce for 12 hours.

Pathophysiology
Adult worms reside within the gastric wall of the definitive host and discharge large quantities of eggs into the stomach. Eggs are excreted with the feces and, if exposed to water, hatch within 7 days. The gnathostome larva matures within the intermediate host, a tiny crustacean of the genus Cyclops. Cyclops is then ingested by a variety of waterborne organisms, including fish, crawfish, and eels.[35] Hearty gnathostomes can encyst within the host until conditions are appropriate for migration or reproduction. Human infection occurs by ingestion of infected water or animals or by introduction of the parasite through skin wounds. Adult gnathostomes reach 2 to 3 cm in length within definitive hosts but are often much smaller in accidental hosts, such as humans. In humans, larval forms do not migrate to the gastric wall as they do in other mammals but continue migrating through subcutaneous and visceral structures. The parasite can also enter the human host through skin wounds produced by rodents, fish, or cats. Once in subcutaneous tissue, the parasite usually migrates to the liver but can migrate to other areas.

Clinical Findings

Initial symptoms depend upon the mode of infection. If the organism was ingested, mild gastrointestinal distress usually occurs.[36] When skin penetration is the cause of infection, a migrating cutaneous swelling will develop.[37] Clinical symptoms are produced by parasite migration, host inflammatory response, and proteolytic and hemolytic toxins secreted by the gnathostome.[38] The classic manifestation of CNS gnathostomiasis is radiculomyelitis, presenting as severe radicular pain and paresthesia.[39] The pain usually lasts from 1 to 5 days and likely represents the time it takes for the organism to migrate from the nerve root to the CNS. Cranial nerves can also be affected but usually only later in the course of disease after the spinal cord has been traversed.[39] Meningitis is uncommon, especially during early infection, but can occur in patients who are less severely affected or who have rapid rates of organism migration. Subarachnoid hemorrhage occurs in up to 25% of infected patients, and in Thailand, some experts suggest that almost one-quarter of hemorrhagic strokes may be caused by gnathostomiasis infection.[40-42]

Diagnosis

CSF examination often reveals a mild eosinophilic pleocytosis with xanthochromia or elevated red blood cell count.[42] History of migratory subcutaneous swellings in a patient with eosinophilic meningoencephalitis or hemorrhagic stroke should suggest the diagnosis of gnathostomiasis. Extraction of the worm from infected tissue can provide the definitive diagnosis and treatment.[28] Serological tests, such as immunoblot detection of the 24-kDa band, are both sensitive and specific.[43]

Neuroimaging

Neuroimaging often reveals intracranial hemorrhage or resultant obstructive hydrocephalus.[40,41] Scattered foci of hyperintensity on T2 MRI are also described, usually bilaterally (Fig. 3). Contrast-enhanced imaging usually demonstrates meningeal involvement.

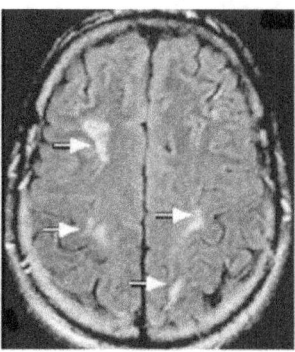

Figure 3 Patient with Gnathostoma infection. Axial FLAIR MRI of the brain showing bilateral clusters of small rounded hyperintensities in deep white matter (arrows). (Reprinted with permission from Hughes AJ, Biggs BA. Parasitic worms of the central nervous system)

Treatment

Mebendazole and ivermectin are equally effective treatments for gnathostomiasis.[44] Gnathostomiasis can persist for up to a decade and may require multiple treatments to achieve total eradication.[36,45] Surgical resection should be performed if an organism is identified. Adjunctive steroids have been useful in some cases.[41] An increase in serum antibodies suggests treatment failure.

Go to:

STRONGYLOIDES
Epidemiology

Strongyloidiasis is a human intestinal infection most often caused by Strongyloides stercoralis. Other subspecies, such as S. fulleborni, although pathogenic in primates, typically cause only minor infections in humans. Historically, strongyloidiasis had been confined to tropical and subtropical regions, but infection is increasingly common in Europe and the United States.[46] In the United States, cases are encountered primarily in tertiary medical centers, especially in the Mid-Atlantic region. In addition, with the advent of HIV infection and more frequent use of immunosuppressant medications, more people in the developed and developing world are at risk for contracting this infection and for developing hyperinfection.[47,48]

Pathophysiology
Strongyloides spp. are capable of living as parasites or free-living organisms. There are three developmental stages: filariform (infective), rhabditiform, and adult. Rhabditoid larvae can become filariform or differentiate into male or female and maintain the rhabditiform cycle indefinitely. Strongyloidiasis is most prevalent in areas of poor sanitation and is usually acquired through contact with the parasite in contaminated water or by direct penetration of the skin by the filariform larvae. In addition, host autoinfection can occur when the parasite completes its life cycle within the host. After entering a human host, the parasite enters the venous circulation, migrates through the lung alveoli, and eventually burrows into the small intestine, where it can reside for up to 50 years.[49] From this site, worms can be released into the stool or develop into the filariform state and reinfect the host. Infection also facilitates coinfection with other agents, sometimes resulting in overwhelming bacteremia with dissemination to the CNS and other organs.[47] Disseminated S. stercoralis infection is more likely to occur in the immunocompromised host.[50] Massive worm burden, known as hyperinfection syndrome, may occur

when the usual parasitic life cycle is accelerated.[51] Hyperinfection is usually limited to the gastrointestinal tract or lungs and is rare in the CNS.

Clinical Findings
Infection may persist for many decades without producing symptoms. Acute disease is limited to the gastrointestinal tract and lungs. Patients often develop wheezing, diarrhea, and postprandial abdominal pain.[52] Transient low-grade fever is common. Chronic disease develops over days to weeks and usually includes a dermatological manifestation called larva currens.[53] The perianal region is the initial site of involvement, but most patients do not notice this early manifestation. The larvae migrate at a rate of up to 5 cm/d and travel subcutaneously or internally to other organs. Disseminated disease can produce infection in other organ systems, including the CNS.[46,54] Alteration in mental status and meningismus are the most common manifestations of CNS involvement, but penetration of vessel walls can produce mycotic aneurysm and intracranial hemorrhage, even vasculitis.[55] If bacterial hyperinfection develops, brain abscess, caused by Escherichia coli in ~30% of cases, may produce focal neurological symptoms.[56]

Diagnosis
Serum eosinophilia is common during primary infection but wanes with dissemination of infection.28Diagnosis can be confirmed by identification of Strongyloides spp. rhabditiform larvae in stool, serum, CSF, or peritoneal fluid. Larvae do not appear in the stool until approximately 1 month after initial infection. In patients with disseminated infection, larvae may also appear in the sputum. Larvae can be detected in duodenal secretions with the Entero-test (Hedero, Palo Alto, CA); a weighted

gelatin capsule is swallowed, the gelatin dissolves allowing the string to pass into the duodenum and 4 hours later the string is removed and examined for larvae. Due to the low sensitivity of direct identification tests, testing of serial samples is recommended, especially for stool specimens. If strongyloidiasis is suspected but not detected by direct identification tests, antibody detection testing should be performed.[57,58] Unfortunately, antibody detection tests cannot distinguish between past or present infection, can be negative in patients with disseminated infection, and may cross-react with other helminthic and filarial infections. Of the available antibody tests, enzyme immunoassay has the highest sensitivity (~90%).[58]

Neuroimaging

In patients with chronic infection, neuroimaging is often nonspecific, but atrophy may be prominent (Fig. 4). Additional abnormalities include abscess formation or mycotic aneurysms, either of which may occur along any vascular distribution but usually spare the extracranial vascular system.[59]

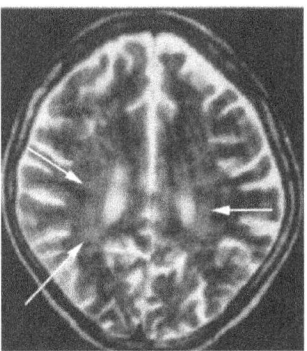

Figure 4 Thirty-five-year-old immunosuppressed patient with Strongyloidesinfection. Axial T2-weighted images reveal global atrophy and patchy periventricular white matter hyperintensities (arrows). (Reprinted with permission from Kothary NN, Muskie JM, Mathur)

Treatment

Ivermectin is the treatment of choice, but thiabendazole, albendazole, and mebendazole are also effective.[60] Steroids should not be used during acute infection, as they may promote dissemination. Disseminated disease carries a mortality rate of almost 80%, so early detection and treatment is imperative.[47,61]

Go to:

TOXOCARA
Epidemiology

Toxocariasis is endemic in all parts of the world.[62] Most human Toxocara spp. infections are caused by T. canis, but T. cati, and T. leonina infections also occur. Recent studies suggest that living in a rural area, ownership of dogs, and dementia are associated with a higher risk for CNS T. canis infection.[63] Children who eat earth (geophagia, pica) are also at higher risk of becoming infected. An infected dog or cat can excrete up to one million eggs each day, and eggs can survive in the environment for many years.[64] Some experts have disputed the role of dogs as vectors of transmission, noting that up to half of patients do not own a pet and cannot recall any close animal contact.[63] In northern industrialized countries, seroprevalence of this infection is 5% in urban adults and up to 40% in children and rural farmers. In the West Indies and Bali, seroprevalence rates approach 80%.[65,66]

Pathophysiology

Introduction into a human host is accidental and occurs by ingestion, most often on contaminated hands.[67] Once in the human gastrointestinal tract, eggs remain in the small bowel for a short period, hatch into second-stage larvae, and then migrate to the liver. Larvae then enter the portal circulation and migrate through small-caliber vessels to the viscera, producing a mild inflammatory response along the migratory path.[28] Chronic inflammation can eventually induce granuloma formation. Migration to the brain is uncommon but usually produces a more dramatic inflammatory response than migration through the periphery.[68]

Clinical Findings

Toxocariasis is almost always a benign self-limited disease, but ocular or cerebral involvement can cause significant morbidity, and infection in the elderly can be fatal.[69] Symptoms depend on the disease burden and system infected, but weakness, lethargy, fever, and headache are common.[68] Visceral larva migrans occurs mainly in children with disseminated infection and can produce granulomas in the liver, lungs, kidneys, heart, muscle, brain, or eye.[70] Ocular involvement, known as ocular larva migrans, can produce symptoms of optic neuritis or blindness and occurs when the parasite migrates to the optic nerve head.[71] Infection can also produce ocular findings similar to retinoblastoma; as retinoblastoma is treated by enucleation, toxocariasis should be excluded as an etiology before such treatment is considered.[72] Although the majority of human Toxocara spp. infections are asymptomatic, subtle cognitive symptoms may not be appreciated or attributed to other behavioral conditions.[73] Unlike other human nematode infections, cognition is affected during almost all chronic Toxocara spp. infections and can range from hyperactive behavior in children to dementia in elderly adults.[73]

Diagnosis

Toxocara spp. larvae are only rarely identified in clinical specimens. Because the parasite enters the human host as a mature adult, eggs are not isolated in stool.[28] Detection of eggs from other organisms, such as Ascaris and Trichuris, suggests exposure to fecal material where Toxocara may also reside.[74] Serum and CSF eosinophilia is a frequent finding, but treatment can reverse this abnormality, and chronic infections may have a blunted eosinophilic response.[67,68] Antibody testing for second-stage T. canis excretory-secretory larval antigens (TESAg) is sensitive and specific for visceral larva migrans provided the serum is pretreated to remove cross-reacting antibodies to organisms such as Ascaris suum.[75] TES-Ag testing can be performed on blood or CSF samples.

Neuroimaging

Contrast-enhanced head CT often demonstrates vasogenic edema and a heterogeneous enhancement pattern resembling malignant gliomas (Fig. 5; personal communication, Dr. Nezih Oktar). MRI imaging can reveal subcortical and white matter disease, resembling small vessel vasculitis. Imaging abnormalities suggestive of small infarctions on FLAIR and T2 sequences often demonstrate microhemorrhages on gradient-echo sequences.[76]

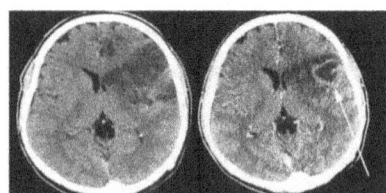

Figure 5 Patient with Toxocara infection. Noncontrast CT imaging demonstrates left frontal hypodensity consistent with edema (left), and contrast-enhanced imaging reveals a ring enhancing lesion (arrow on right). (Reprinted with permission from Oktar N, Barçin)

Treatment
Although diethylcarbamazine is the treatment of choice, mebendazole and albendazole are also effective against toxocariasis.[77] Suggested length of treatment is 3 to 4 weeks. In patients with ocular involvement, steroids should be administered and an ophthalmologist consulted.[78]

Go to:

CONCLUSION
Nematodal infection of the CNS includes a large and diverse variety of parasites. Although many of the published cases are from tropical and subtropical countries, the incidence of many parasitic infections is increasing throughout the world, due to a combination of increased global travel and immunosuppression. In addition, some nematodal infections, such as Baylisacaris procyonis, have caused infections mainly within the United States. The indolent course of many of the nematodal infections make identification difficult, but prompt recognition and diagnosis of some of these infections can prevent additional morbidity and mortality.

Treatment for nematodal infection varies according to the organism (Table 2) but is often limited to management of symptoms. Once a nematodal infection has been identified, a tropical medicine expert should be consulted to assist with determining the appropriate treatment, as treatment regimens do change and newer investigative medications may be available. Several online references are useful for obtaining assistance with diagnosis and expert consultation:
  • The World Health Organization Fact Sheet, available at http://www.who.int/inf-fs/en/index.html

• Centers for Disease Control, Division of Parasitic Diseases, available at http://www.dpd.cdc.gov/dpdx/
• The Medical Letter, available at http://www.medletter.com/index.html

Parasite	Medication	Dosage	Precautions	Potential Side Effects
Angiostrongylaisis	Symptomatic care			
Baylisascariasis	Symptomatic care			
Gnathostomiasis	Albendazole	400 mg PO bid for 21 days; steroid use in certain cases	Use of concurrent steroids or praziquantel may cause toxicity	Abdominal pain, jaundice, alopecia
Strongyloidiasis	Ivermectin (Steroids may cause dissemination)	200 mcg/kg d PO for 2 days; may repeat in 14 d	Avoid use as first line of pregnancy	Mild, generally very well tolerated
Toxocariasis	Mebendazole	25 mg/kg d PO single dose for 4 weeks	Caution in patients on anticonvulsants or medications metabolized by the p450 system	Jaundice, abdominal pain, headache, alopecia

Table 2 Treatment of Selected Nematode Infections of the CNS

ACKNOWLEDGMENTS

Supported by NIH Grants K23-AI01600 and University of Washington Center for AIDS Research (CFAR) Grant AI27757.

REFERENCES

1. Jindrak K. Angiostrongyliasis cantonensis (eosinophilic meningitis, Alicata's disease). Contemp Neurol Ser. 1975;12:133–164. [PubMed]

2. Chau TT, Thwaites GE, Chuong LV, et al. Headache and confusion: the dangers of a raw snail supper. Lancet. 2003;361:1866. [PubMed]

3. Andersen E, Gubler DJ, Sorensen K, et al. First report of Angiostrongylus cantonensis in Puerto Rico. Am J Trop Med Hyg. 1986;35:319–322. [PubMed]

4. Slom TJ, Cortese MM, Gerber SI, et al. An outbreak of eosinophilic meningitis caused by Angiostrongylus cantonensis in travelers returning from the Caribbean. N Engl J Med. 2002;346:668–675.[PubMed]

5. Weir E. Travel warning: eosinophilic meningitis caused by rat lungworm. CMAJ. 2002;166:1184.[PMC free article] [PubMed]

6. Prociv P, Spratt DM, Carlisle MS. Neuro-angiostrongyliasis: unresolved issues. Int J Parasitol. 2000;30:1295–1303. [PubMed]

7. Hulbert TV, Larsen RA, Chandrasoma PT. Abdominal angiostrongyliasis mimicking acute appendicitis and Meckel's diverticulum: report of a case in the United States and review. Clin Infect Dis. 1992;14:836–840. [PubMed]

8. Patikulsila D, Ittipunkul N, Theerakittikul B. Intravitreal angiostrongyliasis: report of 2 cases. J Med Assoc Thai. 2003;86:981–985. [PubMed]

9. Alto W. Human infections with Angiostrongylus cantonensis. Pac Health Dialog. 2001;8:176–182.[PubMed]

10. Clouston PD, Corbett AJ, Pryor DS, Garrick R. Eosinophilic meningitis: cause of a chronic pain syndrome. J Neurol Neurosurg Psychiatry. 1990;53:778–781. [PMC free article] [PubMed]

11. Punyagupta S, Bunnag T, Juttijudata P, Rosen L. Eosinophilic meningitis in Thailand: epidemiologic studies of 484 typical cases and the etiologic role of Angiostrongylus cantonensis. Am J Trop Med Hyg. 1970;19:950–958. [PubMed]

12. Lo Re V, III, Gluckman SJ. Eosinophilic meningitis. Am J Med. 2003;114:217–223. [PubMed]

13. Wang X, Huang H, Dong Q, et al. A clinical study of eosinophilic meningoencephalitis caused by angiostrongyliasis. Chin Med J (Engl) 2002;115:1312–1315. [PubMed]

14. Chye SM, Yen CM, Chen ER. Detection of circulating antigen by monoclonal antibodies for immunodiagnosis of angiostrongyliasis. Am J Trop Med Hyg. 1997;56:408–412. [PubMed]

15. Ellis-Pegler R, Parry G. Eosinophilic meningitis due to Angiostrongylus cantonensis. Clin Infect Dis. 2002;35:777–778. [PubMed]

16. Tsai HC, Liu YC, Kunin CM, et al. Eosinophilic meningitis caused by Angiostrongylus cantonensis associated with eating raw snails: correlation of brain magnetic resonance imaging scans with clinical findings. Am J Trop Med Hyg. 2003;68:281–285. [PubMed]

17. Kuberski T, Wallace GD. Clinical manifestations of eosinophilic meningitis due to Angiostrongylus cantonensis. Neurology. 1979;29:1566–1570. [PubMed]

18. Sorvillo F, Ash LR, Berlin OG, Morse SA. Baylisascaris procyonis: an emerging helminthic zoonosis. Emerg Infect Dis. 2002;8:355–359. [PMC free article] [PubMed]

19. Roussere GP, Murray WJ, Raudenbush CB, et al. Raccoon roundworm eggs near homes and risk for larva migrans disease, California communities. Emerg Infect Dis. 2003;9:1516–1522. [PMC free article][PubMed]

20. Park SY, Glaser C, Murray WJ, et al. Raccoon roundworm (Baylisascaris procyonis) encephalitis: case report and field investigation. Pediatrics. 2000;106:E56. [PubMed]

21. Kazacos KR. Raccoon ascarids as a cause of larva migrans. Parasitol Today. 1986;2:253–255.[PubMed]

22. Gavin PJ, Shulman ST. Raccoon roundworm (Baylisascaris procyonis). Pediatr Infect Dis J. 2003;22:651–652. [PubMed]

23. Fox AS, Kazacos KR, Gould NS, et al. Fatal eosinophilic meningoencephalitis and visceral larva migrans caused by the raccoon ascarid Baylisascaris procyonis. N Engl J Med. 1985;312:1619–1623.[PubMed]

24. Kazacos KR, Boyce WM. Baylisascaris larva migrans. J Am Vet Med Assoc. 1989;195:894–903.[PubMed]

25. Boschetti A, Kasznica J. Visceral larva migrans induced eosinophilic cardiac pseudotumor: a cause of sudden death in a child. J Forensic Sci. 1995;40:1097–1099. [PubMed]

26. Huff DS, Neafie RC, Binder MJ, et al. Case 4: the first fatal Baylisascaris infection in humans—an infant with eosinophilic meningoencephalitis. Pediatr Pathol. 1984;2:345–352. [PubMed]

27. Mets MB, Noble AG, Basti S, et al. Eye findings of diffuse unilateral subacute neuroretinitis and multiple choroidal infiltrates associated with neural larva migrans due to Baylisascaris procyonis. Am J Ophthalmol. 2003;135:888–890. [PubMed]

28. CDC . DPDx Laboratory diagnosis of parasites of public health concern. Vol. 2003. Centers for Disease Control and Prevention; 2003.

29. Rowley HA, Uht RM, Kazacos KR, et al. Radiologicpathologic findings in raccoon roundworm (Baylisascaris procyonis) encephalitis. AJNR Am J Neuroradiol. 2000;21:415–420. [PubMed]

30. Cunningham CK, Kazacos KR, McMillan JA, et al. Diagnosis and management of Baylisascaris procyonis infection in an infant with nonfatal meningoencephalitis. Clin Infect Dis. 1994;18:868–872.[PubMed]

31. Ching HL, Leighton BJ, Stephen C. Intestinal parasites of raccoons (Procyon lotor) from southwest British Columbia. Can J Vet Res. 2000;64:107–111. [PMC free article] [PubMed]

32. Rusnak JM, Lucey DR. Clinical gnathostomiasis: case report and review of the English-language literature. Clin Infect Dis. 1993;16:33–50. [PubMed]

33. Ogata K, Nawa Y, Akahane H, et al. Short report: gnathostomiasis in Mexico. Am J Trop Med Hyg. 1998;58:316–318. [PubMed]

34. Sugaroon S, Wiwanitkit V. Gnathostoma infective stage larvae in swamp eels (Fluta alba) at a metropolitan market in Bangkok, Thailand. Ann Clin Lab Sci. 2003;33:94–96. [PubMed]

35. Chen QQ, Lin XM. A survey of epidemiology of Gnathostoma hispidum and experimental studies of its larvae in animals. Southeast Asian J Trop Med Public Health. 1991;22:611–617. [PubMed]

36. Moore DA, McCroddan J, Dekumyoy P, Chiodini PL. Gnathostomiasis: an emerging imported disease. Emerg Infect Dis. 2003;9:647–650. [PMC free article] [PubMed]

37. Crowley JJ, Kim YH. Cutaneous gnathostomiasis. J Am Acad Dermatol. 1995;33:825–828. [PubMed]

38. Saksirisampant W, Chawengkiattikul R, Kraivichain K, Nuchprayoon S. Specific IgE antibody responses to somatic and excretory-secretory antigens of third stage G. spinigerum larvae in human gnathostomiasis. J Med Assoc Thai. 2001;84(suppl 1):S173–S181. [PubMed]

39. Boongird P, Phuapradit P, Siridej N, et al. Neurological manifestations of gnathostomiasis. J Neurol Sci. 1977;31:279–291. [PubMed]

40. Brant-Zawadzki M, Wofsy CB, Schechter G. CT-evidence of subarachnoid hemorrhage due to presumed gnathostomiasis. West J Med. 1982;137:65–67. [PMC free article] [PubMed]

41. Germann R, Schachtele M, Nessler G, et al. Cerebral gnathostomiasis as a cause of an extended intracranial bleeding. Klin Padiatr. 2003;215:223–225. [PubMed]

42. Punyagupta S, Bunnag T, Juttijudata P. Eosinophilic meningitis in Thailand: clinical and epidemiological characteristics of 162 patients with myeloencephalitis probably caused by Gnathostoma spinigerum. J Neurol Sci. 1990;96:241–256. [PubMed]

43. Nopparatana C, Setasuban P, Chaicumpa W, Tapchaisri P. Purification of Gnathostoma spinigerum specific antigen and immunodiagnosis of human gnathostomiasis. Int J Parasitol. 1991;21:677–687.[PubMed]

44. Nontasut P, Bussaratid V, Chullawichit S, et al. Comparison of ivermectin and albendazole treatment for gnathostomiasis. Southeast Asian J Trop Med Public Health. 2000;31:374–377. [PubMed]

45. Parola P. Gnathostomiasis. Lancet. 2001;358:332. [PubMed]

46. Morgello S, Soifer FM, Lin CS, Wolfe DE. Central nervous system Strongyloides stercoralis in acquired

immunodeficiency syndrome: a report of two cases and review of the literature. Acta Neuropathol (Berl) 1993;86:285–288. [PubMed]

47. Simpson WG, Gerhardstein DC, Thompson JR. Disseminated Strongyloides stercoralis infection. South Med J. 1993;86:821–825. [PubMed]

48. McLarnon M, Ma P. Brain stem glioma complicated by Strongyloides stercoralis. Ann Clin Lab Sci. 1981;11:546–549. [PubMed]

49. Thompson JR, Berger R. Fatal adult respiratory distress syndrome following successful treatment of pulmonary strongyloidiasis. Chest. 1991;99:772–774. [PubMed]

50. Gompels MM, Todd J, Peters BS, et al. Disseminated strongyloidiasis in AIDS: uncommon but important. AIDS. 1991;5:329–332. [PubMed]

51. Kothary NN, Muskie JM, Mathur SC. Strongyloides stercoralis hyperinfection. Radiographics. 1999;19:1077–1081. [PubMed]

52. Robinson J, Ahmed Z, Siddiqui A, et al. A patient with persistent wheezing, sinusitis, elevated IgE, and eosinophilia. Ann Allergy Asthma Immunol. 1999;82:144–149. [PubMed]

53. Arthur RP, Shelley WB. Larva currens: a distinctive variant of cutaneous larva migrans due to Strongyloides stercoralis. AMA Arch Derm. 1958;78:186–190. [PubMed]

54. Igra-Siegman Y, Kapila R, Sen P, et al. Syndrome of hyperinfection with Strongyloides stercoralis. Rev Infect Dis. 1981;3:397–407. [PubMed]

55. Wachter RM, Burke AM, MacGregor RR. Strongyloides stercoralis hyperinfection masquerading as cerebral vasculitis. Arch Neurol. 1984;41:1213–1216. [PubMed]

56. Smallman LA, Young JA, Shortland-Webb WR, et al. Strongyloides stercoralis hyperinfestation syndrome with Escherichia coli meningitis: report of two cases. J Clin Pathol. 1986;39:366–370.[PMC free article] [PubMed]

57. Silva LP, Barcelos IS, Passos-Lima AB, et al. Western blotting using Strongyloides ratti antigen for the detection of IgG antibodies as confirmatory test in human strongyloidiasis. Mem Inst Oswaldo Cruz. 2003;98:687–691. [PubMed]

58. Siddiqui AA, Berk SL. Diagnosis of Strongyloides stercoralis infection. Clin Infect Dis. 2001;33:1040–1047. [PubMed]

59. Masdeu JC, Tantulavanich S, Gorelick PP, et al. Brain abscess caused by Strongyloides stercoralis. Arch Neurol. 1982;39:62–63. [PubMed]

60. Gann PH, Neva FA, Gam AA. A randomized trial of single- and two-dose ivermectin versus thiabendazole for treatment of strongyloidiasis. J Infect Dis. 1994;169:1076–1079. [PubMed]

61. Genta RM. Global prevalence of strongyloidiasis: critical review with epidemiologic insights into the prevention of disseminated disease. Rev Infect Dis. 1989;11:755–767. [PubMed]

62. Magnaval JF, Galindo V, Glickman LT, Clanet M. Human Toxocara infection of the central nervous system and neurological disorders: a case-control study. Parasitology. 1997;115:537–543. [PubMed]

63. Overgaauw PA. Aspects of Toxocara epidemiology: human toxocarosis. Crit Rev Microbiol. 1997;23:215–231. [PubMed]

64. Wolfe A, Wright IP. Human toxocariasis and direct contact with dogs. Vet Rec. 2003;152:419–422.[PubMed]

65. Chomel BB, Kasten R, Adams C, et al. Serosurvey of some major zoonotic infections in children and teenagers in Bali, Indonesia. Southeast Asian J Trop Med Public Health. 1993;24:321–326. [PubMed]

66. Bundy DA, Thompson DE, Robertson BD, Cooper ES. Age-relationships of Toxocara canis seropositivity and geohelminth infection prevalence in two communities in St. Lucia, West Indies. Trop Med Parasitol. 1987;38:309–312. [PubMed]

67. Despommier D. Toxocariasis: clinical aspects, epidemiology, medical ecology, and molecular aspects. Clin Microbiol Rev. 2003;16:265–272. [PMC free article] [PubMed]

68. Del Prete G, Ricci M, Romagnani S. T cells, IgE antibodies, cytokines and allergic inflammation. Allerg Immunol (Paris) 1991;23:239–243. [PubMed]

69. Pawlowski Z. Toxocariasis in humans: clinical expression and treatment dilemma. J Helminthol. 2001;75:299–305. [PubMed]

70. Schochet SS. Human Toxocara canis encephalopathy in a case of visceral larva migrans. Neurology. 1967;17:227–229. [PubMed]

71. Komiyama A, Hasegawa O, Nakamura S, et al. Optic neuritis in cerebral toxocariasis. J Neurol Neurosurg Psychiatry. 1995;59:197–198. [PMC free article] [PubMed]

72. Shields JA, Parsons HM, Shields CL, Shah P. Lesions simulating retinoblastoma. J Pediatr Ophthalmol Strabismus. 1991;28:338–340. [PubMed]

73. Hill IR, Denham DA, Scholtz CL. Toxocara canis larvae in the brain of a British child. Trans R Soc Trop Med Hyg. 1985;79:351–354. [PubMed]

74. Boes J, Helwigh AB. Animal models of intestinal nematode infections of humans. Parasitology. 2000;121(suppl):S97–S111. [PubMed]

75. Magnaval JF, Fabre R, Maurieres P, et al. Evaluation of an immunoenzymatic assay detecting specific anti-Toxocara immunoglobulin E for diagnosis and post treatment follow-up of human toxocariasis. J Clin Microbiol. 1992;30:2269–2274. [PMC free article] [PubMed]

76. Xinou E, Lefkopoulos A, Gelagoti M, et al. CT and MR imaging findings in cerebral toxocaral disease. AJNR Am J Neuroradiol. 2003;24:714–718. [PubMed]

77. Magnaval JF. Comparative efficacy of diethylcarbamazine and mebendazole for the treatment of human toxocariasis. Parasitology. 1995;110:529–533. [PubMed]

78. Taylor MR. The epidemiology of ocular toxocariasis. J Helminthol. 2001;75:109–118. [PubMed]

—

Proc Natl Acad Sci U S A. 2007 Jan 30; 104(5): 1627–1630. Published online 2007 Jan 18. doi: 10.1073/pnas.0610193104

PMCID: PMC1785286

From the Cover

Medical Sciences

Urocanic acid is a major chemoattractant for the skin-penetrating parasitic nematode Strongyloides stercoralis

Daniel Safer,* Mario Brenes,** Seth Dunipace,** and Gerhard Schad***

Author information • Article notes • Copyright and License information •

See commentary "Chemical trails and the parasites that follow them" in volume 104 on page 1447.
This article has been cited by other articles in PMC.

Goto:

ABSTRACT

From both a medical and socioeconomic standpoint, skin-penetrating nematodes are among the most important helminth parasites of humans (1–3). The hookworms Ancylostoma duodenale and Nector americanus parasitize >600 million people globally and contribute significantly to widespread iron-deficiency anemia in the tropical and subtropical world. Hookworms are the causative agents of ill health, diminished work capacity, depressed physical and cognitive development in children, and poor school performance. Consequently, these parasites have a major socioeconomic and medical impact (2, 4). The threadworm Strongyloides stercoralis parasitizes 300 million people globally (5). It is sometimes an HIV-associated nematode. In patients who are immunosuppressed, either as a result of intercurrent disease or intentionally, as a consequence of treatment, the parasite can multiply internally to fatal levels of abundance. Thus, fatalities occur even in sophisticated hospital facilities in highly developed countries (6, 7).

Even though soilborne, skin-penetrating nematode parasites cause ill health throughout much of the world and have the adverse socioeconomic effects described above, little is known about the sequence of biological and physicochemical events that constitute the infective process (1), the process one would wish to interrupt to prevent infection. The host-finding behavior of the free-living infective larvae of the two major hookworms of humans has only recently been analyzed and described in detail (8); the host-provided chemical signals involved in skin penetration have been identified, but those involved in host-finding remain unknown, as do the signal transduction systems resulting in parasite growth and development. These systems, however, are being described in S. stercoralis, a parasitic nematode that is more easily maintained in the laboratory. Neurons that detect thermal gradients and some chemical signals have been identified and are considered to be important in host-finding (9, 10); however, the specific chemical signals that attract skin-penetrating infective larvae to the host have yet to be determined. Here we report the isolation and identification of a chemoattractant that, when provided either as a natural product or as a reagent chemical, attracts infective larvae in an in vitro system.

Go to:

RESULTS

Because dogs, along with humans and other primates, are natural hosts of S. stercoralis, the infective larvae of this parasite are attracted to a crude aqueous extract of canine skin. Inspection of the tracks left by larvae as they migrate toward a well containing crude or purified attractant showed that, even from a distance of 30 mm, migration is strongly directed toward the sample well (Fig. 1). Fig. 2 shows a family of dose–response curves illustrating larval attraction to such an extract at a series of dilutions. Preliminary experiments showed that attractant activity was retained after heating of the attractant for 10 min at 80°C or digestion with trypsin (0.25% for 30 min). Attractant activity was recovered in the filtrate after ultrafiltration through Amicon membranes (Millipore, Billerica, MA) with nominal molecular weight cut-offs from 30,000 to 500 Da. In these preliminary experiments, the larvae also responded positively to an aqueous extract of skin from gerbils, which are a permissive experimental host for S. stercoralis; felines, in contrast, are rarely infected by S. stercoralis, and larvae were not attracted to an extract of feline origin.

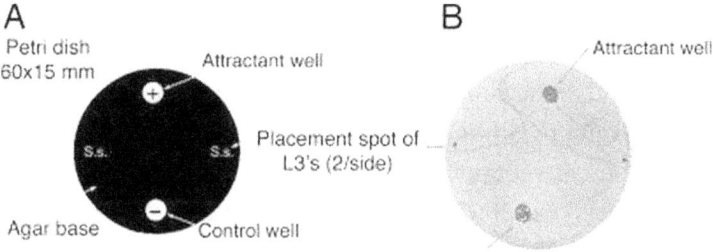

Fig. 1. The chemoattractant assay. (A) Diagram of the plates used to assay chemoattraction. (B) Tracks made by L3 larvae in response to unfractionated canine skin extract.

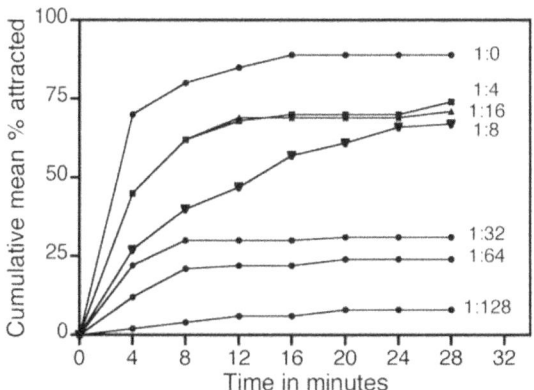

Fig. 2. Dose–response curves for chemoattraction, using serial dilutions of unfractionated canine skin extract. Dilutions are indicated on the graph.

The chemoattractant was isolated from the crude extract of canine skin by three successive chromatographic steps: anion exchange (Fig. 3A), gel filtration (Fig. 3B), and hydrophobic adsorption (Fig. 3C). The purified material consisted of a single component on RP-HPLC (Fig. 3D).

Analysis by GC-MS showed a major component at 138 Da, and comparison of its mass spectrum with the National Institute for Standards and Technology database identified it as urocanic acid (Fig. 4A). The purified attractant and a commercial sample of urocanic acid (Sigma–Aldrich, St. Louis, MO) showed identical UV absorbance spectra (Fig. 4B). 1H NMR (Fig. 4C) was consistent with published results (11). A second component, of mass 94 Da, was also found in the isolated chemoattractant and was identified as 3-aminopyridine (data not shown). Because the chemoattractant activity behaved as an anionic compound, it was concluded that this second component was a contaminant.

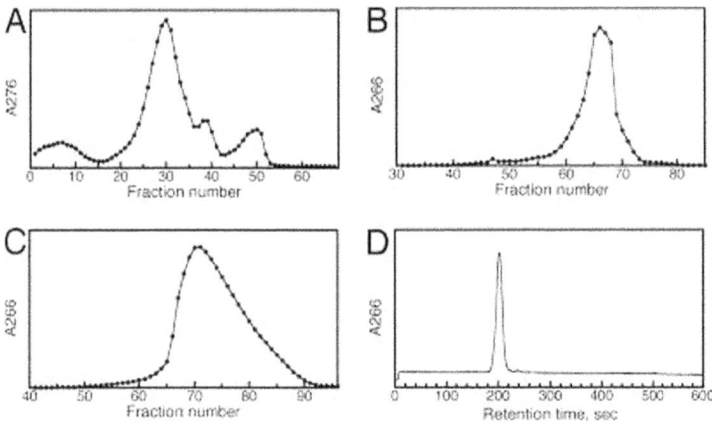

Fig. 3. Chromatographic isolation and analysis of chemoattractant. (A) Anion-exchange chromatography of the crude extract on DEAE-cellulose. The chemoattractant was predominantly in fractions 25–35. (B) Gel filtration chromatography of DEAE fractions 25–35 on Sephadex G25. The chemoattractant was predominantly in fractions 55–70. (C) Hydrophobic adsorption chromatography of G25 fractions 55–70 on AmberChrom CG-71S. The chemoattractant was found in fractions 66–90. (D) Analytical RP-HPLC of the purified chemoattractant after chromatography on AmberChrom CG-71S. All fractions throughout the chemoattractant peak showed a single component, eluting at 200 sec.

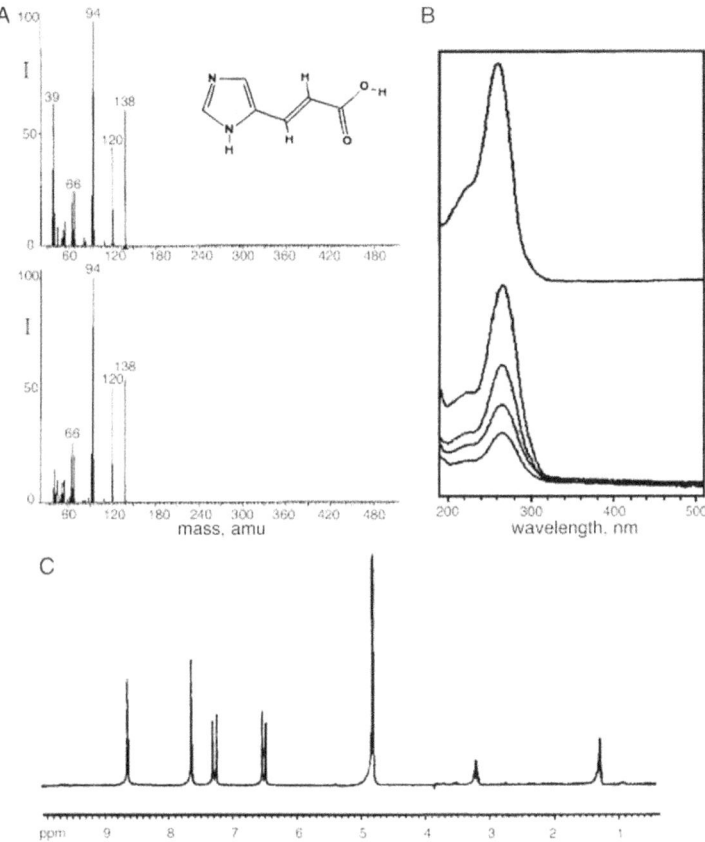

Fig. 4. Spectroscopic characterization of the isolated chemoattractant. (A) Mass spectrum of isolated chemoattractant (Lower) and reference spectrum of urocanic acid (Upper). (Inset) Structure of urocanic acid [3-(4-imidazolyl)acrylic acid]. The relative intensity, I, of the 39-atomic mass unit (amu) fragment (NAn external file that holds a picture, illustration, etc. Object name is cjs0807.jpgCHAn external file that holds a picture, illustration, etc. Object name is cjs0808.jpgN) is lower in the experimental spectrum than in the reference spectrum. (B) UV absorbance spectra of reagent-grade urocanic acid (upper trace) and chemoattractant-containing fractions from the CG71 column (lower traces). (C) 1H NMR spectrum of the purified chemoattractant. Chemical shifts are stated in ppm relative to tetramethylsilane. The major resonances are assigned based on published data (11): imidazole C2, 8.6373 ppm; imidazole C5, 7.6405 ppm; Cα, 7.3010–7.1796 ppm; Cβ, 6.5340–6.4798 ppm.

Because urocanic acid is known to bind metal ions (12), chemoattractant activity was assayed in the presence of equimolar calcium, magnesium, and manganese. All three of these physiologically important metals inhibited chemoattraction: the response of larvae to urocanic acid was reduced by ≈50% by equimolar magnesium and by ≈75% by equimolar calcium or manganese (Fig. 5). Conversely, the response to purified urocanic acid (both isolated from skin and in the form of commercial preparations) was elevated by pretreatment with Chelex to remove residual metal ions. A maximal response, equivalent to the response to unfractionated skin extract, was observed at 150–200 mM urocanic acid (Fig. 6). Migration is strongly directed toward the sample well (Fig. 7), as is the case when the unfractionated extract is used (Fig. 1B).

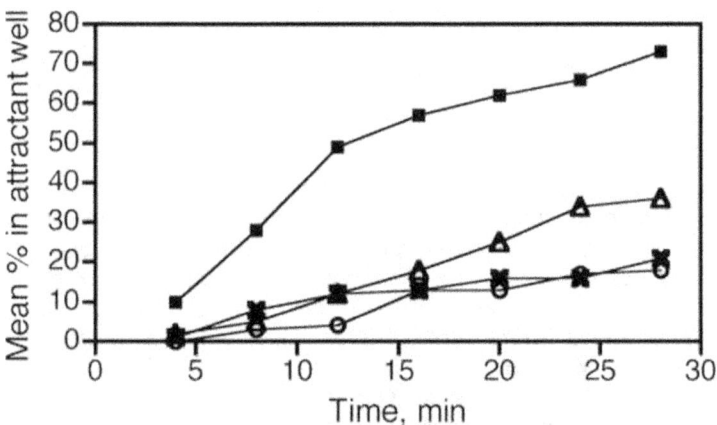

Fig. 5. Inhibition of the chemoattractant activity of 150 mM urocanic acid by equimolar metal ions, assayed as described in Fig. 1 and in the text. Filled squares, no metal added; open triangles, equimolar $MgCl_2$; crosses, equimolar $MnCl_2$; open circles, $CaCl_2$.

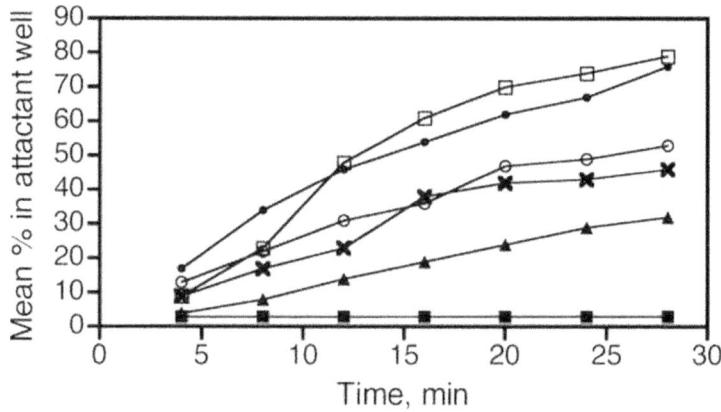

Fig. 6. Dose–response curves for chemoattraction to Chelex-treated urocanic acid. Filled squares, control (deionized water). Urocanic acid concentrations are indicated as follows: filled triangles, 25 mM; crosses, 50 mM; open circles, 100 mM; filled circles, 150 mM; open squares, 200 mM.

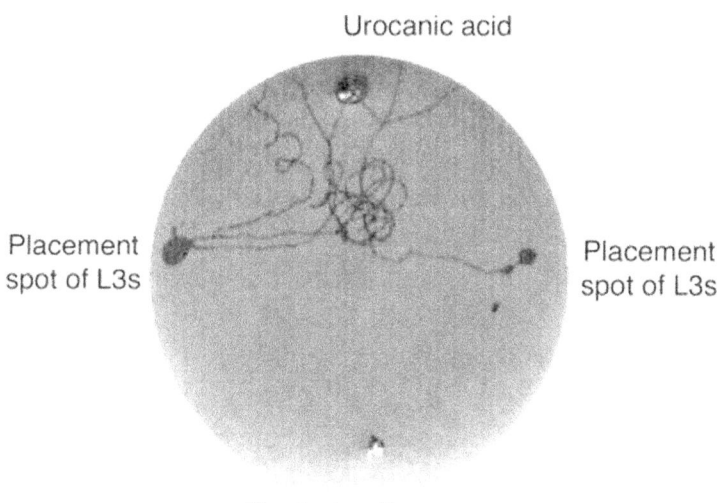

Fig. 7. Tracks made by larvae in response to Chelex-treated urocanic acid. As in Fig. 1, the larvae were placed at the left and right edges of the plate; the well at the top contained urocanic acid, whereas the control well contained deionized water.

Go to:

DISCUSSION

S. stercoralis infective larvae respond positively to several physicochemical attractants. They are attracted to warmth, showing a strong response to temperatures in the range of avian and mammalian body temperature (9). They also respond positively to 3.3–4% carbon dioxide (13) and to sodium chloride (10), both nonspecific attractants produced by terrestrial vertebrates. Although urocanic acid is too widespread a component of mammalian skin to be a host-specific attractant, it may well bias penetration behavior to a limited group of mammals in preference to other species and, in combination with other physical and/or chemical factors, it could be one factor in determining host specificity. Whether host specificity is determined by external physicochemical attractants, internal nutritional requirements, or other physiological factors or by immunological compatibility remains unknown for helminth parasites.

Urocanic acid is produced by deamination of histidine (14) and is abundant in mammalian skin (15). The concentration in the stratum corneum varies between different individuals and at different sites on the body. Most of the reported values are in the range of 6–12 nmol/cm2, except for the sole of the foot, where the observed concentration was ≈60 nmol/cm2 (16). Given the approximate thickness of the stratum corneum as 10 μm, the values for human skin correspond to 6–12 mM and 60 mM, respectively. In isolating urocanic acid from canine skin, the amount recovered was ≈20 nmol/cm2, and it is likely that a significant fraction was lost during purification. Thus, the concentrations of pure urocanic acid that elicit a response in the bioassay are within the physiological range for sloughed-off epidermis. For a soil-dwelling parasite, the high concentrations on the sole of the foot may be particularly relevant to the infective process, attracting larvae to unprotected skin in contact with the ground.

The photochemical activity of urocanic acid has been described by numerous investigators and is metal-dependent (12), which suggested that its chemoattractant activity might also be metal-dependent. Somewhat surprisingly, the converse was found to be true: the activity of both reagent urocanic acid and urocanic acid isolated from skin extract was increased by removal of contaminating metal ions, which resulted in chemoattractant activity equal to that of the crude attractant. Thus, the active form of the attractant appears to be free, rather than metal-bound, urocanic acid. It is possible that, during purification, removal of other metal-binding compounds from the crude extract increased the availability of uncomplexed metal ions, thus promoting the formation of urocanic acid–metal complexes.

The observation that metal ions inhibit chemoattraction suggests that it may be possible to develop an inexpensive, practical, topical preventative for use on exposed body surfaces in persons at risk of infection with the skin-penetrating larvae of S. stercoralis. Such a strategy would be consistent with the current emphasis on "appropriate technology" to prevent parasitic disease in poor developing countries, as advocated by leading nongovernmental organizations such as the Carter Center, the Gates Foundation, and the World Health Organization.

Go to:

MATERIALS AND METHODS
Parasites.
Parasites were obtained as described by Forbes et al. (10).

Preparation of the Extract.

Canine skin from laboratory animals euthanized for purposes of another investigation was generously provided by Mark Haskins (School of Veterinary Medicine, University of Pennsylvania) through an Animal Byproducts Transfer Protocol, as approved by the Institutional Animal Care and Use Committee of the University of Pennsylvania. A 15 × 25-cm rectangle of skin was excised, and the outer layer was removed in strips, which were reduced to a paste with a meat grinder. Portions (5 g each) of the paste were extracted with 10 ml chloroform/methanol/water, 2:1:0.2 (vol/vol) (17). Phase separation was accelerated by centrifugation at 1,800 × g for 15 min. The aqueous phase was partially dried by rotary evaporation to remove residual organic solvent, then lyophilized to dryness. The lyophilized material was redissolved with deionized water, using 0.2 ml/g of macerated skin.

Isolation of the Attractant.

Redissolved extract (50 ml) was incubated with 20 g Amberlite XAD-16 (Sigma–Aldrich) to remove hydrophobic components, without loss of chemoattractant activity. Subsequent chromatographic steps were performed at 4°C, and fractions were screened for attractant activity as described below. The Amberlite-treated extract was loaded onto a DEAE-cellulose column (DE-52, 2.5 × 22 cm; Whatman, Florham Park, NJ) and eluted with a 350 × 350-ml gradient of 0–0.4 M triethylammonium bicarbonate at 40 ml/h; fractions were collected at 10-min intervals. Active fractions were pooled, lyophilized, redissolved in 2.5 ml of deionized water, and applied to a 1.5 × 55-cm column of Sephadex G25-Fine (Amersham Pharmacia Biotech, Piscataway, NJ). The column was eluted with deionized water at 12 ml/h, and fractions were collected at 10-min intervals. Active fractions were again lyophilized, redissolved in 1.5 ml of deionized water, and applied to a 1.5 × 54-cm column of AmberChrom CG-71S (Tosoh Bioscience, Tokyo, Japan). The column was eluted with deionized water at 40 ml/h, and fractions were collected at 2-min intervals.

Analytical Methods.
RP-HPLC was performed using a polar-embedded reverse-phase column (RP-Amide C16, 5 μm, 4.6 × 150 mm; Supelco, Bellefonte, PA); elution was isocratic at 1 ml/min, using deionized water as the mobile phase. 1H NMR spectroscopy was performed at the Center for Biomedical NMR of the University of Pennsylvania School of Medicine, under the direction of Krzysztoff P. Wroblewski, using a Bruker (Billerica, MA) AMX-500 spectrometer at 500 MHz. Analysis by GC-MS was performed by M-Scan (West Chester, PA).

Reagent-grade urocanic acid (Sigma–Aldrich) was suspended in deionized water and neutralized with 1 M Tris(hydroxymethyl) aminomethane base. The final concentration was determined from its absorbance at 277 nm, using the extinction coefficient $18,800 \, M-1cm-1$ (18). To remove trace divalent metal ions, the solution was incubated with 0.2 g Chelex-100 resin (BioRad, Hercules, CA) per ml for 4 h.

Assay for Chemoattractant Activity.
Assays were performed in 60 × 15-mm plastic Petri dishes containing 5 ml of 0.7% Bacto-Agar (Becton Dickinson, Franklin Lakes, NJ) in deionized water. Two wells, 3 mm in diameter, were punched into the agar layer, opposite each other near the edge of the dish and ≈40 mm apart (Fig. 1A). The wells were filled with 15 μl of either test or control solution, and the solutions were allowed to diffuse into the

303

agar for 2 h. Thereafter, two groups of three larvae were introduced into each dish, as shown in Fig. 1; one group was placed about halfway between the two wells near one side of the dish, and the other group was placed opposite the first group, near the other side of the dish, and again approximately halfway between the two wells. The distance between the placement spots and each of the wells was ≈35 mm. The presence of larvae in either of the wells was recorded at 4-min intervals for 28 min. Their response was considered positive when the larvae entered the sample well and remained there during successive observations. Duplicate plates were used for each assay; thus, each experimental point in an assay represents the behavior of 12 larvae. An unfractionated aqueous extract of canine skin was used as a positive control in all assays. To check for external factors that might influence the direction of migration, plates were set up without attractant and in various orientations, and the migration of L3 larvae was monitored. When the tracks were to be recorded photographically, a filter membrane (black, gridded HABG, 47 mm; Millipore) was placed on top of the agar layer. Holes were punched through the membrane over the wells in the agar, and the filter was allowed to absorb the fluid layer. Larvae were then placed on the filter as described above, and their now easily visible tracks were observed to confirm a chemotactic response and were documented photographically (Fig. 1B).

Go to:

ACKNOWLEDGMENTS
We thank Dr. Krzysztoff Wroblewski for invaluable help in interpreting the spectroscopic data; Patricia O'Donnell (School of Veterinary Medicine, University of Pennsylvania) for help with securing the needed canine

materials; Drs. James Lok and Edward Pearce for critical review of the manuscript; and our colleague, Dr. Francis T. Ashton, for initiating our collaboration. This work was supported by National Institutes of Health Grants R01 AI 22662 (to G.S.) and RR 02512 (to M. Haskins).

Go to:

FOOTNOTES

The authors declare no conflict of interest.

See Commentary on page 1447.

Go to:

REFERENCES

1. Hotez PJ, Bethony J, Bottazzi ME, Brooker S, Diemert D, Loukas A. Trends Parasitol. 2006;22:327–331. [PubMed]

2. Lammie PJ, Fenwick A, Utzinger J. Trends Parasitol. 2006;22:313–321. [PubMed]

3. Molyneux DH, Hotez PJ, Fenwick A. PLoS Med. 2005;2:e336. [PMC free article] [PubMed]

4. Bleakly H. J Europ Econ Assoc. 2003;1:376–386.

5. Siddiqui AA, Berk SL. Clin Infect Dis. 2001;33:1040–1047. [PubMed]

6. Bradley SL, Dines DE, Brewer NS. Mayo Clin Proc. 1978;53:332–335. [PubMed]

7. Keiser PB, Nutman TB. Clin Microbiol Rev. 2004;17:208–217. [PMC free article] [PubMed]

8. Haas W, Haberl B, Idris SI, Kallert D, Kersten S, Stiegler P. Parasitol Res. 2005;95:30–39. [PubMed]

9. Lopez PM, Boston R, Ashton FT, Schad GA. Int J Parasitol. 2000;30:1115–1121. [PubMed]

10. Forbes WM, Ashton FT, Boston R, Zhu X, Schad GA. Vet Parasitol. 2004;120:189–198. [PubMed]

11. Halle J-C, Pichon C, Terrier F. J Biol Chem. 1984;259:4142–4146. [PubMed]

12. Menon EL, Perera R, Kuhn RJ, Morrison H. Photochem Photobiol. 2003;78:567–575. [PubMed]

13. Sciacca J, Forbes WM, Ashton FT, Lombardini E, Gamble HR, Schad GA. Parasitol Int. 2002;51:53–62. [PubMed]

14. Mehler AH, Tabor H. J Biol Chem. 1953;201:775–784. [PubMed]

15. Young AR. Phys Med Biol. 1997;42:789–802. [PubMed]

16. Kavanagh G, Crosby J, Norval M. Br J Dermatol. 1995;133:728–731. [PubMed]

17. Folch J, Lees M, Sloane Stanley GH. J Biol Chem. 1957;226:497–509. [PubMed]

18. Dawson RMC, Elliott DC, Elliott WH, Jones KM. Data for Biochemical Research. 2nd Ed. Oxford: Oxford Univ Press; 1969. pp. 60–61.

—

List of parasites of humans

From Wikipedia, the free encyclopedia

Main article: Human parasite

Contents

[show]

ENDOPARASITES[edit]

Protozoan organisms[edit]

Common name of organism or disease	Latin name (sorted)	Body parts affected	Diagnostic specimen	Prevalence	Source/Transmission (Reservoir/Vector)
Granulomatous amoebic encephalitis and *Acanthamoeba* keratitis (eye infection)	*Acanthamoeba* spp.	eye, brain, skin	culture	worldwide	contact lenses cleaned with tap water
Granulomatous amoebic encephalitis (skin infection)	*Balamuthia mandrillaris*	brain, skin	culture	worldwide	via respiratory tract or skin lesion
Babesiosis	*Babesia B. divergens*, *B. bigemina*, *B. equi*, *B. microfti*, *B. duncani*	red blood cells	Giemsa-stained thin blood smear	New York, Martha's Vineyard, Nantucket (different species have worldwide distribution)	tick bites, e.g. *Ixodes scapularis*
Balantidiasis	*Balantidium coli*	intestinal mucosa, may become invasive in some patients	stool (diarrhea=ciliated trophozoite; solid stool=large cyst with horseshoe shaped nucleus)		ingestion of cyst, zoonotic infection acquired from pigs (feces)
Blastocystosis	*Blastocystis* spp.	intestinal	direct microscopy of	• worldwide: one of the	eating food contaminated

Common name of organism or disease	Latin name (sorted)	Body parts affected	Diagnostic specimen	Prevalence	Source/Transmission (Reservoir/ Vector)
			stool (PCR, anti body)	most common human parasites[1][2] • United States: infected ~23% of the population during year 2000[1][3] • Developing regions: infects 40–100% of the total populations[1][2][4]	with feces from an infected human or animal
Cryptosporidiosis	_Cryptosporidium_ spp.	intestines	stool	widespread	ingestion of oocyst (sporulated), some species are zoonotic (e.g. bovine fecal contamination)
Cyclosporiasis	_Cyclospora cayetanensis_	intestines	stool	United States	ingestion of oocyst thru contaminated food
Dientamoebiasis	_Dientamoeba fragilis_	intestines	stool	up to 10% in industrialized countries	ingesting water or food contaminated with feces
Amoebiasis	_Entamoeba histolytica_	Intestines (mainly Large, can go to extraintestinal sites)	stool (fresh diarrheic stools have amoeba, solid stool has cyst)	areas with poor sanitation, high population density and tropical regions	fecal-oral transmission of cyst, not amoeba
Giardiasis	_Giardia lamblia_	lumen of the	stool	widespread	ingestion of

Common name of organism or disease	Latin name (sorted)	Body parts affected	Diagnostic specimen	Prevalence	Source/Transmission (Reservoir/Vector)
		small intestine			cysts in fecal contaminated water or food, can be zoonotic (deer, beavers)
Isosporiasis	*Isospora belli*	epithelial cells of small intestines	stool	worldwide – less common than *Toxoplasma* or *Cryptosporidium*	fecal oral route – ingestion of sporulated oocyst
Leishmaniasis	*Leishmania* spp.	cutaneous, mucocutaneous, or visceral	visual identification of lesion or microscopic stain with Leishman's or Giemsa's stain	Visceral leishmaniasis – Worldwide; Cutaneous leishmaniasis – Old World; Mucocutaneous leishmaniasis – New World	*Phlebotomus*, *Lutzomyia* – bite of several species of phlebotomine sandflies
Primary amoebic meningoencephalitis(PAM)[5][6]	*Naegleria fowleri*	brain	culture	rare but deadly	Nasal insufflation of contaminated warm fresh water, poorly chlorinated swimming pools, hot springs, soil
Malaria	*Plasmodium falciparum*(80% of cases), *Plasmodium vivax*, *Plasmodium ovale curtisi*, *Plasmodium ovale wallikeri*, *Plasmodium*	red blood cells, liver	Blood film	tropical – 250 million cases/year	Anopheles mosquito, bites at night

Common name of organism or disease	Latin name (sorted)	Body parts affected	Diagnostic specimen	Prevalence	Source/Transmission (Reservoir/ Vector)
	malariae, *Plasmodium knowlesi*				
Rhinosporidiosis	*Rhinosporidium seeberi*	nose, nasopharynx	biopsy	India and Sri Lanka	nasal mucosa came into contact with infected material through bathing in common ponds
Sarcocystosis	*Sarcocystis bovihominis,S arcocystis suihominis*	intestine, muscle	muscle biopsy	widespread	ingestion of uncooked/undercooked beef/pork with *Sarcocystis* sarcocysts
Toxoplasmosis (Acute and Latent)	*Toxoplasma gondii*	eyes, brain, heart, liver	blood and PCR	worldwide: one of the most common human parasites; estimated to infect between 30–50% of the global population.[7][8]	ingestion of uncooked/undercooked pork/lamb/goat with *Toxoplasma* bradyzoites, ingestion of raw milk with *Toxoplasma* tachyzoites, ingestion of contaminated water food or soil with oocysts in cat feces that is more than one day old
Trichomoniasis	*Trichomonas vaginalis*	female urogenital tract (males asymptomatic)	microscopic examination of genital swab	worldwide	sexually transmitted infection – only trophozoite

Common name of organism or disease	Latin name (sorted)	Body parts affected	Diagnostic specimen	Prevalence	Source/Transmission (Reservoir/ Vector)
					form (no cyst)
Sleeping sickness	Trypanosoma brucei	blood lymph and central nervous systems	microscopic examination of chancre fluid, lymph node aspirates, blood, bone marrow	50,000 to 70,000 people only found in Africa	tsetse fly, day biting fly of the genus Glossina
Chagas disease	Trypanosoma cruzi	colon, esophagus, heart, nerves, muscle and blood	Giemsa stain – blood	Mexico, Central America, South America – 16-18 million	Triatoma/Reduviidae – "Kissing bug" Insect Vector, feeds at night

HELMINTHS ORGANISMS (WORMS)[edit]

Helminth organisms (also called helminths or intestinal worms) include:

Tapeworms[edit]

Common name of organism or disease	Latin name (sorted)	Body parts affected	Diagnostic specimen	Prevalence	Transmission /Vector
Tapeworm – Tapeworm infection	Cestoda, Taenia multiceps	intestine	stool	rare worldwide	
Diphyllobothriasis– tapeworm	Diphyllobothrium latum	intestines, blood	stool (microscope)	Europe, Japan, Uganda, Peru, Chile	ingestion of raw fresh water fish
Echinococcosis – tapeworm	Echinococcus granulosus, Echinococcus multilocularis, E. vogeli, E. oligarthrus	liver, lungs, kidney, spleen	imaging of hydatid cysts in the liver, lungs, kidney and spleen	Mediterranean countries	as intermediate host, ingestion of material contaminated by feces from a carnivore; as definite host, ingestion of uncooked meat (offal) from a herbivore
Hymenolepiasis[9]	Hymenolepis nana, Hymenolepis diminuta				ingestion of material contaminated by flour beetles, meal worms, cockroaches
Beef tapeworm	Taenia saginata	Intestines	stool	worldwide distribution	ingestion of undercooked beef
Cysticercosis -Pork	Taenia solium	Brain, muscle, Eye	stool, blood	Asia, Africa, South	ingestion of undercooked

Common name of organism or disease	Latin name (sorted)	Body parts affected	Diagnostic specimen	Prevalence	Transmission /Vector
tapeworm		(Cysts in conjuntiva/anterior chamber/sub-retinal space)		America, Southern Europe, North America.	pork
Bertielliasis	*Bertiella mucronata, Bertiella studeri*	Intestines	Stool	Rare	Contact with non human primates
Sparganosis	*Spirometra erinaceieuropaei*				ingestion of material contaminated with infected dog or cat faeces (humans: dead-end host)

Flukes[edit]

Common name of organism or disease	Latin name (sorted)	Body parts affected	Diagnostic specimen	Prevalence	Transmission /Vector
Clonorchiasis	*Clonorchis sinensis*; *Clonorchis viverrini*	gall bladder ducts and inflammation of liver		East Asia	ingestion of under prepared fresh water fish
Lancet liver fluke	*Dicrocoelium dendriticum*	gall bladder		rare	ingestion of ants
Liver fluke – Fasciolosis[10]	*Fasciola hepatica*, *Fasciola gigantica*	liver, gall bladder	stool	*Fasciola hepatica* in Europe, Africa, Australia, the Americas and Oceania; *Fasciola gigantica* only in Africa and Asia, 2.4 million people infected by both species	freshwater snails
Fasciolopsiasis – intestinal fluke[11]	*Fasciolopsis buski*	intestines	stool or vomitus (microscope)	East Asia – 10 million people	ingestion of infested water plants or water (intermediate host:amphibic snails)
Metagonimiasis – intestinal fluke	*Metagonimus yokogawai*		stool	Siberia, Manchuria, Balkan states, Israel, Spain	ingestion of undercooked or salted fish
Metorchiasis	*Metorchis conjunctus*			Canada, US, Greenland	ingestion of raw fish
Chinese liver fluke	*Opisthorchis viverrini*, *Opisthorchis felineus*, *Clonorchis sinensis*	bile duct		1.5 million people in Russia	consuming infected raw, slightly salted or frozen fish

Common name of organism or disease	Latin name (sorted)	Body parts affected	Diagnostic specimen	Prevalence	Transmission /Vector
Paragonimiasis, lung fluke	*Paragonimus westermani*; *Paragonimus africanus*; *Paragonimus caliensis*; *Paragonimus kellicotti*; *Paragonimus skrjabini*; *Paragonimus uterobilateralis*	lungs	sputum, feces	East Asia	ingestion of raw or undercooked freshwater crabs crayfishes or other crustaceans
Schistosomiasis– bilharzia, bilharziosis or snail fever (all types)	*Schistosoma* sp.			Africa, Caribbean, eastern South America, east Asia, Middle East – 200 million people	skin exposure to water contaminated with infected fresh water snails
intestinal schistosomiasis	*Schistosoma mansoni* and *Schistosoma intercalatum*	intestine, liver, spleen, lungs, skin,rarely infects the brain	stool	Africa, Caribbean, South America, Asia, Middle East – 83 million people	skin exposure to water contaminated with infected *Biomphalaria*fresh water snails
urinary schistosomiasis	*Schistosoma haematobium*	kidney, bladder, ureters, lungs, skin	urine	Africa, Middle East	skin exposure to water contaminated with infected *Bulinus* sp. snails
Schistosomiasisby *Schistosoma japonicum*	*Schistosoma japonicum*	intestine, liver, spleen, lungs, skin	stool	China, East Asia, Philippines	skin exposure to water contaminated with infected *Oncomelania*sp. snails
Asian intestinal	*Schistosoma mekongi*			South East Asia	skin exposure to water

Common name of organism or disease	Latin name (sorted)	Body parts affected	Diagnostic specimen	Prevalence	Transmission /Vector
schistosomiasis					contaminated with infected *Neotricula aperta* – fresh water snails
	Echinostoma echinatum	small intestine		Far East	ingestion of raw fish, mollusks, snails
Swimmer's itch	*Trichobilharzia regenti*, Schistosomatidae			worldwide	skin exposure to contaminated water (snails and vertebrates)

Roundworms[Edit]

Common name of organism or disease	Latin name (sorted)	Body parts affected	Diagnostic specimen	Prevalence	Transmission /Vector
Ancylostomiasis/Hookworm	*Ancylostoma duodenale*, *Necator americanus*	lungs, small intestine, blood	stool	common in tropical, warm, moist climates	penetration of skin by L3 larva
Angiostrongyliasis	*Angiostrongylus costaricensis*	intestine	stool		ingestion of infected faeces or infected slugs
Anisakiasis[12]	*Anisakis*	allergic reaction	biopsy	incidental host	ingestion of raw fish, squid, cuttlefish, octopus
Roundworm – Parasitic pneumonia	*Ascaris* sp. *Ascaris lumbricoides*	Intestines, liver, appendix, pancreas, lungs, Löffler's syndrome	stool	common in tropical and subtropical regions	
Roundworm – Baylisascariasis	*Baylisascaris procyonis*	Intestines, liver, lungs, brain, eye		rare: North America	stool from raccoons
Roundworm-lymphatic filariasis	*Brugia malayi*, *Brugia timori*	lymph nodes	blood samples	tropical regions of Asia	Arthropods
Dioctophyme renalis infection	*Dioctophyme renale*	kidneys (typically the right)	Urine	Rare	Ingestion of undercooked or raw freshwater fish
Guinea worm – Dracunculiasis	*Dracunculus medinensis*	subcutaneous tissues, muscle	skin blister/ulcer	South Sudan (eradication ongoing)	
Pinworm – Enterobiasis	*Enterobius vermicularis*, *Enterobius gregorii*	intestines, anus	stool; tape test around anus	widespread; temperate regions	
Gnathostomia	*Gnathostoma*	subcutaneous	physical	rare –	ingestion of

Common name of organism or disease	Latin name (sorted)	Body parts affected	Diagnostic specimen	Prevalence	Transmission /Vector
sis[13]	*spinigerum*, *Gnathostoma hispidum*	tissues (under the skin)	examination	Southeast Asia	raw or undercooked meat (e.g., freshwater fish, chicken, snails, frogs, pigs) or contaminated water
Halicephalobiasis	*Halicephalobus gingivalis*	brain			soil contaminated wounds
Loa loa filariasis, Calabar swellings	*Loa loa filaria*	Connective tissue, lungs, eye	blood (Giemsa, haematoxylin, eosin stain)	rain forest of West Africa – 12-13 million people	Tabanidae – horse fly, bites in the day
Mansonelliasis, filariasis	*Mansonella streptocerca*	subcutaneous layer of skin			insect
River blindness, onchocerciasis	*Onchocerca volvulus*	skin, eye, tissue	bloodless skin snip	Africa, Yemen, Central and South America near cool, fast flowing rivers	Simulium/Black fly, bite during the day
Strongyloidiasis – Parasitic pneumonia	*Strongyloides stercoralis*	Intestines, lungs, skin (Larva currens)	stool, blood		skin penetration
Thelaziasis	*Thelazia californiensis*, *Thelazia callipaeda*	Eyes	ocular examination	Asia, Europe	*Amiota (Phortica) variegata*, *Phortica okadai*
Toxocariasis	*Toxocara canis*, *Toxocara cati*	liver, brain, eyes (Toxocara canis – Visceral larva migrans, Ocular larva	blood, ocular examination	worldwide distribution	pica, unwashed food contamined with Toxocara eggs, undercooked

Common name of organism or disease	Latin name (sorted)	Body parts affected	Diagnostic specimen	Prevalence	Transmission /Vector
		migrans)			livers of chicken
Trichinosis	*Trichinella spiralis*, *Trichinella britovi*, *Trichinella nelsoni*, *Trichinella nativa*	muscle, periorbital region, small intestine	blood	more common in developing countries due to improved feeding practices in developed countries.	ingestion of undercooked pork
Whipworm	*Trichuris trichiura*, *Trichuris vulpis*	large intestine, anus	stool (eggs)	common worldwide	accidental ingestion of eggs in dry goods such as beans, rice, and various grains or soil contaminated with human feces
Elephantiasis – Lymphatic filariasis	*Wuchereria bancrofti*	lymphatic system	thick blood smears stained with hematoxylin.	Tropical and subtropical	mosquito, bites at night

OTHER ORGANISMS[edit]

Common name of organism or disease	Latin name (sorted)	Body parts affected	Diagnostic specimen	Prevalence	Transmission /Vector
Acanthocephaliasis	Archiacanthocephala, *Moniliformis moniliformis*	Gastrointestinal tract, peritoneum, eye	Faeces, parasite itself	worldwide	ingestion of intermediate hosts
Halzoun syndrome	*Linguatula serrata*	nasopharynx	physical examination	Mid East	ingestion of raw or undercooked lymph nodes (e.g., meat from infected camels and buffalos)
Myiasis	Oestroidea, Calliphoridae, Sarcophagidae	dead or living tissue			
Screwworm, Cochliomyia	*Cochliomyia hominivorax* (family Calliphoridae)	skin and wounds	visual	North America (eradicated), Central America, North Africa	direct contact with fly
Chigoe flea	*Tunga penetrans*	Subcutaneous tissue	physical examination	Central and South America, Sub-Saharan Africa	

Common name of organism or disease	Latin name (sorted)	Body parts affected	Diagnostic specimen	Prevalence	Transmission /Vector
Bedbug	Cimicidae: *Cimex lectularius*	skin	visual	Worldwide	sharing of clothing and bedding
Human botfly	*Dermatobia hominis*	Subcutaneous tissue	physical examination	Central and South America	Mosquitoes and biting flies

ECTOPARASITES[edit]

Common name of organism or disease	Latin name (sorted)	Body parts affected	Diagnostic specimen	Prevalence	Transmission/ Vector
Head louse – Pediculosis	Pediculus humanus	hair follicles	visual identification under magnification	Common worldwide	head-to-head contact
Body louse – Pediculosis	Pediculus humanus corporis		visual identification under magnification (Vagabond's disease)	Worldwide	skin-to-skin contact such as sexual activity and via sharing clothing or bedding
Crab louse – Pediculosis	Pthirus pubis	pubic area, eyelashes	visual identification under magnification	Worldwide	skin-to-skin contact such as sexual activity and via sharing clothing or bedding
Demodex – Demodicosis	Demodex folliculorum/brevis/canis	eyebrow, eyelashes	Microscopy of eyelash or eyebrow hair follicle	Pandemic, worldwide	prolonged skin-to-skin contact
Scabies	Sarcoptes scabiei	skin	microscopy of surface scrapings	Worldwide	skin-to-skin contact such as sexual activity and via sharing clothing or bedding
"Chiggers" (Trombiculidae) – Trombiculosis	Arachnida: Trombiculidae	skin	visual identification under magnification, microscopy	worldwide (mesichabitats)	High grass, weeds
Flea, Siphonaptera	Pulex irritans	skin	visual identification under magnification	Worldwide	environment
Tick	Arachnida: Ixodidaeand	skin	visual	Worldwide	High grass, leaf litter, weeds

Common name of organism or disease	Latin name (sorted)	Body parts affected	Diagnostic specimen	Prevalence	Transmission/ Vector
	Argasidae				

References[Edit]

1. Boorom KF, Smith H, Nimri L, Viscogliosi E, Spanakos G, Parkar U, Li LH, Zhou XN, Ok UZ, Leelayoova S, Jones MS (2008). "Oh my aching gut: irritable bowel syndrome, Blastocystis, and asymptomatic infection". Parasit Vectors. 1(1): 40. PMC 2627840 . PMID 18937874. doi:10.1186/1756-3305-1-40. Blastocystis is now by far the most prevalent mono-infection in symptomatic patients in the United States [14] and was found 28.5 times more often than Giardia lamblia as a mono-infection in symptomatic patients in a 2000 study [14].

2. Figure 4: Prevalence of IBS and Blastocystosis by country

3. Roberts T, Stark D, Harkness J, Ellis J (May 2014). "Update on the pathogenic potential and treatment options for Blastocystis sp". Gut Pathog. 6: 17. PMC 4039988 . PMID 24883113. doi:10.1186/1757-4749-6-17. Blastocystis is one of the most common intestinal protists of humans. ... A recent study showed that 100% of people from low socio-economic villages in Senegal were infected with Blastocystis sp. suggesting that transmission was increased due to poor hygiene sanitation, close contact with domestic animals and livestock, and water supply directly from well and river [10]. ...

4. Table 2: Summary of treatments and efficacy for Blastocystis infection

5. Amin OM (2002). "Seasonal prevalence of intestinal parasites in the United States during 2000" (PDF). Am. J. Trop. Med. Hyg. 66 (6): 799–803. PMID 12224595. Retrieved 3 January 2016. Parasitologic investigations of large patient populations are rarely

conducted in the United States, where the illusion of freedom from parasitic infections still predominates. Such investigations are considerably more common in third-world countries where endemic parasitoses are more readily documented.1 In an attempt to address this problem we reported the results of routine examination of fecal specimens for parasites from 644 patients in the United States during the summer of 1996. ...

6. Prevalence. Nine hundred sixteen (32%) of 2,896 tested patients were infected with 18 species of intestinal parasites in the year 2000 (Table 1) in 48 states and the District of Columbia as follows ... Blastocystis hominis was the most frequently detected parasite in single and multiple infections, with Cryptosporidium parvum and Entamoeba histolytica/E. dispar ranking second and third, respectively.

7. El Safadi D, Gaayeb L, Meloni D, Cian A, Poirier P, Wawrzyniak I, Delbac F, Dabboussi F, Delhaes L, Seck M, Hamze M, Riveau G, Viscogliosi E (March 2014). "Children of Senegal River Basin show the highest prevalence of Blastocystis sp. ever observed worldwide". BMC Infect. Dis. 14: 164. PMC 3987649 . PMID 24666632. doi:10.1186/1471-2334-14-164.

8. Cogo PE, Scaglia M, Gatti S, Rossetti F, Alaggio R, Laverda AM, et al. Fatal Naegleria fowleri Meningoencephalitis, Italy Emerging Infectious Diseases [serial on the Internet]. 2004 Oct; accessed Jan 2009

9. Bennett, Nicholas John State University of New York Upstate Medical University Domachowske, Joseph; Khan, Asad A Louisiana State UniversityHealth Science Center; King, John W; Cross, J Thomas Naegleria eMedicine; accessed Jan 2009

10. Flegr J, Prandota J, Sovičková M, Israili ZH (March 2014). "Toxoplasmosis--a global threat. Correlation of latent toxoplasmosis with specific disease burden in a set of 88 countries". PLoS ONE. 9 (3): e90203. PMC 3963851 . PMID 24662942. doi:10.1371/journal.pone.0090203. Toxoplasmosis is

becoming a global health hazard as it infects 30-50% of the world human population. Clinically, the life-long presence of the parasite in tissues of a majority of infected individuals is usually considered asymptomatic. However, a number of studies show that this 'asymptomatic infection' may also lead to development of other human pathologies. ... The seroprevalence of toxoplasmosis correlated with various disease burden. Statistical associations does not necessarily mean causality. The precautionary principle suggests however that possible role of toxoplasmosis as a triggering factor responsible for development of several clinical entities deserves much more attention and financial support both in everyday medical practice and future clinical research.

11. Pappas, G; Roussos, N; Falagas, ME (October 2009). "Toxoplasmosis snapshots: global status of Toxoplasma gondii seroprevalence and implications for pregnancy and congenital toxoplasmosis.". International Journal for Parasitology. 39 (12): 1385–94. PMID 19433092. doi:10.1016/j.ijpara.2009.04.003.

12. Tolan, Robert W Jr Hymenolepiasis eMedicine; updated Feb 2008

13. Yılmaza, Hasan; Gödekmerdan, Ahmet Human fasciolosis in Van province, Turkey doi:10.1016/j.actatropica.2004.04.009

14. Centers for Disease Control and Prevention Fasciolopsiasis

15. Anisakiasis

16. Tolan, Robert W Gnathostomiasis eMedicine, updated Feb 2008

Strongyloides stercoralis

From Wikipedia, the free encyclopedia

This article is about the organism. For the infection, see
Strongyloidiasis.

Threadworm

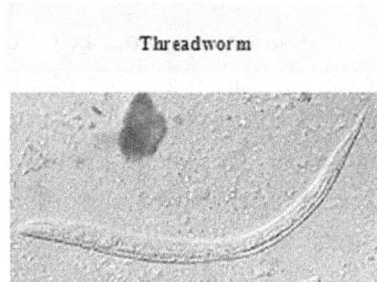

First stage larva (L1) of *S. stercoralis*

Scientific classification

Kingdom:	Animalia
Phylum:	Nematoda
Class:	Secernentea
Order:	Rhabditida
Family:	Strongyloididae
Genus:	*Strongyloides*
Species:	*S. stercoralis*

Binomial name

Strongyloides stercoralis

Bavay, 1876

Strongyloides stercoralis is a human pathogenic parasitic roundworm causing the disease strongyloidiasis. Its common name is threadworm. In the UK and Australia, however, the term threadworm can also refer to nematodesof the genus Enterobius, otherwise known as pinworms.[1]

The Strongyloides stercoralis nematode can parasitize humans. The adult parasitic stage lives in tunnels in the mucosa of the small intestine. The genus Strongyloides contains 53 species,[2][3] and S. stercoralis is the type species. S. stercoralis has been reported in other mammals, including cats and dogs. However, it seems that the species in dogs is typically not S. stercoralis, but the related species S. canis. Non-human primates are more commonly infected with S. fuelleborni and S. cebus, although S. stercoralis has been reported in captive primates. Other species of Strongyloides, naturally parasitic in humans, but with restricted distributions, are S. fuelleborni in central Africa and S. kellyi in Papua New Guinea.

Contents
[show]

Geographic distribution[edit]
S. stercoralis has a very low prevalence in societies where fecal contamination of soil or water is rare. Hence, it is a very rare infection in developed economies. In developing countries, it is less prevalent in urban areas than in rural areas (where sanitation standards are poor). S. stercoralis can be found in areas with tropical and subtropical climates.[4]

Strongyloidiasis was first described in the 19th century in French soldiers returning home from expeditions in Indochina. Today, the countries of the old Indochina (Vietnam, Cambodia, and Laos) still have endemic strongyloidiasis, with the typical prevalences being 10% or less. Regions of Japan used to have endemic strongyloidiasis, but control programs have eliminated the disease. Strongyloidiasis appears to have a high prevalence in some areas of Brazil and Central America. It is endemic in Africa, but the prevalence is typically low (1% or less). Pockets have been reported from rural Italy, but current status is unknown. In the Pacific islands, strongyloidiasis is rare, although some cases have been reported from Fiji. In tropical Australia, some rural and remote Australian Aboriginalcommunities have very high prevalences of strongyloidiasis.[5]

In some African countries (e.g., Zaire), S. fuelleborni was more common than S. stercoralis in parasite surveys from the 1970s, but current status is unknown. In Papua New Guinea, S. stercoralis is endemic, but prevalence is low. However, in some areas, another species, S. kellyi,[6] is a very common parasite of children in the New Guinea Highlands and Western Province.[6]

Knowledge of the geographic distribution of strongyloidiasis is of significance to travelers who may acquire the parasite during their stays in endemic areas.

Because strongyloidiasis is transmittable by textiles, such as bedclothes and clothing, care must be taken never to use hotel bed sheets in endemic areas. Personal sleeping bags and using plastic slippers when showering are very important when travelling in tropical regions.

Life Cycle[edit]
The strongyloid's life cycle is heterogonic—it is more complex than that of most nematodes, with its alternation between free-living and parasitic cycles, and its potential for autoinfection and multiplication within the host. The parasitic cycle is homogonic, while the free-living cycle is

heterogonic. The heterogonic life cycle is advantageous to the parasite because it allows reproduction for one or more generations in the absence of a host.

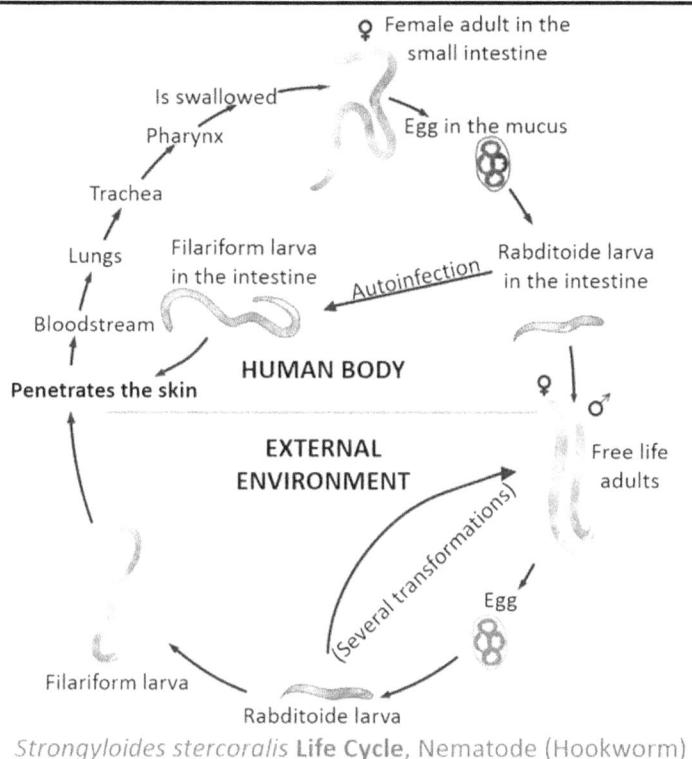

Strongyloides stercoralis **Life Cycle,** Nematode (Hookworm)

In the free-living cycle, the rhabditiform larvae passed in the stool can either molt twice and become infective filariform larvae (direct development) or molt four times and become free-living adult males and females that mate and produce eggs from which rhabditiform larvae hatch. In the direct development, first-stage larvae (L1) transform into infective larvae (IL) via three molts. The indirect route results first in the development of free-living adults that mate; the female lays eggs, which hatch and then develop into IL. The direct route gives IL faster (three days) versus the indirect route (seven to 10 days). However, the indirect route results in an increase in the number of IL produced. Speed of development of IL is traded for increased numbers. The free-living males and females of S. stercoralis die after one generation; they do not persist in the soil. The latter, in turn, can either develop into a new generation of free-living adults or develop into infective filariform larvae. The filariform larvae penetrate the human host skin to initiate the parasitic cycle.

The infectious larvae penetrate the skin when it contacts soil. While S. stercoralis is attracted to chemicals such as carbon dioxide or sodium chloride, these chemicals are not specific. Larvae have been thought to locate their hosts via chemicals in the skin, the predominant one being urocanic acid, a histidine metabolite on the uppermost layer of skin that is removed by sweat or the daily skin-shedding cycle.[7] Urocanic acid concentrations can be up to five times greater in the foot than any other part of the human body. Some of them enter the superficial veins and are carried in the blood to the lungs, where they enter the alveoli. They are then coughed up and swallowed into the gut, where they parasitise the intestinal mucosa of the duodenum and jejunum. In the small intestine, they molt twice and become adult female worms. The females live threaded in the epithelium of the small intestine and, by parthenogenesis, produce eggs, which yield rhabditiform larvae. Only females will reach reproductive adulthood in the intestine. Female strongyloids reproduce through parthenogenesis. The eggs hatch in the intestine and young larvae are then excreted in the feces. It takes about two weeks to reach egg development from the initial skin penetration. By this process, S. stercoralis can cause both respiratory and gastrointestinal symptoms. The worms also participate in autoinfection, in which the rhabditiform larvae become infective filariform larvae, which can penetrate either the intestinal mucosa (internal autoinfection) or the skin of the perianal area (external autoinfection); in either case, the filariform larvae may follow the previously described route, being carried successively to the lungs, the bronchial tree, the pharynx, and the small intestine, where they mature into adults; or they may disseminate widely in the body. To date, occurrence of autoinfection in humans with helminthic infections is recognized only in Strongyloides stercoralis and Capillaria philippinensis infections. In the case of Strongyloides, autoinfection may explain the possibility of persistent infections for many years in persons not having been in an endemic area and of hyperinfections in immunodepressed individuals.

Morphology[edit]
Whereas males grow to only about 0.9 mm (0.04 in) in length, females can grow from 2.0 to 2.5 mm (0.08 to 0.10 in). Both sexes also possess a tiny buccal capsule and cylindrical esophagus without a posterior bulb.[8] In the free-living stage, the esophagi of both sexes are rhabditiform. Males can be distinguished from females by two structures: the spicules and gubernaculum.

Autoinfection[edit]
An unusual feature of S. stercoralis is autoinfection. Only one other species in the Strongyloides genus, S. felis, has this trait. Autoinfection is the development of L1 into small infective larvae in the gut of the host. These autoinfective larvae penetrate the wall of the lower ileum or colon or the skin of the perianal region, enter the circulation again, travel to the lungs, and then to the small intestine, thus repeating the cycle. Autoinfection makes strongyloidiasis due to S. stercoralisan infection with several unusual features.

Persistence of infection is the first of these important features. Because of autoinfection, humans have been known to still be infected up to 65 years after they were first exposed to the parasite (e.g., World War II or Vietnam War veterans). Once a host is infected with S. stercoralis, infection is lifelong unless effective treatment eliminates all adult parasites and migrating autoinfective larvae.

Symptoms[edit]
Main article: Strongyloidiasis
Many people infected are asymptomatic at first. Symptoms include dermatitis: swelling, itching, larva currens, and mild hemorrhage at the site where the skin has been penetrated. Spontaneous scratch-like lesions may be seen on the face or elsewhere. If the parasite reaches the lungs, the chest may feel as if it is burning, and wheezing and coughing may result, along with pneumonia-like symptoms (Löffler's syndrome). The intestines could eventually be invaded, leading to burning pain, tissue damage, sepsis, and ulcers. Stools may have yellow mucus with a recognizable smell. Chronic diarrhea can be a symptom.[9] In severe cases, edema may result in obstruction of the intestinal tract, as well as loss of peristaltic contractions.[10]

Strongyloidiasis in immunocompetent individuals is usually an indolent disease. However, in immuno-compromised individuals, it can cause a hyperinfective syndrome (also called disseminated strongyloidiasis) due to the reproductive capacity of the parasite inside the host. This hyperinfective syndrome can have a mortality rate close to 90% if disseminated.[11][12][13]

Immunosuppressive drugs, especially corticosteroids and agents used for tissue transplantation, can increase the rate of autoinfection to the point where an overwhelming number of larvae migrate through the lungs, which in many cases can prove fatal. In addition, diseases such as human T-lymphotropic virus 1, which enhance the Th1 arm of the immune system and lessen the Th2 arm, increase the disease state.[12] Another consequence of autoinfection is the autoinfective larvae can carry gut bacteria back into the body. About 50% of people with hyperinfection present with bacterial disease due to enteric bacteria. Also, a unique effect of autoinfective larvae is larva currens due to the rapid migration of the larvae through the skin. Larva currens appears as a red line that moves rapidly (more than 5 cm or 2 in per day), and then quickly disappears. It is pathognomonic for autoinfective larvae and can be used as a diagnostic criterion for strongyloidiasis due to S. stercoralis.

Diagnosis[edit]
Locating juvenile larvae, either rhabditiform or filariform, in recent stool samples will confirm the presence of this parasite.[14] Other techniques used include direct fecal smears, culturing fecal samples on agar plates, serodiagnosis through ELISA, and duodenal fumigation. Still, diagnosis can be difficult because of the day-to-day variation in juvenile parasite load.

Treatment[edit]
Ideally, prevention, by improved sanitation (proper disposal of feces), practicing good hygiene (washing of hands), etc., is used before any drug regimen is administered.

Ivermectin is the drug of first choice for treatment because of higher tolerance in patients.[5] Thiabendazole was used previously, but, owing to its high prevalence of side effects (dizziness, vomiting, nausea, malaise) and lower efficacy, it has been superseded by ivermectin and as second-line albendazole. However, these drugs have little effect on the majority of these autoinfective larvae during their migration through the body. Hence, repeated treatments with ivermectin must be administered to kill adult parasites that develop from the autoinfective larvae. This means at least two weeks treatment, then a weeks pause, then again treatment. Follow-up treatment and blood tests are necessary for decades following infection.

In the UK, mebendazole and piperazine are currently (2007) preferred.[15] Mebendazole has a much higher failure rate in clinical practice than albendazole, thiabendazole, or ivermectin.[16]

Chemoattractant[edit]

This parasite depends on chemical cues to find a potential host. It uses sensor neurons of class AFD to identify cues excreted by the host.[17]S. stercoralis is attracted to nonspecific attractants of warmth, carbon dioxide, and sodium chloride. Urocanic acid, a component of skin secretions in mammals, is a major chemoattractant. Larvae of S. stercoralis are strongly attracted to this compound.[7] This compound can be suppressed by metal ions, suggesting a possible strategy for preventing infection.

See also[edit]

- Larva currens
- List of parasites (human)

References[edit]

1. Vanderkooi, M. (2000). Village Medical Manual (5th ed.). Pasadena: William Carey Library. ISBN 0878087788.

2. Speare, R. (1989). "Identification of species of Strongyloides". In Grove, D. I. Strongyloidiasis: a major roundworm infection of man. London: Taylor & Francis. pp. 11–83. ISBN 0850667321.

3. Skerratt, L. F. (1995). "Strongyloides spearei n. sp. (Nematoda: Strongyloididae) from the common wombat Vombatus ursinus (Marsupialia: Vombatidae)". Systematic Parasitology. 32 (2): 81–89. doi:10.1007/BF00009506.

4. Segarra-Newnham, M. (2007). "Manifestations, diagnosis, and treatment of Strongyloides stercoralis infection". Ann Pharmacother. 41 (12): 1992–2001. PMID 17940124. doi:10.1345/aph.1K302.

5. Johnston, F. H.; Morris, P. S.; Speare, R.; McCarthy, J.; Currie, B.; Ewald, D.; Page, W.; Dempsey, K. (2005). "Strongyloidiasis: A review of the evidence for Australian practitioners". The Australian Journal of Rural Health. 13 (4): 247–54. PMID 16048468. doi:10.1111/j.1440-1584.2005.00710.x.

6. Dorris, M.; Viney, M. E.; Blaxter, M. L. (2002). "Molecular phylogenetic analysis of the genus Strongyloides and related nematodes". International Journal for Parasitology. 32 (12): 1507–17. PMID 12392916. doi:10.1016/s0020-7519(02)00156-x.

7. Safer, D.; Brenes, M.; Dunipace, S.; Schad, G. (2007). "Urocanic acid is a major chemoattractant for the skin-penetrating parasitic nematode Strongyloides stercoralis". Proceedings of the National Academy of Sciences. 104 (5): 1627. PMC 1785286 . PMID 17234810. doi:10.1073/pnas.0610193104.

8. Roberts, L.; Janovy, J., Jr. (2005). Foundations of Parasitology (7th ed.). Boston: McGraw Hill. p. 412. ISBN 0071112715.

9. Thamwiwat, Alisa; Mejia, Rojelio; Nutman, Thomas B.; Bates, Jeffrey T. (6 July 2014). "Strongyloidiasis as a Cause of Chronic Diarrhea, Identified Using Next-Generation Strongyloides stercoralis-Specific Immunoassays". Current Tropical Medicine Reports. 1 (3): 145–147. doi:10.1007/s40475-014-0026-7.

10. Roberts, L.; Janovy, J., Jr. (2005). Foundations of Parasitology (7th ed.). Boston: McGraw Hill. pp. 414–415. ISBN 0071112715.

11. Igra-Siegman, Y; Kapila, R; Sen, P; Kaminski, ZC; Louria, DB (1981). "Syndrome of hyperinfection with Strongyloides stercoralis". Reviews of infectious diseases. 3 (3): 397–407. PMID 7025145. doi:10.1093/clinids/3.3.397.

12. Marcos, L. A.; Terashima, A.; Dupont, H. L.; Gotuzzo, E. (2008). "Strongyloides hyperinfection syndrome: An emerging global infectious disease". Transactions of the Royal Society of

Tropical Medicine and Hygiene. 102 (4): 314–318. PMID 18321548. doi:10.1016/j.trstmh.2008.01.020.

13. Newberry, AM; Williams, DN; Stauffer, WM; Boulware, DR; Hendel-Paterson, BR; Walker, PF (Nov 2005). "Strongyloides hyperinfection presenting as acute respiratory failure and gram-negative sepsis.". Chest. 128 (5): 3681–4. PMC 1941746 . PMID 16304332. doi:10.1378/chest.128.5.3681.

14. Roberts, L.; Janovy, J., Jr. (2005). Foundations of Parasitology (7th ed.). Boston: McGraw Hill. p. 415. ISBN 0071112715.

15. NHS Direct Health Encyclopedia by: Dr. Dave Cheever

16. Boulware, DR; Stauffer, WM; Hendel-Paterson, BR; Rocha, JL; Seet, RC; Summer, AP; Nield, LS; Supparatpinyo, K; Chaiwarith, R; Walker, PF (June 2007). "Maltreatment of Strongyloides infection: case series and worldwide physicians-in-training survey.". The American Journal of Medicine. 120 (6): 545.e1–8. PMC 1950578 . PMID 17524758. doi:10.1016/j.amjmed.2006.05.072.

17. Forbes, WM; Ashton, FT; Boston, R; Zhu, X; Schad, GA (2004). "Chemoattraction and chemorepulsion of Strongyloides stercoralis infective larvae on a sodium chloride gradient is mediated by amphidial neuron pairs ASE and ASH, respectively". Veterinary parasitology. 120 (3): 189–98. PMID 15041094. doi:10.1016/j.vetpar.2004.01.005.

—

(on next page)
Overview of taxonomy of Strongyloides genus.
[hide]

Infectious diseases
Parasitic disease: helminthiases
B65–B83
120–129

View this graphic online at:
https://en.wikipedia.org/wiki/Template:Helminthiases

[hide]

Infectious diseases · Parasitic disease: helminthiases (B65–B83 · 120–129)

Flatworm/ platyhelminth infection	Fluke/trematode (Trematode infection)		Blood fluke		Schistosoma mansoni/japonicum/mekongi/haematobium (Schistosomiasis) · Trichobilharzia regenti (Swimmer's itch)
			Liver fluke		Clonorchis sinensis (Clonorchiasis) · Dicrocoelium dendriticum/Dicrocoelium hospes (Dicrocoeliasis) · Fasciola hepatica/gigantica (Fasciolosis) · Opisthorchis viverrini/Opisthorchis felineus (Opisthorchiasis)
			Lung fluke		Paragonimus westermani/Paragonimus kellicotti (Paragonimiasis)
			Intestinal fluke		Fasciolopsis buski (Fasciolopsiasis) · Metagonimus yokogawai (Metagonimiasis) · Heterophyes heterophyes (Heterophyiasis)
	Cestoda (Tapeworm infection)		Cyclophyllidea		Echinococcus granulosus/Echinococcus multilocularis (Echinococcosis) · Taenia saginata/Taenia asiatica/Taenia solium (pork) (Taeniasis/Cysticercosis) · Hymenolepis nana/Hymenolepis diminuta (Hymenolepiasis)
			Pseudophyllidea		Diphyllobothrium latum (Diphyllobothriasis) · Spirometra erinaceieuropaei (Sparganosis) · Diphyllobothrium mansonoides (Sparganosis)
Roundworm/ Nematode infection	Secernentea	Camallanida		Dracunculus medinensis (Dracunculiasis)
		Spirurida	Filarioidea (Filariasis)		Onchocerca volvulus (Onchocerciasis) · Loa loa (Loa loa filariasis) · Mansonella (Mansonelliasis) · Dirofilaria repens · Dirofilaria immitis (Dirofilariasis) · Wuchereria bancrofti/Brugia malayi/Brugia timori
				(Lymphatic filariasis)	
			Thelazioidea		Gnathostoma spinigerum/Gnathostoma hispidum (Gnathostomiasis) · Thelazia (Thelaziasis)
			Spiruroidea		Gongylonema
		Strongylida (hookworm)			Hookworm infection · Ancylostoma duodenale/Ancylostoma braziliense (Ancylostomiasis · Cutaneous larva migrans) · Necator americanus (Necatoriasis) · Angiostrongylus cantonensis (Angiostrongyliasis) · Metastrongylus (Metastrongylosis)
		Ascaridida			Ascaris lumbricoides (Ascariasis) · Anisakis (Anisakiasis) · Toxocara canis/Toxocara cati (Visceral larva migrans/Toxocariasis) · Baylisascaris · Dioctophyme renale (Dioctophymosis) · Parascaris equorum
		Rhabditida			Strongyloides stercoralis (Strongyloidiasis) · Trichostrongylus spp. (Trichostrongyliasis) · Halicephalobus gingivalis
		Oxyurida			Enterobius vermicularis (Enterobiasis · Pinworm)
	Adenophorea				Trichinella spiralis (Trichinosis) · Trichuris trichiura (Trichuriasis · Whipworm) · Capillaria philippinensis (Intestinal capillariasis) · Capillaria hepatica

Taxon identifiers: Wikidata: Q244111 ↗ · Wikispecies: Strongyloides stercoralis ↗ · ADW: Strongyloides_stercoralis ↗ · EoL: 292658 ↗ · EPPO: STGYST ↗ · Fauna Europaea (new): 06de9931 3bc5-4929-88f6-ed0bfd8e30a ↗ · GBIF: 2283792 ↗ · iNaturalist: 417544 ↗ · IRMNG: 10709807 ↗ · NCBI: 6248 ↗ · NZOR: 6a1aa0a3-c192-4aa3-a1f9-528ce191a9-9 ↗

Categories   Rhabditida   Parasitic nematodes of humans   Parasitic nematodes of mammals   Conditions diagnosed by stool test   Animals described in 1876

CHAPTER 27

PROBIOTICS AND PREBIOTICS

Probiotics are finally starting to get the recognition they deserve, but they still have a long way to go before the western world realizes just how truly essential they are. With the increasing prevalence of the over prescribing of anti-biotics combined with processed, outright *dead* food that is standard fare in the American diet, probiotics are needed now more than ever.

They are more than just good bacteria. They comprise the entire eco-culture and microbiome of the human gastrointestinal tract. It should be emphasized that approximately **80% of the human immune system lives in the G.I. tract.** It's also now been well established that there is a strong brain-gut connection and many of the brain's neurotransmitters (serotonin, dopamine, etc) begin formation in the gut. The gut has a "mind" of its own, a.k.a. the **enteric nervous system.** This neural network sends/receives impulses, registers/archives experiences, and reacts to emotions. The gut can upset the brain just as the brain can upset the gut, and there is an entirely new field of medicine emerging known as *neurogastroenterology*. There are so many important biological functions dependent on the microbiome that the body has a seemingly redundant system of maintaining the levels of these bacteria. The appendix (yes, science has finally figured out its purpose) functions as a backup reservoir of good bacteria, and re-seeds the gut after times of illness (or in modern times, antibiotics) that periodically wipe out the established colonies of these important flora.

There are several beneficial brands of probiotics on the market, however there are a lot of junk or useless brands on the market that are a complete waste of money. A general rule of thumb is that if you can find it at an average grocery store or convenience store like CVS/Walgreens (i.e. brands like Align or Culturelle), *they are absolute rubbish and should be avoided at all costs* if you expect to get any sort of actual benefit from them. Also, contrary to popular myth, if your gastrointestinal flora has been wiped out after a heavy course of anti-biotics, eating a little bit of yogurt is practically useless for the purposes of true colony re-establishment.

The most complete, most robust formula we've found as of the writing of this book is **Primal Defense Ultra** by the Garden of Life company. It's generally available at most health food stores and on Amazon.com. (Garden of Life also produces an excellent doctor-formulated **pre-biotic fiber**, which is a type of fiber that can feed your existing pro-biotic reserve and accelerate the bacteriological proliferation process.) Primal Defense Ultra contains 13 different non-competing strains of beneficial micro-organisms, including *saccharomyces boulardii*, which directly competes metabolically against candida yeast. We also like to alternate Primal Defense with **ProbioMax DF *100 Billion CFU***, which is a practitioner-grade offering from Xymogen that drastically boosts 4 key strains (*lactobacillus acidophilus, lactobacillus plantarum, Bifidobacterium longum, and Bifidobacterium lactis HN019*). Lastly, we use the "pre-biotic" **ProbioPhage DF** from Designs for Health. ProbioPhage DF has 5 strains of probiotics, but more importantly it contains a special blend of helpful **bacteriophages**, which are benevolent viruses that exclusively infect bacteria, never human cells. Bacteriophages have been studied from the early 1900's, have the unique advantage of providing a non-host derived immunity, and are still widely used in Russia today for gut health, immune boosting, and for the treatment of infectious diseases.

We've have had the good fortune over the years to be able to leverage the synergy and power of these multi-spectral pro-, pre-, and phage biotics to help patients achieve optimal gut health. One of the biggest hurtles we face in the medical field today is that more patients than ever now suffer from G.I. issues... most notably leaky gut, Celiac, Chrohn's disease, IBS, ulcers, acid reflux, nutrient malabsorption, gastritis, constipation etc...

Dietary changes are key, but when patients are willing to make those changes, i.e. eating living, organic foods, taking pro-biotics, throwing away the microwave (and resolving to *never* use this cancer-causing device again), completely abandoning chemical-laden GMO franken-foods like McDonalds, eliminating candida, and generally overhauling their previously toxic lifestyle, we are able to radically reverse these disease states and help the patients heal themselves. And that is quite an exciting thing to see!

Patients that really *want* to make that change, *can* make that change. But the process is one of commitment, not simple involvement. Before we go down that path with anyone, we like to be very honest and upfront with them with regard to the long road ahead to recovery they must face in order achieve true gut restoration. We tell everyone that there is no simple/temporary 'diet' to follow, there is only the option of a fundamental lifestyle change. There are no "cheat" days. KFC, McDonalds, Taco Bell, Arby's, DQ, Whataburger, China WOK, Steak-n-Shake, Burger King, Sonic, Checkers, Wendy's, Krystal, Hardee's, etc., all have to go, *permanently*. You have to be willing to value yourself enough to say "I'm never again going to put the toxic chemical-laden sludge produced by these corporations in my body again, not even once, *not for the rest of my life. I'm never going to drink a diet coke again. I'm going to choose not only life, but I'm going to choose to live well and thrive and become completely free of the chemical dependency under which I was previously subjugated.*" That's a very powerful intention, it often ruffles a lot of feathers, and man is it hard to stick to (at first). But the results are undeniable, and at about the 4 to 6-week point, the patients who've truly made it begin to feel outright superhuman. They're happier, healthier, hornier, they've lost weight, they sleep better, their allergies are gone, their depression is gone, and they have a new zest and appreciation for life. They no longer crave/desire/are addicted to the GMO Franken-food that imprisoned them in their own bodies for years. They have a new zen, a new peace, and a razor-sharp cognitive focus that becomes a self-sustaining singularity of limitless energy.

The ancient Chinese philosopher Lao Tzu (Laozi) (604 B.C.—531 B.C.) is famous for the expression *"A journey of a thousand miles begins with the first step."* This also holds true in the world of gastrointestinal health. Our western culture is based on instant gratification. If you've read this far into the book, you might be thinking 'ok, probiotics, got it, no problem, I'll put them on the list, I'll get through the bottle in a month, and everything will be back to normal.' Sadly, this isn't the case.

I always make it a well-driven point to all of my patients suffering from G.I. issues, that yes, we will get some initial improvement in short order with our therapies. But while we do have access to the best probiotics and synergy thereof known to man, it still takes a *full two years to rebuild the gastro-intestinal tract, the stomach lining, and microbiome* in the sense of restoring optimal function. Whether it's IBS, Chrohn's, damaged stomach lining, weakened/wiped-out microbiome, etc., it takes some time, vigilance, and dedication. This sort of chronic ailment did not suddenly appear overnight, nor is there a simple fix that's going to resolve it instantaneously. We can certainly accelerate the process in some cases with more advanced therapies like stem cell, as well as practitioner grade oral formulas like **RepairVite** from Apex Energetics, but it still takes time. (We recommend RepairVite because it has aloe vera, L-glutamine, deglycyrrhizinated licorice, and several other potent ingredients which help the body sooth and repair the gastrointestinal lining.) But there is no magic 'Pepto-Bismol' fix. (Although we do put patients suffering from stomach ulcers on a temporary regimen of 50/50 mixed Pepto-Bismol/Argentyn23 colloidal silver drink to shrink the ulcers for a couple weeks.) Also, one of the single most powerful healing/detox practices that can be done on a daily basis for both gastro-intestinal and whole-body health is drinking raw, organic celery juice. Doing this a minimum of 5 days week, even by itself, can yield a tremendous improvement in both gut and liver function.

As a side note, the over-prescription of anti-biotics is one of the primary causes of obesity in America today. We get prescribed a 'Z-Pack' (Azithromycin) for the common cold, which by the way does *nothing* to reduce the severity or duration of the cold (rhino-virus), and as a side effect we absolutely wreck our biological eco-culture in the gut. (We also begin to propagate anti-biotic resistant strains of bacteria, but that's an entirely separate problem). Once our good bacteria/microbiome is damaged, we open the doors for a cascade failure of opportunistic infections, most notably the fungal infection candida, to proliferate, which leads to weight gain. We need to completely re-evaluate the role of anti-biotics and drastically scale back the inappropriate usage and over-prescribing that is running rampant in our healthcare system today.

CHAPTER 28

SLEEP/INSOMNIA

We all have to sleep. Go long enough without it and you begin to hallucinate, have impulsive thoughts, lose muscle coordination, experience immune system impairment, you can't heal, and you generally begin to experience a breakdown of core functions, and eventually fall into psychosis.

So what causes insomnia? If you ask ten people who suffer from it, there is a decent chance that you would get ten different answers. There are many known triggers…stress, anxiety, pain, an overactive mind, stimulants (caffeine/nicotine), not disconnecting from our electronic devices, etc. But these vicious cycles we find ourselves in (and whether or not they are self-inflicted) are all causative of the same root issue, which is the disruption of the natural **circadian rhythm**. For thousands of years, our bio-rhythms and circadian rhythms were always in sync and in tune with nature. We awoke when the sun rose, and we slept when the sun set. We were able to effectively heal from any minor injuries, recharge our endocrine and immune systems, and wake up alert with razor sharp cognitive function after a night of deep, *restorative* sleep. This is obviously no longer the case. Our natural melatonin production and release ceases to function properly, thanks in part to artificially sourced lights and smartphone/pc/tablet use late at night, the never-ending stresses of work deadlines, medication side effects, etc.

Before we can address this issue, let's first examine how the sleep cycle naturally works. Here is a quick explanatory read from psychologist Diana L. Walcutt, PhD:

Do you ever wonder why you don't dream when you sleep? The truth is, if you are getting proper amounts of sleep in proper time periods, and not taking medications or using alcohol or illegal substances, you are dreaming. You just don't remember them unless they wake you.

Stages of Sleep
Wakefulness includes Gamma, High Beta, Mid Beta, Beta Sensory Motor Rhythm, Alpha, and Theta brain waves. Our composite brain wave, that is, what you would see if you had an EEG (electro-encephalo-graph, or picture of the electrical activity in your brain), would be made up of many of the brain waves named above, all at the same time.

Stage One
When we are preparing to drift off, we go through Alpha and Theta, and have periods of dreaminess, almost like daydreaming, except we are beginning to fall asleep. These are interesting states, in that we experience them throughout the day and some people may have more of these waves than others.

Those who practice meditation, or deep prayerfulness, often kinda "hang out" in Alpha. It's a restful place. During this stage, it's not unusual to experience strange and extremely vivid sensations or a feeling of falling followed by sudden muscle contractions. These are known as hypnogogic hallucinations. You may even feel like you are hearing someone call your name, or the phone ringing. Recently, I thought I heard the doorbell, but realized that it was a hypnogogic hallucination and went back to sleep.

We then begin to enter Theta, which is still a relatively light period between being awake and asleep. This usually lasts for 5-10 minutes. Research has shown that the average sleeper takes about 7 minutes to fall asleep. You may fall asleep sooner, or take longer.

Stage Two

The second stage of sleep lasts about 20 minutes. Our brain begins to produce very short periods of rapid, rhythmic brain wave activity known as Sleep Spindles. Body temperature begins dropping and heart rate starts slowing down.

Stage Three

Deep, slow brain waves known as Delta Waves begin to emerge during this stage. It is a transitional period between light sleep and a very deep sleep.

Stage Four

This is sometimes referred to as Delta Sleep because of the delta waves that occur during this time. Stage Four is a deep sleep that lasts for about 30 minutes. Sleepwalking and bed-wetting typically happen at the end of Stage Four sleep. (This does not include the problems that can happen with sleep medications like Ambien and Lunesta).

Stage Five: REM

Most dreaming occurs during Stage Five, known as REM. REM sleep is characterized by eye movement, increased respiration rate and increased brain activity. REM sleep is also referred to as paradoxical sleep because, while the brain and other body systems become more active, your muscles become more relaxed, or paralyzed. Dreaming occurs because of increased brain activity, but voluntary muscles become paralyzed. Voluntary muscles are those that you need to move by choice, for example, your arms and legs. Involuntary muscles are those that include your heart and gut. They move on their own.

Rapid eye movement, or REM sleep, is when you typically dream. You may have images float by in earlier stages, particularly when you are going through Alpha or Theta, but the actual dream state occurs in REM.

This period of paralyzation is a built-in protective measure to keep you from harming yourself. When you are paralyzed, you can't leap out of bed and run. Do you ever feel like you can't escape during a dream? Well, the truth is, you can't. You can breathe, and your heart is working, but you really can't move.

Cycles

Sleep does not progress through all of these stages in sequence, however. Sleep begins in Stage One and progresses into stages 2, 3, and 4. Then, after Stage Four sleep, Stages Three, then Two are repeated before going into REM sleep. Once REM is over, we usually return to Stage Two sleep. Sleep cycles through these stages approximately 4 or 5 times throughout the night.

We typically enter REM approximately 90 minutes after falling asleep. The first cycle of REM often lasts only a short amount of time, but each cycle becomes longer. This is why we need long periods of sleep each night. If we get short periods of sleep, we can't really get through the stages we need to heal and stay healthy. REM can last up to an hour as our sleep progresses. In case you are wondering, if you feel like a dream is taking a long period of time, it really is. Contrary to what was once believed, dreams take as long as they actually seem.

Getting sleepy? OK, sleep well, perchance to dream....

Ok! Now that we understand the sleep cycle, how do we repair it and *reactivate* the ability to get deep, truly regenerative sleep? Glad you asked!

Step one (as with any other ailment) is always to eliminate the *distractors*. In this case, these are classified as any potentially disruptive elements that might impede or disturb otherwise peaceful slumber. We need to remove:

- **All major electronics** from the bedroom during sleeping hours. Power down your cellphones, tablets, tv's, laptops, kindles, video games, etc, and completely relocate them to another room. This may seem excessive, but the electromagnetic field(s) emitted by these electronic devices are extremely disruptive to our cells, and most of them still emit a low-level field even *when they are turned off.* All modems/routers/wi-fi within a 15 yard/meter radius of the bedroom should be *unplugged* so as to be completely disconnected. (Sound crazy? Do some research on the cellular disruption caused by wi-fi and then get back to me. This issue is going to become about a hundred times worse if the proposed 5G networks get rolled out in the near future with repeater towers placed every 500 meters throughout all major metropolitan areas.) Watching TV at night might seem relaxing, but from a neuro-chemical standpoint, it creates a stimulatory/excitatory effect. One of the single most harmful things you can do, not just for sleep, but for your health and your bio-electric energy field in general, is to sleep with a cell phone right next to your head on your nightstand, or next to you in general. This is before we even take into consideration the obvious, that if it rings/chimes/bings/chirps or lights up when you are at any stage of sleep, it can completely disrupt not just those few minutes of sleep, but that entire 90-minute cycle of sleep. Furthermore, as we enter the ever-increasing power output of the aforementioned "5G" cell signal era, studies have shown that even a 2-minute phone call can suppress delta wave function (the type of brain wave needed for sleep) for well over an hour, and that longer phone calls can measurably alter the very structure of our brain, creating an ever-worsening progression of the phenomenon known as "cell phone insomnia." But even this startling information pales in comparison to what some of the longer term studies are showing us with regard to behavioral alteration and the development of certain types of cancer from long term cell phone use/exposure.

- **Stimulants**—most notably caffeine and nicotine are psychoactive substances that can make us feel wired. They cause vasoconstriction, an increase in blood pressure/heart rate, and put a chronic strain on our central nervous system. Everyday use is a more subtle equivalent of sticking your finger in an electrical socket. In moderation a little caffeine *on occasion* (like with the bulletproof coffee example in a previous chapter) can be helpful, but a daily dependency just to get going is unhealthy. More specifically if we consume stimulants after approximately 2 pm, it has the potential to interfere with our ability to get to sleep *on time*.

- **Disharmonious Environment**—Let's focus on what makes a restful environment now that we've removed the electronics and artificial lights. Positive elements include keeping the room quiet, dark, and cool. Use a sleeping mask or 'black-out' curtains to eliminate any remaining ambient light. Wear as little clothing as possible to allow your skin to breathe. Take a relaxing shower and come to bed clean. Consciously breathe deeply (see the breath-work chapter) and actively let the stresses of the day fall away. As is mentioned in Ephesians, 'never let the sun go down on your wrath.' Invest in a high-quality bed (my personal favorite is the Tempur-Pedic). They can be a little pricey, but we spend a third of our lives resting upon them, it may be worth stretching the budget a little to maximize the comfort and support we receive from them night after night. I highly recommend either wearing a Q-Link srt-3 necklace or similar product to help shield against EMF/wi-fi and to use an earthing/grounding mat. The bedroom should also be a place of tranquility, of peace, of harmony, free of any clutter or work-related items or cat litter boxes or spare car parts (I only mentioned these utterly random items because I've seen it in person before). It's also very healthy to have 3 or 4 living house plants (ferns, dracenas, bonzais, etc) in the bedroom.

- **Sub-Optimal Timing**—There is an optimal amount of sleep for each one of us, and the overwhelming majority of us need somewhere between 7½ to 9 hours of *undisturbed* sleep. (This number may drop to 6 hours as we get older and less active.) Due to the demands of life, most of us don't get anywhere near that much. But just as important as the quantity of sleep is the *timing* of sleep. The optimal hours for brain restorative sleep are roughly between the hours of 10pm to 2am. Let's hear from Kulreet Chaudhary, MD on the importance of *when* you get to sleep:

  > Getting a good night's sleep is an effortless technique to create longevity and health. Deep rest during the night helps you fight stress, maintain a healthy weight, and keeps your energy levels high. Timing your sleep is like timing an investment in the stock market – it doesn't matter how much you invest, it matters *when* you invest.
  >
  > The deepest and most regenerative sleep occurs between 10 p.m. – 2 a.m. After 2am, your sleep becomes more superficial. If you are not getting the deep, regenerative sleep that occurs between 10 p.m. – 2 a.m., then you may wake up between 2 a.m. – 3 a.m., when the sleep cycle naturally becomes more superficial, and have trouble falling back to sleep. If your body is chronically deprived of the regenerative sleep between 10 p.m. – 2 a.m., then

you may still feel fatigued when you wake up in the morning.

You have an internal clock lodged deep within the brain that regulates your sleep – the pineal gland. The pineal gland receives information about the sun through your eyes via the optic nerve. As the sun sets, the pineal gland is able to sense the change in light transmitted through your eyes and it begins to secrete a hormone, melatonin, to prepare your body for sleep.

Exposure to bright light prevents the secretion of melatonin and darkness promotes it. Typically, within one to two hours after the sunset, you will begin to feel drowsy as the melatonin levels rise. This is the body's signal to go to sleep. By midnight your melatonin levels have peaked and there is a gradual decline in melatonin levels after midnight.

At 10 p.m., your body goes through a transformation following the rise in melatonin production. This transformational phase of sleep is associated with an increase in the "internal" metabolic activity that is responsible for the repair and restoration of your body. A reduction of your mental and physical activity is necessary for this 10 p.m. shift to occur. If you are still awake, the "second wind" phenomenon occurs at 10 p.m. because there is a rise in mental activity and energy at this time. However, the true value of the "second wind" can only be experienced if you are asleep by 10 p.m.

Scientists are just beginning to discover the antioxidant role of melatonin. Your body produces numerous natural antioxidants that prevent cellular and DNA damage, which ultimately causes disease.

One of the powerful nocturnal antioxidants produced is melatonin. As you sleep, your body is removing the effects of free radicals that have been produced by stress throughout the day. This natural, nocturnal clean-up crew maintains physical balance without any effort. All you need to do to benefit from this process is to sleep when your pineal gland sends the melatonin signal.

If you are awake past 10 p.m., this process of free radical removal becomes interrupted, and your body's ability to remove the effects of free radicals is significantly impaired. First of all, most people who stay awake past 10 p.m. are usually working on the computer, watching TV or reading. All of these activities result in an exposure to light and therefore interrupt the production of melatonin. Secondly, the metabolic energy that becomes available at 10 p.m. for the removal of free radicals is expended and now unavailable. It gets dissipated in the "second wind" phenomenon and is lost as mental energy rather than used as metabolic energy for the purpose of removing free radicals. So rather than allowing our bodies to maximize its natural cycle of repair during sleep, we interfere with it. This results in a state of night vigilance where you are alert during the night and groggy during the day. This cycle is extremely harmful to health.

Typically, if you miss the 10 p.m. bedtime, it will take much longer to fall asleep. The quality of sleep will also be less refreshing and there will still be a sense of fatigue in the morning. Even adjusting your bedtime from 11 p.m. to 10 p.m. will make an enormous difference in the quality of your sleep and enhance your feeling of wakefulness the following day. The reason for this is that you are taking advantage of the natural wave of neurochemistry that is already well on its way before 10pm and you get the added support of the metabolic changes that occur at the 10 p.m. mark.

If you are currently falling asleep well past 10 p.m., make it a goal to sleep earlier by 15-30 minutes each week until you hit the 10 p.m. goal. If you are also waking up after 6 a.m., it is important to wake up 15-30 minutes earlier so you feel ready for bed by 10 p.m. If you are having problems with insomnia, there are several things you can do to help reset your sleep cycle.

—Chaudhary, 2011

If you are anything like me, i.e. a 'nite owl,' it can seem nearly impossible to simmer down enough to want to go to sleep anywhere before 2am. There is simply too much stuff to do! I'm having too much fun, I'm hanging out with friends, I'm reading, learning, exercising, paying bills online, reviewing patient charts, watching a movie, or writing this book! My mind is naturally more alert in the evening hours. Cheerful morning people mostly chap my ass by sheer virtue of the fact that they find it to be a completely logical, rational, and reasonable state of being to be up and productive before 9am. (I'm pretty sure the Sun doesn't even come up until at least 8:30ish, but I could be wrong!) We are learning more and more that this may be a function of our genetic make-up as opposed to just poor habit patterns. Thanks to a gene-insertion study at Vanderbilt University done on mice, biologists have begun to understand the role of a part of the brain called the Suprachiasmatic Nucleus (SCN), which is the home to the body's 'master clock.' The SCN works as a two-way street. According to the experiment:

One group of mice had neurons that would fire more often when exposed to light; another group had neurons that would fire more often when light was suppressed. That meant the researchers were able to control the neuron's firing rate, and they were able to show by manipulating the firing rate, they could actually stimulate the SCN. This suggests that SCN firing rate is fundamental to circadian pace-making as both an input to and output of the molecular clockworks. In other words, triggering or suppressing the right neurons effectively reset the SCN, rebooting the biological clock.

So how does this affect us? We most likely aren't going to turn to sensory altering gene-insertion therapy to modify our sleep cycles, at least not yet. The field of Optogenetics (yes, that's a thing) is still in its infancy, and it would be preferable and more pragmatic to try the natural route first anyways. The important part we can take from this relatively complex data set is a better understanding of ourselves and how our circadian biorhythms operate. A problem well-defined is a problem half solved. What this means to those individuals (myself included) whose SCN/brain function is wired to be more alert at night is that we need to take a more proactive approach when it comes to helping rewire our minds/bodies to be in a more restful state of being when the Sun goes down. This most certainly won't happen overnight (pun intended), but over the course of 3 to 4 weeks it is possible to retrain our bodies to remember that 'hey, night time is for sleeping!.' For those of us that are (again, myself included) in the middle of actively trying to rewire our sleep patterns, we do have some options at our disposal to help. After removing the distractors, creating a comfortable sleep environment, taking measures to relax in the evenings, and deploying the proper EMF shielding, it's time to work on ourselves internally. There are a few amazing supplements that can help us with that. My personal favorite is the practitioner grade **Kavinace Ultra PM** by

NeuroScience. It has a combination of melatonin, 5-HTP, and phenylbut, a derivative of the neurotransmitter GABA that acts as a gentle but effective central nervous system depressant. I also recommend having a warm glass of **CALM**, which is a pure magnesium citrate and has a muscle relaxing, vasodilating, and anxiety reducing effect on the body. A short term regimen of supplements like these are helpful in augmenting and returning us to a more beneficial sleep cycle, and do not produce any type of dependency. (In addition to supplements, one might also integrate the specific acupuncture points for deep, restorative sleep—I'm personally a fan of the ShenMin point in the ears—as well as listening to Delta-Wave Binaural Beats via surround-sound, noise-cancelling head phones.)

This type of approach is directly opposite of the pharmaceutical approach, which can clearly produce dependency and adverse side effects. Let's briefly touch on both OTC and prescription sleep medications and why we want to avoid them:

One common over the counter remedy is to simply take an anti-histamine such as Benedryl. Many OTC sleep aids (i.e. ZzzQuil) are nothing more than repackaged Benedryl/diphenhydramine with different marketing. This is a very poor sleep solution, and there have been several studies, including one published in *JAMA Internal Medicine* that show a clear link between the long-term use of anticholinergic medications like Benedryl and dementia. These drugs cause brain fog and compound fatigue issues by giving you 'drugged' sleep, not restful, brain-restoring sleep. We are by no means demonizing Benedryl here, merely advocating its use only on rare occasion for a mild allergic reaction or anaphylaxis, *not* as a sleep aid.

Common prescription sleep meds like Ambien (zolpidem) and Lunesta (eszopiclone) are also rife with their own side effects. We aren't going to fill up two whole pages listing them off here, but go to WebMD or Drugs.com if you want to see the whole catalog. The biggest problem with them (other than their use resulting in dependency) is that they can produce what many call the 'zombie' effect. This is the feeling you get when you slept for several hours but you still feel like you've just completed running a marathon or being run over by a bus. You feel depleted, lethargic, tranquilized. This occurs because of one key factor: when you go to sleep naturally (or with the aid of a more natural supplement like melatonin/Kavinace Ultra), a specific part of your central nervous system goes to sleep with you. It's only then that you can get to a state of deep rest and recovery. This is what is supposed to happen. With drugs like Ambien, this *doesn't* happen. That component of your nervous system is still spooled up, tooled up, and often running full steam ahead. For this very reason there have been many humorous, but scary documented stories of people sleep-walking on these drugs, doing everything from having sex and not remembering it, to eating buttered cigarettes, to getting into a car and driving a hundred miles only to wake up wondering where they are and why they are getting their pajamas dry-cleaned. This is problematic on many levels.

As a western society, we need to re-establish the value of solid, regenerative sleep as one of the foundational pillars of optimal health and wellness. Sleep is the fountain of youth. We often push our bodies and brains well beyond their natural limits, which comes at a huge premium in the long run. Treat yourself, your body, and your mind right and structure your life around getting quality sleep. You deserve it, and you'll be glad you did.

CHAPTER 29

QUANTUM PHYSICS AND THE MATRIX EFFECT

We are just now beginning to understand the true capacity of what we can tap into with our minds. We already know in the study of quantum physics (via the famous 'double slit' phenomenon taught in every Physics 101 class) that observing a scientific experiment can influence the outcome. We know that the power of prayer is real. We know that the mind has the power to heal the body. We know that a large part of reality is subjective, the question is, how much? How many of the 'rules' are real and how many of them are imagined? How many of them can be bent, and how many of them can be broken? How much of the movie *The Matrix* was more than just a cinematic experience? (*The Matrix* is absolutely critical watching btw if you haven't seen it. It's probably the most important movie ever made.)

Everything and everyone is connected, and everyone we see around us as 'individuals' that come into our lives are also reflections of elements of ourselves. As we begin to raise our spiritual awareness, entirely new possibilities and realities will emerge within us and within our world. There is a deeper reason the Christ commanded that we 'do unto others as we would have them do unto us.'

One of my close personal friends, mentors, spiritual guides James 'Jimmy Mack' Mckeown would say, "It's time to access all that is and bring in the ethereal rain that can make a difference in your life." For those who want to know what the holographic diagram of what certain elements of your personal future and health holds, I would encourage you to check out his website jimmymackhealing.com.

For the future of medicine and medical diagnosis that is happening *right now*, the reader is encouraged to read the book *Medical Medium* by Anthony William. (MedicalMedium.com)

For those actively seeking the presence and state of true mindfulness, to better understand themselves, and to pursue the real calling of why we are on this planet, the reader is encouraged to read the book *The Yoga of Jesus*, by Paramahansa Yogananda.

This isn't so much a chapter as it is an acknowledgement and a suggestion that after thousands (perhaps millions?) of years of existence, we may only just now be beginning to scratch the surface of what it means to be human beings. We (Consciousness) are more than the sum of our parts and no form of current science has any idea how to quantify that. Recognizing this absolute, and anything this chapter alludes to, even from the space and perspective of a clear, rational mind, is often ridiculed and met with cynicism by those who eat, sleep, and breathe academia and mock what is seen as "woo-woo." But there are things that cannot and will never be explained by modern science. With that in mind, this chapter promises you nothing, but it invites you to explore for yourself what might be possible when we cast off old conventions, old ways of thinking, and old suppressive constructs, and exchange them for the aim of accessing true consciousness, higher self, and the Creator's purpose for our lives.

CHAPTER 30

ACUPUNCTURE, FIRE CUPPING, AND SEXUAL ENERGY/HEALTH

Acupuncture

Say that word alone and you will get a wildly diverse range of reactionary responses depending upon the company you keep. This modality is one of my personal favorites because even as a holistically minded person I was initially a firm skeptic. (Emphasis on the word *was*.) It just didn't make any sense, all this mumbo jumbo about "meridians" and qi/chi. Surely, turning someone into a pin-cushion with needles to balance out some esoteric variance of 'yin' and 'yang' energy produced (at best) a placebo effect. Look up acupuncture on Wikipedia and in the first paragraph, it quickly gets thrown under the bus as being squarely in the category of pseudoscience.

Yet nothing could be further from the truth. After grasping the way acupuncture really works, experiencing it myself to address certain ailments, and understanding the power, safety, and efficacy of it, I'm now convinced.......no, 'convinced' isn't a strong enough word...I *know* with absolute certainty that this practice is the very definition of true science, of sound understanding of the human body. It's the personification and embodiment of the highest level of comprehension of the body electric, and the culmination of over 8,000 years of knowledge, rooted in the ancient Daoist tradition, which pre-dates most of recorded human history.

Everything in the body is voltage. Healing is therefore the manipulation, modulation, amplification, and transduction of that voltage. Your brain and central nervous system run on electricity, and they issue commands to the entire rest of the body via bio-electrical signaling. Your heart produces, and is enveloped by, its own electromagnetic field. That's what they are measuring on an EKG. Every one of the trillions of living cells in your body holds within it a small micro-current of electrical charge (measured in milliamps). Even the Schumann Resonance, the global electromagnetic resonance which composes a set of spectrum peaks in the extremely low frequency (E.L.F.) portion of the Earth's electromagnetic field, correlates directly to the alpha rhythm of human brainwaves and has been described as the 'tuning fork of life.' The planet we live on literally charges us up. Would it not then be a natural and rational conclusion that our bodies have within them bio-electrical conduits, pathways, or *meridians* by which the electrical signaling occurs and travels? Or does it make more sense that we are incoherent blobs of flesh, just meat suits that hold organs and bones together? I would argue that not only do such meridians (obviously) exist, but they are extensively and comprehensively well-mapped, and have been so since well before modern medicine, anti-biotics, and germ theory even existed. I would argue that if we wanted to, we could allocate the funding and research necessary to quantify and confirm it in western fashion. But why? We already know that it works and it has always worked. Western science is just now coming around to the inevitable actualization of some these truths. They readily admit now that an infected molar in the mouth can correlate with, and possibly cause certain heart problems. Even certain forward-thinking insurance companies (HMO's, PPO's, etc) are beginning to cover acupuncture under the 'preventative care' elements of their plans because they realize the tremendous amount of money it's going to save them in the long run. With or without the confirmation of western science, acupuncture is going to maintain its prevalence and presence as it has for millennia. Why? Because it works...but the healthcare system as a whole will become more manageable, more navigable and more efficient once the official stamp of approval is handed down and the 'bean counters' stop fighting against the inevitable. Thankfully, we are making some progress. Here in the state of Florida where I live, a D.O.M. (Doctor of Oriental Medicine) can actually function as a primary care physician and hold all the privileges therein (they just can't prescribe controlled substances.)

The real issue once again isn't the science, it's the philosophy and perhaps the cultural differences that plague and stymie the progress. So let's get around that, let's transcend that. Just because your primary care physician may not feel comfortable throwing words like chi, yin, yang, and chakra around, he or she should be able to grasp and accept the concept that if we place a conductive material (i.e. stainless steel, gold, or silver acupuncture needles) at the end points of these known bio-electrical pathways, then we can stimulate them. If we can stimulate them and increase/potentiate/amplify the signal, then we elicit a physiological response which facilitates healing via the bio-electric pathways. We've already clinically proven that inducing a specific low-frequency micro-current drastically increases the speed at which a bone fracture heals, let's open our eyes to seeing what it can do for the rest of the body. Let's strip the mysticism out of it, update the nomenclature, and pragmatically integrate it into our modern healthcare system (and make a procedural/ICD-10 code for it too just so it rustles everyone's jimmies properly).

The paradox is that our current model of medicine doesn't even require that we know how a drug works, only that it does work and is relatively (and we use the term loosely) safe. When a drug works but we aren't sure how, we simply say, "The mechanism of action is *unknown*."

Wait, huh? Yes, you read that correctly. There is an extensive list of medications approved by the FDA to which we have *no idea* how they work, most notably Tylenol (acetaminophen), Flexeril (cyclobenzaprine), Metformin, Robaxin (methocarbamol), and Provigil (modafinil) to name a few common ones. If we as a medical community have somehow signed off on the daily usage of something like Tylenol, which has well-known damaging side effects to the liver and has been linked with long term hepatic failure, and we have no idea what its mechanism of action is or how it actually works, then why such a high threshold and barrier to entry to something that actually heals and often precludes the need for drugs like Tylenol? I'll repeat it many, many more times; we don't need to update our science so much as we need to update our thinking.

As a continuance of the theme of this chapter, I'll briefly touch on Reflexology/Acupressure and Fire Cupping. I think it would be a fair joke to say most people in the know think 'reflexology' is a Latin term for 'extremely painful foot massage!' And they wouldn't be entirely wrong, it can be very intense, but is also a very effective healing modality. It operates on the same type of meridian principles as acupuncture, however it diverges slightly with a focus on using manual manipulation(s) as opposed to needles, and with an end goal of organ detox. We don't pierce any organs with acupuncture needles, nor do we pierce the end points of the organ meridians on the bottom of the feet during reflexology. But we can promote healing, detoxification, immune boosting, increased circulation, and bio-electric energy rebalancing with respect to certain types of blockages with this wonderful modality.

Fire Cupping

Here is yet another modality that has been around for thousands of years in TCM (traditional Chinese medicine), as well as in ancient Egypt. The *Ebers Papyrus*, one of the oldest (dating to 1550 B.C.) known medical textbooks describes the usage of cupping therapy. But it has recently returned to the limelight, most notably because of the Olympic swimmer and gold medalist Michael Phelps. He has drawn quite the media spotlight to fire cupping due to the telltale hickey/octopus sucker marks being clearly visible on his back during his high profile swimming competitions.

The technique is second to none when it comes to inducing blood flow to a specific area. More blood flow = faster, more efficient, more complete healing. I personally like it better and find it more effective than even deep tissue massage with regard to myofascial release, breaking up adhesions in the fascia (especially in older patients) and getting other miscellaneous stubborn musculoskeletal issues to heal.

The way it works begins with a small fire being lit just inside of a glass cup (usually which has been pre-swabbed with rubbing alcohol) and a vacuum is created. The cup is quickly transferred to the intended area on the skin and powerful suction occurs. This suction forces new blood into the tissue(s) and pulls stagnant blood away. The vacuum induces the separation of several layers of tissue and stagnant interstitial fluid, and causes micro trauma, as well as phenomenon known as 'sterile inflammation.' It sounds like a bad deal, but it's a very short term and isolated type of positive inflammation which signals the influx of white blood cells, platelets, cytokines, fibroblasts, and other healing co-factors to the area to begin the regenerative process. Neovascularization also begins, which allows new blood vessels to form and creates a better, permanent ability to transport more oxygen and micro-nutrients to the tissues. Over time and over the course of multiple treatments, the increased blood flow combined with the stretching of the fascia and tissue yields much better movement and range of motion in addition to injury healing.

Sexual Energy/Sexual Health

Sexual Energy and Libido is function of a combination of the bio-electric pathways and the endocrine system. In the eastern cultures, it has always been well-known that sexual energy = bio-electric energy = *spiritual* energy. Regardless of the nomenclature system, if you can learn to tune that energy up to optimal *capacitance*, then you can heal. In the indigenous tribes of South America, they've always known that a decline in libido directly relates with a decline in health. In males specifically, the lack of a "morning wood" (similar to what happens to just about every 16 to 22-year-old male every morning upon rising) is indicative of a cause for concern. The lack thereof means circulation is sub-optimal, it means testosterone is declining, it means the bio-electric pathways are not optimally circulating at full gain. This was typically not an issue for the males of those South American indigenous tribes, because the testosterone level and circulation of the 70-year-old males was still at the same level of the 20-year-old males...i.e. it never declined because they maintained it with optimal health practices and with herbal medicines like Maca. (More on this in the hormone/endocrine chapter.) Unfortunately, that concept of sexual health is mostly lost in western medicine, not because of a lack of science, but because of cultural differences, most notably the fear/guilt/shame mechanism that's baked in to what most western organized religion teaches when it comes to human sexuality as a whole. This has to end. Sexual engagement, bio-electric energy recirculation, and release are core components of and have a staggering amount of influence on being a healthy human being. This is true on every level—biochemical, mental, emotional, physical, spiritual. As taboo as it sounds, very specific sexually therapeutic protocols have been used to heal for thousands of years, and those traditions are still academically taught to this day in certain Asian cultures at the masters' degree level. I won't delve any further into that at this time, however I would highly encourage the reader (if the interest is there) for you to pick up the books *The Multi-Orgasmic Man, The Multi-Orgasmic Woman, and The Multi-Orgasmic Couple.* (Cheap copies can be found on Amazon.com). They are, at first glance, classified under the genre of self-help/couple's therapy books, but they do *begin* to explore the concepts and practices of ***micro-cosmic orbit***, deep breathing and sexual energy recirculation to help maintain optimal health.

CHAPTER 31

AYAHUASCA: THE ULTIMATE MEDICINE

I saved the best for last. To be deemed the most powerful medicine on the planet, a medicine would have to come *from* the planet. It would have to be able to activate our DNA, and bridge the gap between worlds by healing mind, body, and spirit. It would have to be able to heal in the same fashion and *intent* as Christ did when he walked the earth 2,000 years ago. The medicine itself would have to be part of a higher sentient intelligence. One of the greatest gifts given to us as humans are the plant medicines of South America. There is *nothing* on the Earth treatment-wise that begins to hold a candle to South American medicine. It will absolutely rock your world (in a good way). I would encourage you to do your own research on this subject, it is not for everyone, it is definitely not for the feint of heart, but it will call to you if and when you're ready. It represents the very pinnacle of true healing, both for us as spiritual beings having a physical experience and for the planet. It is the model by which all medicine should follow. You can go to AyahuascaChurches.org for more information. For now, I'll leave you with a brief overview/excerpt (borrowed with permission from the Ayahuasca Church) of the major 'teacher' plants:

Ayahuasca— The word Aya is derived from two Quechua words: aya meaning "spirit," "soul," or "ancestor," and huasca meaning "vine" or "rope." Thus, Aya is revered as "the vine of the soul."

What is Aya?

Aya is an Amazonian plant mixture with an ancient history of use as a medicine and shamanic means of communication, dating back at least 2,500 years. It has long been a central part of the spiritual and cultural traditions of South America and the Amazon. A powerful teacher, Aya is a medicine capable of bringing about great physical, emotional, mental, and spiritual healing. She is reverently referred to as "Mother Aya" by those whose lives she has touched. As such, Aya is not intended for recreational use. She should be treated seriously and consumed in a ceremonial environment under the guidance of an experienced drinker.

What makes up the Aya brew?

The Aya tea is primarily made from the Banisteriopsis caapi vine, which is combined with either chacruna (Psychotria viridis) or chagropanga (Diplopterys cabrerana), other medicinal plants that contain a high amount of the psychedelic substance N-Dimethyltryptamine, known as DMT. DMT is a tryptamine found in nearly every living thing on earth and is released in our bodies during birth and death, though scientists do not fully understand its purpose. Many believe that, because of DMT's release at the start and end of our lives, it puts us closer in touch with the unexplained forces of life that create and embody our universe. Because of the profound feelings of connectedness and personal transcendence that DMT can produce, it has been called "the spirit molecule."

How is the Aya brew made?

To make the Aya tea brew, the Banisteriopsis caapi vine is cut into 8- to 12-inch pieces, then pounded with a hard wooden mallet to separate the fibers. The pounded mixture of vine and leaves is then added to a pot, covered with water, and boiled and reduced for several hours. Other plants or tree barks may also be added to the brew to modify its healing and visionary effects, such as mapacho for cleansing, bobinsana for opening the heart, toe for clearer visions, or ajo-sacha for clearing negative energies. When the liquid in the pot has boiled down to just a few inches, it is drained off and transferred to another vessel where it is further reduced to the desired concentration. The final product is usually a very dark brown color, with a slightly sticky consistency similar to molasses. Preparing Aya is much more than just chemistry, and the intention and state of mind of the person making the tea has a significant impact on the experience of those who drink it. This is why it is very important that an experienced shaman prepare the Aya brew, so that they are able to channel their inner energy and intentions into the tea by keeping healing, positive intentions in mind and pushing away all negativity. The shaman also sings icaros (songs sung during healing ceremonies) while making the Aya tea, asking the spirits for good healings and visions in the ceremonies for which it will be used.

How does the Aya medicine work?

Aya should not be viewed or treated as a drug. It is a medicine capable of inducing altered states of consciousness that usually last between four to eight hours after ingestion. Results vary among individuals and can range from mildly stimulating to extremely visionary. For some, it can offer profound realizations and physical and psychological healing; for others, it can open one's heart to the beauty of the world and that which connects all living and non-living things on earth. And then for others, the experience may be in part entirely unique. Aya heals in a variety of ways. One primary way is by collecting energies that do not belong and then purging them from the individual, which may include vomiting, diarrhea, shaking, yawning, crying, and/or sweating. However, it is important to understand that this is the medicine doing its work and surrendering to it will result in the best healing. Thus, this work should not be entered into lightly and without firm, true intention and respect for what Mother Aya provides. One should feel a strong calling to the medicine, not be looking for amusement or fulfilling mere curiosity. Even more, the healing process requires courage, commitment, and trust in the medicine and in what Aya intends for you. You must be willing to surrender to faith that the medicine is doing what you need, for it to work best, even if there are parts that are unpleasant.

Will Aya cure me of my worries or illness?
While a very large number of issues have been successfully addressed with Aya and other medicinal plants, ranging from physical ailments like diabetes to psychological issues such as addiction, Aya does not promise to be a cure-all for every individual. It is a medicine, and as with all treatments, individuals will respond differently with varying results.

Other powerful South American plant medicines:

Kambo—A very carefully titrated dose of dart frog poison used in shamanic cleansing of the body. Researchers have called it 'one of the strongest natural antibiotics and anesthetics in the world.' Kambô contains several peptides that trigger extreme reactions in human beings, and which scientific studies have shown to be beneficial to the body. Some of these peptides traverse the blood-brain barrier and stimulate the brain's endocrine glands, resulting in a strengthened immune response and a deep cleanse of the body. The reported effects of Kambô cover a wide range of potential medical uses: treatment of depression, migraines, blood circulation problems, vascular insufficiency, organ diseases, cancer, female fertility problems, AIDS, hepatitis, brain diseases such as Alzheimer's and Parkinson's, and more.[2] Kambô also has antibiotic properties and strengthens the immune system while physically destroying pathogenic microorganisms. Other uses and benefits of Kambô include:

- Works as a prophylactic against malaria
- Boosts strength and stamina
- Strengthens the immune system to aid the destruction of pathogenic microorganisms
- Has analgesic and anti-inflammatory effects
- Acts as an antibiotic that aids in healing infections
- Helps regulate blood pressure
- Detoxifies the liver, intestine, and entire digestive system
- Treats a variety of other conditions such as depression, migraines, blood circulation problems, Alzheimer's and Parkinson's diseases, vascular insufficiency, organ diseases, cancer, female fertility problems, hepatitis, and AIDS

What are the specific peptides found in Kambô?
When scientists analyzed the chemical makeup of the Phyllomedusa bicolor's sapo venom,they found that it contained many peptides with clear benefits to the human body, including:

- Dermorphin: This potent mu-opioid receptor agonist is 4000 times stronger than morphine
- Deltorphin: This potent delta-opioid receptor agonist is 4000 times stronger than morphine
- Phyllomedusin: This tachykinin affects the salivary glands, tear ducts, intestines, and bowels, contracts the smooth muscles, and contributes to violent purging.
- Phyllokinin and Phyllomedusin: These potent blood-essel dilators increase the permeability of the blood-brain barrier.
- Phyllocaerulein: This peptide stimulates the adrenal cortex and the pituitary gland, causes a fall in blood pressure and tachycardia,has a potent action on the gastrointestinal smooth muscle, and stimulates gastric, biliary, and pancreatic secretions.
- Sauvagine: This peptide stimulates the adrenal cortex, causing a long-lasting fall in blood pressure and intense tachycardia.
- Adenoregulin: This peptide acts on the adenosine receptors.
- Dermaseptin: This potent antimicrobial works on both Gram-positive and Gram-negative bacteria, and acts as antiviral for the herpes simplex virus.

Rapé—(pronounced "ha-peh" or "rapay") is sacred shamanic snuff medicine. It is legal, usually made of tobacco powder and various Amazonian medicinal plants, trees, leaves, seeds, and other sacred ingredients that are ground into a fine, aromatic powder. Rapé is a rare and profoundly healing and cleansing miracle medicine that has been used since ancient times.

How is Rapé administered?

Rapé is traditionally blown through each nostril on both sides using a pipe made from bamboo or bone. It can be self-administered using a V-shaped self-applicator pipe (Kuripe) that connects the mouth to the nostrils. More often, though, Rapé is administered by another person using a blow pipe (Tepi) that connects the blower's mouth to the other person's nostrils. To respect the spiritual healing it offers, Rapé should be used only in a quiet, sacred space, with sacred music playing if you'd like. After each application, you should breathe slowly and with intention, with your eyes closed.

What can I expect from the Rapé experience?

You may experience purging, vomiting, bowel movements, and/or excess saliva after a Rapé, application. This is normal, however, and indicates that negative energy, toxins, and sickness are being released from your body. You may need a bucket, toilet tissue, and drinking water close to hand.

What are the healing effects of Rapé?

The intense blow of the Rapé immediately focuses the mind. By quieting the noise that fills our mind, it opens us up, and intensifies our connection with the world and the universe. Rapé profoundly helps to realign and open all your chakras or energy channels, including the third eye. It helps clear negativity and confusion, which can improve your spiritual and emotional grounding. This paves the way for releasing emotional, physical, and spiritual illnesses and eases from our minds and bodies, including helping to detoxify the body. In this way, it can relieve one of all excess mucus, toxins, and bacteria, thereby even assisting in fighting colds and snuffles. For these many healing effects, Rapé is often used in conjunction with an

Aya ceremony or Sananga medicine to help with purging, releasing sickness, moving any stuck energy flows, and clearing one's mind.

Sananga—is a very powerful, healing eye medicine made from the roots and bark of a shrub called Apocynaceae that grows in the Amazon jungle. The bark of this special shrub's root is used to make these sacred eye drops, which have been traditionally used by indigenous peoples to lift panama, or negative energetic influences that can promote bad luck, depression, difficulties, and disease.

What are the healing powers of Sananga?

Sananga was traditionally used in the Amazonian cultures for sharpening sensory perceptions and awareness. But Sananga's greatest healing power is in its ability to deeply cleanse us on the energetic, physical, emotional, and spiritual level by unblocking stuck energy flows and realigning and opening up the chakras. This can aid in healing mental and physical sickness. Sananga profoundly helps to cleanse the physical, emotional, and energetic fields of our bodies. It opens up the inner sight, and deeply cleanses the whole aura from the inside out. Other benefits of Sananga include:

- Improves the vision that connects us to the spiritual realm
- Opens up the "third eye" chakra
- Helps to decalcify and activate the pineal gland
- Clears negative thought patterns and mental confusion

San Pedro—(from The Encyclopedia of Psychoactive Substances by Richard Rudgley, Little, Brown and Company 1998) — The San Pedro cactus is the name given to psychoactive species of the genus Trichocereus (T. pachanoi, T. peruvianus) which comprises about thirty species, mainly found in the Andes. It is a large columnar cactus that grows up to heights of twenty feet and it contains mescaline, as does the well-known peyote cactus. The San Pedro cactus has also been found to have other psychoactive alkaloids. The mescaline seems to be most highly concentrated in the skin, which can be peeled, dried and made into a powder for consumption.

The usual native preparation of the cactus involves boiling slices of the stem for a number of hours and then, once cooled, the resulting liquid is drunk. Sometimes the San Pedro is used in conjunction with other psychoactive plants, such as coca, tobacco, Brugmansia and Anadenanthera. The hallucinogenic properties of its traditional use, including aguacolla, cardo, cuchuma, giganton, hermoso, huando and, of course, San Pedro.

Like many other of the entheogenic substances used in the aboriginal religions of the Americas, the use of the hallucinogenic San Pedro cactus is ancient, and its use has been a continuous tradition in Peru for over 3,000 years. The earliest depiction of the cactus is a carving which shows a mythological being holding the San Pedro. It belongs to the Chavín culture (c. 1400-400 BC) and was found in an old temple at Chavín de Huantar in the northern highlands of Peru, and dates about 1300 BC. A particularly surprising discovery was made by a Peruvian archaeologist named Rosa Fung in a pile of ancient refuse at the Chavín site of Las Aldas near Casma; namely what seem to be remnants of cigars made from the cactus. Artistic renderings of it also appear on later Chavín artefacts such as textiles and pottery (ranging from about 700-500 BC). The San Pedro is also a decorative motif of later Peruvian ceramic traditions, such as the Salinar style

(c. 400-200 BC), the Nasca urns (c. 100 BC-AD 700). It has also been proposed that a recurrent snail motif in Moche art represents a mescaline-soaked snail which has partaken of the San Pedro. If this is the case then the snail may be added to the list of animals having psychoactive properties.

Not surprisingly, considering their general contempt for native life and particularly the use of psychoactive plants, European missionaries were very negative when reporting the use of the San Pedro. Yet a Spanish missionary, cited by Christian Rätsch, grudgingly admitted the cactus' medicinal value in the midst of a tirade reviling it:

> It is a plant with whose aid the devil is able to strengthen the Indians in their idolatry; those who drink its juice lose their senses and are as if dead; they are almost carried away by the drink and dream a thousand unusual things and believe that they are true. The juice is good against burning of the kidneys and, in small amounts, is also good against high fever, hepatitis, and burning in the bladder.

An account of the cactus by a shaman is in radical contrast to this rather contemptuous view:

> The drug first... produces... drowsiness or a dreamy state and a feeling of lethargy... a slight dizziness... then a great 'vision,' a clearing of all the faculties... it produces a light numbness in the body and afterward a tranquility. And then comes detachment, a type of visual force... inclusive of all the senses... including the sixth sense, the telepathic sense of transmitting oneself across time and matter... like a kind of removal of one's thought to a distant dimension.

The entheogenic status of the cactus remains as strong today as it always was. Not only do its uses in shamanic trances and healing sessions continue but it is also used to combat more recent problems such as alcoholism. The peyote cactus used widely by the North American Indians is also considered a medicine against alcoholism and this parallel is all the more striking as both cacti contain mescaline.

Ibogaine—There are currently over 2.5 million Americans who have an opioid use disorder. Those who receive medication-assisted treatment for opioid addiction are prescribed methadone, buprenorphine, or naltrexone. While these medications have been proven to be effective treatments for opioid addiction, they do have side effects and are not completely risk-free. Is there another medication out there that can treat opioid addiction without such risks? Is there a quick fix to help relieve the withdrawal symptoms? Some in the medical subculture believe the psychedelic drug ibogaine may be a potential treatment for opioid addiction.

What is ibogaine?
Ibogaine is a powerful psychoactive substance, extracted from the iboga plant found in central Africa. The plant has been used by the indigenous people of Cameroon and Gabon for centuries during healing ceremonies and spiritual rituals.

Howard Lotsof inadvertently discovered ibogaine as a potential treatment for opioid addiction in 1962. Lotsof, who at the time was addicted to heroin, wanted a psychedelic high and ingested ibogaine. After the effects from ibogaine wore off, Lotsof noticed he no longer had the desire to take heroin and did not experience withdrawal symptoms. This led Lotsof to examine ibogaine as a possible treatment for drug addiction. While scientists and health professionals are still learning exactly how ibogaine affects the human body, it is believed to impact the neurotransmitters in the brain and block neurotransmitter receptors that are involved with addiction. The drug also causes hallucinations and a wide array of other side effects that can last up to 24 hours or longer after an initial dose.

What studies are out there?
Because no traditional clinical trials have been conducted in the United States, proponents of ibogaine primarily use preclinical studies, animal testing, and a large amount of anecdotal evidence to support the use of ibogaine as a treatment for opioid addiction. Some of this research has produced promising results.

There have been case studies demonstrating long term abstinence from opioids after receiving ibogaine. One study described the case of a 37 year old female with a long history of opioid addiction who abstained from opioids for 18 months after using ibogaine. Her previous longest period of abstinence was for only two months while she was on methadone maintenance treatment.

There are several other reports from around the world about individuals experiencing successful abstinence from opioids following ibogaine treatment, including individuals from New Jersey and South Africa. Additionally, observational studies conducted in countries where ibogaine is legal show some positive results of ibogaine treatment. For example, a study in New Zealand concluded that ibogaine treatment reduced opioid withdrawal symptoms and improved individuals' chances of opioid abstinence in the months following ibogaine treatment.

This is just a brief exposure to only a small fraction of the many powerful medicines from South America. As we enter into a brave new world, the paradigm of truly *adaptive* medicine must incorporate *all* healing modalities to usher in the new synergy of true healing.

CHAPTER 32

CONCLUSION

It's been a joy and an adventure to write this book. I hope that you enjoyed reading it and that it benefits your life in one way or another. A big thank you to those who encouraged me along the way and to those who've allowed me to utilize some of your writings for reference. I do not claim authorship or credit from any of those borrowed excerpts, articles, or the referenced medical research herein. The intent behind this labor of love is not to pontificate as some health guru or expert. I am neither of those things, and I only wish to continue to ask questions and learning something new via seeking the truth. The purpose of this writing is simply to bring this information together in one place and make it more easily accessible to everyone, practitioners and patients alike...to provoke a new dialogue, to encourage critical thinking, to give hope, to spark synergy, to make progress, and to make humanity at large aware of the progress that's already being achieved. It is time for a radical shift to take hold in the *consciousness* of medicine. The future of healing is here...***now!***

www.ingramcontent.com/pod-product-compliance
Lightning Source LLC
Chambersburg PA
CBHW072046230526
45468CB00019B/40